COMPLETE CANDIDA YEAST GUIDEBOOK

Revised 2nd Edition

EVERYTHING YOU NEED TO KNOW ABOUT PREVENTION, TREATMENT & DIET

JEANNE MARIE MARTIN
with ZOLTAN P. RONA, M.D.

THREE RIVERS PRESS • NEW YORK

Published by Three Rivers Press, New York, New York.
Member of the Crown Publishing Group, a division of Random House, Inc.
www.crownpublishing.com

THREE RIVERS PRESS and the Tugboat design are registered trademarks of Random House, Inc.

Originally published by Prima Publishing, Roseville, California, in 2000.

All products mentioned in this book are trademarks of their respective companies.

Medical Disclaimer

The advice and information contained herein is not intended to replace or contradict any advice given to you by your doctor or health-care specialist. This book is a source of information and reference and is meant to complement your doctor's advice. Either you or the professional who examines and treats you must take responsibility for any use made of the data in this volume.

Choose a qualified doctor, holistic if possible, whom you trust; his or her recommendations for your Candida albicans should supercede recommendations given in this book. Your health-care practitioner knows you personally and is responsible for making recommendations based on his or her knowledge of your unique circumstances and present state of health.

Printed in the United States of America

Library of Congress Cataloging-in-Publication Data

Martin, Jeanne Marie
    Complete candida yeast guidebook : everything you need to know about prevention, treatment & diet / by Jeanne Marie Martin with Zoltan Rona.—Rev. 2nd ed.
        p.   cm.
    Includes bibliographical references and index.
    1. Candidiasis—Popular works. I. Title. II. Rona, Zoltan.
RC123.C3 M37   2000
616.9'69—dc21   00-062355
                                                                                          CIP

ISBN 0-7615-2740-0

10 9 8 7 6
Second Edition

Dedicated to the 90 percent or more of Americans and Canadians who knowingly or unknowingly suffer from the minor or major mental, emotional, and physical discomforts of Candida yeast overgrowth.
May you find peace, healing, and renewed vitality!

Other Books by Jeanne Marie Martin

For the Love of Food: The Complete Natural Foods Cookbook

All Natural Allergy Cookbook

Hearty Vegetarian Soups and Stews

Eating Alive (with Dr. Jonn Matsen)

Vegan Delights: Gourmet Vegetarian Specialties

201 Fat-Burning Recipes (with Cathi Graham)

*Return to the Joy of Health: Natural Medicine and Alternative Treatment for
All Your Health Complaints* (with Dr. Zoltan Rona)

Light Cuisine: Seafood, Poultry & Egg Recipes for Healthy Living

The Power of Superfoods (with Sam Graci)

Your Natural Medicine Chest: Natural Remedies for 101 Ailments

Recipes for Romance: Passionate Poetry, Aphrodisiacs and Menus for Loving

Contents

Foreword

COMPLETE CANDIDA YEAST GUIDEBOOK IS A REAL
treasure. There are many yeast infection books on the market; while some offer
valuable information, others offer confusing and contradictory information.
Jeanne Marie Martin's newest book stands alone as the most up-to-date, comprehensive, and down-to-earth book on Candida written so far.

The *Complete Candida Yeast Guidebook* starts off with a detailed descrip-
tion of Candida yeast infections by a well-known holistic doctor, Zoltan Rona.
The book's first half is a thorough and in-depth discussion of the underlying
causes of Candida. As Rona states in Part I, fungi are everywhere and exist in a
balanced state in the human body until we disrupt the balance through the use
of antibiotics, the use of cortisone, or excess sugar consumption—only a few
of many potential culprits.

Dr. Rona writes a fascinating section on mycotoxins—that is, the toxins
secreted by fungi—based on research done by Dr. A. V. Constantini. These
mycotoxins are found in large amounts in such common foods as corn,
peanuts, barley, and dried coconut.

The thorny question of how to make the diagnosis of Candida is adeptly
addressed. Dr. Rona maintains, as I do, that the best way to make the diagnosis
is through a trial therapy based on the signs and symptoms (which are thoroughly detailed in this book) and a high index of suspicion.

In another unique section, Dr. Rona outlines other conditions that may
be related to Candida, such as prostate cancer, breast cancer, heart disease,

gout, psoriasis, low platelet count, rheumatoid arthritis, multiple sclerosis, inflammatory bowel disease, and other ailments.

This book provides an absolutely excellent and comprehensive section on treatment, including an exhaustive list of natural antifungals, supplements, natural digestive aids, and the newest drugs. Chapters on how to boost the immune system naturally and case histories from both authors are informative reading.

Then, in her unique style, well-known author and nutritional counselor Jeanne Marie Martin guides you through every detail you need to follow a Candida diet, which is by far the most important part of therapy. She has really thought of everything.

Martin discusses controversial foods for Candida such as apple cider vinegar, soy sauce, milk, and more. She gives invaluable shortcuts for preparing meals, special cooking tips, information on how to travel and eat in a restaurant, and instructions for how to shop for Candida diets. The book contains over 200 tasty recipes, mainly vegetarian, a few with fish and poultry, and all corn-free, potato-free, and wheat-free. She focuses positively on what you can eat rather than bemoaning what must be eliminated.

An amazingly detailed section on substitutions for ingredients is provided, which is helpful for Candida sufferers and essential for those with allergies. A highly useful summary of nutrition guidelines is also included.

As any health practitioner knows, trying to get a patient to follow and stay on the Candida diet for long periods of time is the most difficult part of treatment. This is the first book I know of that offers a detailed four-phase diet that answers the varying diet concerns for all types of Candida treatments. The Phase I diet offers a way for those unaccustomed to wholesome natural foods to ease gradually into the required diet. Phase II, the strictest, is for average to severe cases of Candida. Phase III is for mild-to-moderate cases of Candida and is suitable, with additions, for children or for healing and recovery diets for many ailments. The Phase IV diet provides base guidelines for maintaining and preventing future Candida recurrences. The Phase III and Phase IV diets may include cooked feta and other occasional cooked cheeses, some whole grain flours, and yeast-free grain products.

Perhaps the best thing about this book is the delicious recipes that Jeanne Marie has perfected in her more than twenty-five years' experience. These delectable recipes are soothing, healing, and digestible for people on restricted diets. In fact, Jeanne Marie has discovered that people who heal fastest from Candida are those who take the time to prepare tasty, exciting meals.

A necessary chapter discussing what to do if your Candida is not healing and how to stay healthy after your Candida treatment is completed rounds off the *Complete Candida Yeast Guidebook*.

This book is invaluable not only to Candida sufferers, but also to the health-care specialist, families, and friends who are looking after them. I highly recommend it.

Carolyn DeMarco, M.D.
Author of *Take Charge of Your Body: Women's Health Advisor*

Dr. DeMarco, an expert on women's health care and holistic medicine, is a much sought-after speaker at conferences, seminars, and on TV shows throughout Canada and the U.S. She writes for a variety of health magazines, including *Wellness M.D.*, *Health Naturally*, *Today's Health*, *Modern Woman*, *Images*, *Healthsharing*, *Alive*, *Herizons*, and *Wedding Bells*.

Acknowledgments

Many thanks to my students, clients, friends, and colleagues who helped inspire this book and contributed to its making.

Special thanks to my coauthor Dr. Zoltan Rona for his professional input, expertise, and confirmation of my nutrition plans and principles.

Heartfelt thanks to my dear adopted parents, Malcolm and Penny Macdonald, for their love and support, without which this book would have taken much longer to write.

Soul-filled thanks to God for infinite inspiration and the endurance required to complete this work.

HOW YOU CAN HEAL CANDIDA

BY JEANNE MARIE MARTIN

CANDIDA ALBICANS, CANDIDIASIS, OR YEAST OVER-growth, as it is commonly called, is a "hidden epidemic" in North America. It is becoming a major disease and an underlying factor in many other diseases. Candida may be what is bothering you when others say that your health problems are "all in your head."

WHAT IS CANDIDA?

Candida yeast is a type of fungus, a microorganism that is not beneficial for the body; therefore, it is called "unfriendly" bacteria. Candida exists everywhere and humans come in contact with it throughout the day on everything they touch, in the air they breathe, and on most of what they consume. It is not generally a problem unless it "overgrows" and then interferes with the balance of friendly bacteria in the body. This overabundance leads to all kinds of health concerns.

WHO HAS CANDIDA AND WHAT ARE ITS EFFECTS?

Many people think yeast infections only occur in females and are primarily a vaginal disease. In fact, Candida affects men, women, and children alike; the main habitat is the digestive tract. Outer physical forms of Candida are dandruff, white flaky skin, vaginal discharge, jock itch, athlete's foot, heavily coated white tongues in adults; and colic and thrush in children. The people most susceptible to Candida are those with allergies; poor digestion; other diseases or illnesses (especially viral infections, chronic fatigue syndrome, AIDS, and cancer); histories of long treatments with antibiotics, birth control pills, or other drugs; or those who are under excessive stress, are overtired, or are overworked. Candida is found often in people with certain personality types—those who are doers, givers, overachievers, or workaholics; who have low self-esteem; who are type-A personalities; and who spread themselves too thin. These health concerns, diseases, and stresses weaken the immune system and throw the body off-balance, making it more susceptible to yeast overgrowth.

As many as 90 percent or more of Americans and Canadians may be suffering the effects of these microscopic "critters," considered also to be a type of parasite. An overabundance of yeast in the body can produce minor or major side effects, such as: anxiety, allergies, asthma, acne, bloating, cystitis, chemical sensitivities, coughs, cramps, constipation, chronic fatigue syndrome (CFS), confusion, trouble concentrating, depression, diarrhea, emotional problems, eczema, fatigue, fuzzy thinking, food cravings and sensitivities, gas, gastritis, headaches, hypoglycemia, hives, hyperactivity, heartburn, irritability, indigestion, intestinal pain, irrational fears, lethargy, low self-esteem, memory loss or poor memory, migraines, sore muscles, nausea, panic, puffiness, PMS, psoriasis, quick anger, rash, sexual problems, skin infections, stiffness, sleep disturbance, sinus pressure, sore throat, thrush, vaginal yeast infections, and/or weight gain.

KEYS TO COMPLETE CANDIDA CURE

If you suspect or know you have Candida yeast problems, this book provides guidelines for diagnosing, understanding, and treating this "disease" with natural remedies, prescription drugs, wholesome foods and recipes, and appropriate lifestyle changes.

With proper treatment and a new diet and lifestyle, Candida albicans can be healed in about six to eight weeks—*unless there are underlying causes.* Some individuals with minor problems may be cured in as little as three to four weeks. Long-term Candida sufferers may require three to four months or more of treatment, depending on the method. Once overabundant Candida yeast has been in the body, it can easily recur if body systems and energy levels reach a low state over a period of time. It is virtually impossible to wipe out all traces of Candida albicans in the body; new yeast organisms enter the body easily from outside sources in day-to-day contact with the environment. Individuals with additional health concerns may have to repeat treatments every few years, until robust health is achieved.

To "cure" Candida albicans, it is necessary to destroy as many "critters" or unfriendly bacteria as possible and restore a healthful balance of friendly bacteria within the body. Yeast must be kept under control and in check by killing the present yeast; avoiding new external contact with yeast (as much as possible); cultivating helpful, friendly bacteria in the body; and consuming foods and water that do not feed the yeast and make them strong.

During the "healing process," body energy levels must be raised and maintained so the body is no longer so susceptible or predisposed toward the yeast. The body must become healthy, able to digest and assimilate foods properly, and so strong that the yeast organisms cannot regain control because the body's restored natural defenses prevent it.

Regular cleansing regimens and treatments can cleanse the body of stored poisons and toxins such as pesticides, preservatives, artificial colors and flavors, chemicals, smoke, air pollution contaminants, and heavy metals, among other substances. Cleansing treatments can be highly beneficial for all individuals living in "modern society." These may significantly reduce intestinal parasites and Candida yeast. Specific intestinal cleansing programs may also help remove old, caked-on fecal matter in the colon that provides a breeding ground for yeast and other bacteria. Employing one or more cleansing programs a year can reduce harmful contaminants in the body that weaken the immune system (the body's natural defense system that protects it from disease) and support Candida yeast overgrowth. Talk to a holistic (whole body) doctor or natural health specialist about cleansing techniques and programs to suit your particular needs. (See also Chapters 4 and 23.)

A variety of other simple methods can reduce yeast growth in the body on a daily basis. These may require taking nutritional supplements and maintaining a reasonably wholesome diet and lifestyle. See Part III.

Important Keys

1. With proper treatment, a wholesome diet, and lifestyle changes, Candida albicans can be healed in about two months (unless there are underlying causes).
2. Candida albicans overgrowth can easily recur any time the body's immune system and energy levels reach a low state for a period of time. A weakened body is the perfect breeding ground for rapid yeast growth.
3. Traces of Candida albicans almost always remain in the body, even after treatment.
4. New yeast can easily enter the body from outside sources daily.
5. A healthy individual maintains enough "friendly bacteria" in the body to counteract or keep yeast growth under control or in check.
6. For successful treatment, one must kill the present yeast, avoid picking up too much new, external yeast, and eat foods that do not feed and help yeast grow and multiply.
7. A person must raise the body's health and wellness levels to avoid reoccurrence of yeast overgrowth. Until one achieves and maintains robust health, treatment may be repeated every one to two years.
8. Cleansing programs can assist the body to heal, boost the immune system, and help remove Candida yeast from the body.
9. Once treatment is successful, yeast growth in the body may be controlled by taking supplements and maintaining a reasonable and wholesome diet and lifestyle.

CANDIDA BOOK HIGHLIGHTS

Most Candida yeast books claim that you must be a meat eater, a carnivore, in order to heal Candida albicans, which is a limited and erroneous point of view. Several of these same books contradict themselves by recommending reduced heavy proteins and fats in the diet because they are hard to digest. In our view, dietary preferences are a matter of choice. Dietary restrictions need only be placed on foods that feed yeast, weaken the body, or aggravate food sensitivities or allergies. Whether you are a vegan (who eats no animal products: meat, eggs, dairy, or honey), a vegetarian (who eats no meat but enjoys dairy and/or eggs), a partial vegetarian (who eats no red meat but enjoys fish and/or poultry), or a meat eater (who eats all kinds of meat and other foods) is your decision.

One wholesome eating program we recommend is *Eat Right for Your Blood Type,* the diet that is the same as the book title, by Peter D'Adamo, N.D. The basic food lists in that book for each blood type can be adapted to this Candida book's diets and menus. Thus, the most important foods for your blood type can be regularly included in your Candida recipes. Certain foods may be avoided because of allergy or preference. Even O+ people can be healthy vegans if they choose. Simply substitute a serving of "Highly Beneficial" beans and whole grains recommended by the book for each meat serving and increase vegetable servings each day to compensate. For information on Dr. D'Adamo's books and diets, contact http://www.dadamo.com or look for his books at book and health stores.

The variety of healthful Candida diets presented in this book work to control the yeast while providing nutrients necessary for a healthful lifestyle. Guidelines suggest options that allow you to make your own treatment and food choices. How you proceed is up to you and your health-care practitioner. Follow your doctor's advice, even if it contradicts this book. If you are not happy with your doctor's advice, get a second or even a third opinion.

The best news is that you do not have to starve on a Candida diet anymore. No more bland, boring recipes so you can "survive" the diet and treatment "ordeal." Instead, you will enjoy wholesome, healing foods! You actually digest foods better when you like them. It is essential to the healing process to include a wide range of healthful, delicious foods. This book provides diet guidelines and a wide assortment of recipes that can be used before, during, and after Candida treatment.

Over 95 percent of these recipes can be prepared dairy-free; some have optional dairy ingredients such as butter or yogurt. The recipes have been thoroughly tested, and they taste delicious even if dairy products are not used. This book contains no recipes using: corn; wheat; grain flours; pasta; peanuts; pickles; mushrooms; green olives; eggplant; potatoes; yellow sweet potatoes; iceberg or head lettuce; baking or nutritional yeast; vinegar; sugar; sweet fruits like bananas, mangoes, melons, oranges, or grapes; miso; tempeh; white peas and beans; dried split peas; sausages; luncheon meats; hot dogs; ground meats; shellfish; or red meats.

The *Complete Candida Yeast Guidebook* does contain helpful recipes for: Mock Tomato Sauce, Mock Tamari Soy Sauce, Homemade Salsa, Homemade Ketchup, Homemade Vegetable Bouillon Cubes, Homemade Vegetable Broth Powder, Mock Meat Gravy, and Mock Meat Balls. There are over 75 main dishes (including soups, hearty appetizers, sauces, and egg recipes in other chapters), mostly vegetarian, with 10 fish and poultry recipes—more than 200 recipes altogether for snacks, party foods, travel foods, lunches, breakfasts, main dishes, beverages, soups, stews, salads, dressings, sauces, gravies, and treats that are not too sweet.

Some of the recipes are time-consuming; however, many of these can be prepared in large batches and frozen to save time. Also, hundreds of easy main dishes can be made using one of the special sauce recipes on plain whole grains and/or legumes (beans). Legumes freeze well, up to three months or more, and both legumes and whole grains keep fresh in the refrigerator for up to eight days. A large pot of one or two can be prepared and eaten throughout the week by reheating. Brown rice can be steamed with vegetables or put into veggie burgers, soups, and stews. Numerous time-saving shortcuts are outlined in this book.

Tips are given for exercise, relaxation, deep breathing, good digestion, food combining, menus, shopping, and dining out. Information on choosing doctors, case histories, and natural ways to boost the immune system is included.

Dr. Zoltan Rona, a renowned holistic medical doctor from Toronto, has contributed an excellent section on Candida treatments, including natural, holistic, herbal, and vitamin supplements, as well as prescription treatments. He provides a rare overview of practically all known modern remedies for yeast overgrowth. He explains fully what the disease encompasses and recommends treatments for Candida-related ailments.

This book offers new, varied options for treatment that make the healing process more comfortable, enjoyable, and rewarding. The fringe benefits are better physical, mental, and emotional health.

PRINCIPLES OF HEALTH

One of the main purposes of this book is not only to cure disease but to teach an understanding of the most important principles of a healthful diet and lifestyle and how to maintain a healthy body.

When you understand the way the body works and can assist the process of helping it function at its optimum best, you possess the knowledge and wisdom you need to take your health into your own hands and preserve, protect, and enhance your physical, mental, and emotional well-being. Your natural instincts will be awakened and better utilized. You must study the Principles of Health and learn to support your body's natural restorative processes.

Healing requires creating health through a positive change of attitude, boosting the immune system, strengthening the body's natural healing capacities, and bringing yourself to a state of harmony with living. As you learn more about the body, you can work with the forces of nature instead of against them. Health is our natural state. Disease takes over when we desert healthful ways of living.

Take responsibility to explore and educate yourself about your own health. Doctors can assist this process, but you must do the work. All men, women, and children must learn to nurture themselves, respect the body and its processes, and allow themselves to function at their best, as they were intended to do by nature. This is the holistic or wholistic (whole body) approach. Holistic healing employs natural remedies and treatments along with wholesome foods, exercise, sunshine, fresh air, positive thinking, fulfilling work, and a balanced lifestyle.

Balanced lifestyle is worth discussing further. Earlier in this introduction, I mentioned that doers, givers, overachievers, workaholics, those who spread themselves too thin, and type-A personalities were among those most likely to have Candida problems. Remember, no matter how good your diet, exercise program, and the rest of your lifestyle is, you have to s-l-o-w d-o-w-n! You can do the Candida treatment and diet successfully and have Candida come back again in a few months or more if you don't learn *how* to live! The world will still revolve on its axis if you do less. Learn to do less—better. You will make fewer mistakes, and the quality of what you do will improve *if* you take time to do things at a slower pace that allows you to be more conscious and fully present in the moment. Let the rest of your family or office learn to take on more responsibilities. You are not on this planet Earth to pick up all the loose ends, family chores, and office projects no one else wants to do. Others won't want to do them when they know they can get you to. They may be on to something. They are not willing to overwork, so why should you be? Learn to say, "*No*, I have enough to do already!"

Choose to create health, and the methods you require will become available. Every disease has a prevention as well as a cure; we just have to find it and utilize it. Many people already know the cure and do not want to use it! Some smokers still smoke even after lung cancer becomes evident. Junk food eaters eat junk food even when they are overweight. Some individuals with clogged arteries eat fatty foods after heart attacks have occurred. Choosing good health means being willing to do what it takes to maintain it or get it back. This book can assist you with this process.

Eating a healthful diet and taking care of your body can be enjoyable! Wholesome foods can be prepared so that they taste delicious. (Despite sour-puss claims that you have to suffer or eat tasteless foods to heal, this is not true!) The recipes in this book will prove that healthful foods can have terrific flavor!

In order to digest foods properly and in order to heal, one has to enjoy eating. If a food tastes good, we salivate more, releasing more digestive enzymes to process food with. So, naturally, we absorb more nutrients when we enjoy our food. Your taste buds do change as your diet, lifestyle, and level of health alter. As children, we have over 7,000 active taste buds, which diminish to 700 by the time many of us are in our sixties. Environmental poisons, toxins, and food additives interfere with the ability to taste, but can be avoided when one lives a healthful lifestyle, eats wholesome foods, and employs some cleansing techniques regularly. Almost no one liked the taste of straight alcoholic beverages at first; they got "used to it." It is far easier to get used to the taste of fresh wholesome foods and vegetables, and that's a promise!

It takes work to create a new, more healthful lifestyle, but the rewards are enormous. While attempting to cure your Candida yeast problem, you may find that your healthful diet and lifestyle may also improve overall health, slow the aging process, reduce symptoms and damage from other diseases, and improve mental and emotional health. Good food preparation and wholesome eating are worth the extra initial effort and become quite easy with time and practice.

MY CANDIDA STORY: SHORT & SWEET

In my childhood I was sickly with colic; thrush; hyperactivity; learning difficulties; memory problems; allergies to dairy products, wheat, and oranges; and, unknown at the time, intestinal parasites from the tropical country where I was born. As a child, I hated all food, except sweets. These health problems mushroomed into anorexia nervosa, constant headaches, stomach problems, mood swings, and, eventually, major memory loss—so severe that I could not read a book or hold a job. I suffered up to eight-hour-long anxiety attacks, screaming fits, sleep disorders, nightmares, hallucinations, and dark depressions.

At age nineteen, I was seeing a psychiatrist three times a week and taking large doses of prescribed Thorazine, with terrible side effects. When I was twenty-one, medical specialists gave me three months or less to live. They said that my liver was beyond repair from poor health, excessive alcohol, and wasteful living. They told me my pancreas, spleen, and lungs were ruined. In the past, I had smoked two and a half packs of cigarettes a day. I had grown up with parents who were both heavy smokers. My daily diet included several donuts or pastries, three to six candy bars, six to eight cans of pop, cookies or cake, one pint of ice cream, french fries, ten cups of coffee with sugar, and a burger, pizza, or steak with a bit of tomatoes, canned corn, or peas.

I refused to accept the doctors' gloomy predictions! I had no intention of dying because I felt I had not yet fully lived. I decided I would do anything, even eat "icky" health foods, to heal. Over the next twenty years, I learned to make health foods taste good, and I explored and experimented with every healing method that appeared beneficial for me. Many of these methods are shared in this book. I spent nearly five years retrieving and healing lost parts of my memory and mind. The way was fraught with pitfalls, mistakes, problems, and health crises. During this time, I suffered from chronic depression, low blood sugar, metal poisonings (lead, copper, and mercury), miscarriages, Epstein-Barr and chronic fatigue syndrome, intestinal parasites, allergies, skin rashes, hormone imbalances, huge ovarian cysts, a host of other diseases, and recurrent bouts of Candida albicans.

I had to laugh when a local allergy association refused to let me write for its newsletter because I was "not sick enough to understand the problems of those with allergies." Some people have more energy invested in remaining ill than they do in embracing health. Despite eight near-death experiences, I kept right on going. I have an iron will (and a soft heart) and am determined to live a healthful, happy, fulfilling life. Each year now is better than the last. I made up for lost time by backpacking through Europe for three months at age forty and by age forty-five had completed 10 books (four co-authored, including this one).

I struggled with seemingly incurable Candida for six years in a row (it was off and on before that). When I was thirty-eight, the underlying cause—intestinal parasites, the "worst case" my doctors had ever seen—was finally discovered and controlled with special treatments. From that point on, Candida was a minor issue, easily dealt with by occasional supplements, cleansing programs, and two-week Candida treatments every one to two years.

My health is good and stable now, and my energy levels are high. I write health books, I teach natural cooking and nutrition classes for Langara College in Vancouver, I provide individual nutritional consultations as a clinical nutritionist, and I also work as a part-time floral designer and gardener for a large church. Between 1994 and 1996, I wrote four new books and rewrote an old one, working up to 100 hours per week. From 1998 to 1999 I toured the United States, vacationing and promoting my books. I now keep my workload down to about 40 to 50 hours a week (sometimes less), which is like working part time for an energetic type like me. I make sure to take time to enjoy life, spend time with friends, play, and rest.

I presently do two to four cleanses per year and fast 12 to 24 days per year. These help keep me young, energetic, and healthy, and do wonders for my digestion and looks. I practice yoga, bike, dance, garden, walk, do deep breathing, meditate, write poetry, and love working as much as I love playing.

One fringe benefit of my near-death experiences is that I have learned to treasure and savor life, with its daily ups and downs. Life is beautiful, exciting, and full of opportunities for growth, expression, and enjoyment. People often say I look ten to twenty years younger than I am. I feel better now than I have in my entire life. Each year gets sweeter, more satisfying and rewarding. I am getting older, healthier, and younger in spirit each year. In writing this story, I hope to inspire any of you who are sick and dismayed by severe health problems and Candida albicans to know that it is possible to heal and enjoy life. It takes work, but it is definitely worth the effort!

One of my favorite quotes about life is from Charles Dickens in *David Copperfield:* "I know your life has been hard, but you are what you are because of it. The best steel must go through the fire. It is not enough to be loving, talented, or beautiful. We must be strong!"

For more information on Jeanne Marie Martin, see her website: www.jeannemariemartin.com.

Part I

WHAT TO DO ABOUT CANDIDA

BY DR. ZOLTAN P. RONA
AND JEANNE MARIE MARTIN

Chapter 1

THE DISEASE THAT DOES NOT EXIST

BY DR. ZOLTAN P. RONA

THE EXISTENCE OF A CANDIDA PROBLEM IS ONLY denied by those not up-to-date on recent medical, microbiological, and biochemical literature. Those who stand to gain financially from this pretense will strongly maintain that the problem does not exist. Everything in this book has been documented by peer-reviewed scientific research and case histories. Just as truth prevailed over the historically denied association between scurvy and vitamin C deficiency or between peptic ulcers and the bacterium *helicobacter pylori,* universal acceptance of Candida-related illness is only a matter of time.

Fungi are everywhere. Whether we like it or not, these single-cell organisms can be found in land, water, and air. They are present in our cleanest waters, soils, food, churches, and hospitals. It is estimated that over 500,000 different species of fungi thrive on this planet, and they can be extremely sturdy life forms, capable of changing from rapidly growing forms to those of no growth for periods of thousands of years. Given the correct stimulus, they can change from a round, benign, yeast-like form to an invasive, budding mycelial form. A single fungus can only be seen under a microscope; colonies can be apparent to the naked eye in the form of mushrooms, toadstools, and mold on leftover food. In the past decade, a great deal of attention has been focused on a single fungus called Candida albicans, but we should expand our awareness of fungi beyond just Candida.

Fungi can enter our bodies through our noses, lungs, and gastrointestinal tracts. At any one time we may have 5,000 different species of fungi living in our bodies as normal inhabitants of the skin, vagina, and gastrointestinal tract. Our immune systems, pH level, and other microorganisms ("friendly bacteria") protect us against major infectious problems that can stem from continuous exposure to fungi. Exceptions are localized fungal skin infections, such as athlete's foot, ringworm, dandruff, jock itch, and vaginal discharge. With increasing immune system debility, fungi can infect the bloodstream, as happens with AIDS, leading to death through general toxemia. Less life-threatening but still serious in terms of functional impairment, other immune system illnesses such as chronic fatigue syndrome (also called myalgic encephalomyelitis) are almost always complicated by fungal infections.

We all have various bacteria and fungi like Candida living in our large bowels, as part of what is called "normal flora." Ideally, there should be a balance between fungi and normal flora. These microorganisms are helpful in digestion, synthesis of vitamins and enzymes, and prevention of infections and cancer. Ordinarily, Candida and other fungi are benign and live in balance with other microbes in the bowel. They become invasive only under special circumstances.

When we disrupt the normal flora balance with such things as antibiotics (penicillin, tetracycline, erythromycin, sulfa drugs, and many others), immunosuppressive drugs such as chemotherapy, steroid drugs such as estrogens, the birth control pill, progesterone, or cortisone, we create an imbalance in the bowel that favors the growth of fungi. Stress, diabetes, hypoglycemia, and other metabolic diseases can be triggers for Candida/fungal proliferation, leading to infection, inflammation, and chronic disease.

Consuming large amounts of refined carbohydrates (candies, chocolate, cakes, cookies, chips, soft drinks, white breads, donuts), alcohol, and caffeine leads to excessive growth of fungi. Even the sugar found in fruits and fruit juices, if consumed in large enough amounts, can favor the overgrowth of gastrointestinal fungi. The consumption of yeast, mold, and fungi found as unwanted growths on healthful foods such as grains, fruits, nuts, and some vegetables leads to a worsening of the problem. Common edible mushrooms are nothing more than a species of fungi that can increase the gut fungal population. Leftovers of formerly healthful foods may be contaminated with fungi and molds. Yeast and fungi thrive in the gastrointestinal tract when provided with large doses of sugar in almost any form and the live or dead bodies of other yeast and fungi.

Diabetics frequently suffer from the effects of an overgrowth of yeast, particularly when blood sugar levels are not under control. Many diseases in which the immune system is compromised are associated with yeast infections. Candida seems to thrive whenever the immune system has been weakened by drugs, disease, or a poor diet. The mercury found in the common black dental filling has been implicated as an immunosuppressive agent. A large number of scientific studies link fungal infections with silver mercury dental amalgam hypersensitivity. Stress, chemical additives, and nutritional deficiencies create an overpopulation of yeast in the colon that spreads up the digestive tract into the small intestine, stomach, esophagus, and oral cavity. In the mouth, Candida infection produces a noticeable white coating of the mucous membranes, known as thrush. The tongue, gums, cheeks, and palate may all be coated with Candida or other fungi.

Benign Candida (the yeast form) can convert into the more invasive form of Candida (the mycelial form) when host defenses are weakened. They can invade the bloodstream and spread to practically all organs and tissues in the body. Overcolonization of Candida in the digestive tract causes changes in the permeability of the bowel (degree of penetrability of substances from the gut to the bloodstream), allowing undigested or partially digested proteins to enter the circulation. Normally, this does not happen. When it does, previously well-tolerated foods may start to behave as allergens. This is one reason why the clearing of a chronic Candida infection from the bowel has such a powerfully beneficial impact on the signs and symptoms of food allergy-related illnesses.

MYCOTOXINS: SOURCE OF THE SYMPTOMS

Candida and other fungi produce a large number of biologically active substances called mycotoxins. These toxins are secreted to serve the fungi by protecting it against viruses, bacteria, parasites like protozoa, insects, animals, and humans. In the human host, these toxins can get into the bloodstream and produce an array of central nervous system symptoms (fatigue, spaciness, confusion, irritability, mental fogginess, memory loss, depression, dizziness, mood swings, headaches, nausea, burning sensations, numbness and tingling, and others). Many of the signs and symptoms thought to be caused by low blood sugar (hypoglycemia) are more often the direct result of fungal mycotoxins.

One example of a Candida mycotoxin is acetaldehyde, a by-product of alcohol. An accumulation of acetaldehyde produces many symptoms of alcohol toxicity and is thought to be the chemical mainly responsible for what has popularly been termed "hangover."

Not all mycotoxins are harmful to human health, however. One example of a beneficial mycotoxin is penicillin. Other mycotoxins, like those produced by poisonous mushrooms, can kill outright. The mycotoxins associated with Candida albicans infestation can produce chronic illness, frequently described as "feeling sick all over."

The end result of Candida/fungal overgrowth, invasion, and the subsequent creation of toxins is the *yeast syndrome*. People may identify themselves as "having Candida," but there is no uniformity of opinion on what to call the syndrome itself. This is because no two people share exactly the same symptoms. Some patients have thirty or more symptoms. Doctors who treat the condition often label the syndrome *Candida-related complex*. Since it remains unclear whether other fungi besides Candida can cause the same signs and symptoms, perhaps we should say *fungal-related complex*.

Fungal problems are usually secondary to other primary imbalances related to the general health of the immune and endocrine system. Treating only the fungal infection may help relieve a great number of symptoms but may not necessarily relieve the primary defect (for example, diabetes; adrenal insufficiency; vitamin and mineral deficiencies; immune dysfunction; toxic heavy metal poisoning, especially with mercury; hydrochloric acid deficiency; pancreatic enzyme deficiency; hypothyroidism; and others). Ideally, this could be sorted out by tests ordered by a qualified health-care practitioner.

A lack (achlorhydria) or insufficiency (hypochlorhydria) of hydrochloric acid production by the stomach predisposes an individual to Candida or fungal overgrowth. In healthy individuals, the high acid content of gastric juices helps kill off most fungi and other potentially harmful microorganisms found in food. As one grows older and the stomach's ability to produce hydrochloric acid diminishes, Candida and other fungi can get past the stomach acid barrier and overpopulate the gut. One of the major inhibitors of hydrochloric acid production is an unsuspected food allergy, especially to wheat or milk and other dairy products. The problem can be reversed by eliminating the offending allergenic foods and augmenting the diet with acidifying nutritional supplements.

Pancreatic enzyme deficiency can cause fungal overgrowth in the gastrointestinal tract. Like hydrochloric acid, pancreatic enzymes (protease, lipase, amylase, and others) help digest and inactivate fungi that enter the body with food. Low stomach acid production and pancreatic enzyme insufficiency can be diagnosed through a comprehensive stool and digestive analysis ordered by a natural health-care practitioner. Acid or pancreatic digestive enzyme supplements can be taken to improve the situation. Examples of acid and other digestive enzyme supplements include glutamic acid, betaine hydrochloride, pepsin, pancreatin, bile salts, papain, bromelain, stomach bitters, and plant enzymes.

Evidence now exists that fungi, through production of mycotoxins, initiate many degenerative diseases: cancer, heart disease, gout, arthritis, and autoimmune disease (thyroiditis, chronic fatigue syndrome, multiple sclerosis, systemic lupus erythematosus, rheumatoid arthritis, myasthenia gravis, scleroderma, and others). The major killer diseases in North America are intimately connected to fungal mycotoxins. Diseases of "unknown etiology" often have a fungal connection. Treatment of the fungal infection can bring about improvement or elimination of that disease.

Many foods typically considered healthful have been discovered to be heavily colonized by fungi and their mycotoxins. These include corn, peanuts, cashews, and dried coconut. To a lesser degree, fungi can also be found in breads of all kinds, barley, rye, wheat, rice, millet, and practically all cereal grains. A diet high in contaminated grains and nuts increases the likelihood of fungal colonization of the gastrointestinal tract. Worse, animals fed mycotoxin-contaminated grains end up with fungal overgrowth; the fat and muscles of most grain-fed animals in North America are loaded with mycotoxins. Animal fat has been well documented to be associated with a greater risk of both heart disease and cancer. According to some researchers, it is not the animal fat that increases cancer and heart disease risk, but the mycotoxin load in the fat itself.

We have all been brought up with the unshakable dogma that cigarette smoking causes lung cancer and that tobacco is a carcinogen. Few realize that all the cigarettes sold in North America are contaminated with yeast or fungi and have had sugar and yeast added to the final product. Sugar increases fungal growth. So does baker's or brewer's yeast. It is conceivable that tobacco itself is harmless and that it is made carcinogenic commercially, partially because of the fungal contamination. The mycotoxin *fusarium,* found in cigarettes, has been linked with lung cancer, esophageal cancer, and cancer of the uterus.

The manufacture of bread, beer, wine, cheese, chewing tobacco, aged and cured meats, and cigarettes involves a fungal fermentation process and increases the likelihood of exposure to mycotoxins. Alcohol is a fungal-produced toxin and has been documented to cause brain and nervous system damage, liver cancer, birth defects, and hundreds of other negative health conditions. The consumption of small amounts of these foods may be tolerated by those with healthy immune systems but deadly to those suffering from chronic illness of any kind.

One well-known mycotoxin called *cyclosporin* is used for organ transplantation to prevent rejection. Unfortunately, cyclosporin causes cancer, high blood fats (hyperlipidemia), and hardening of the arteries (atherosclerosis) in anyone who receives it. An astounding 100 percent of all cyclosporin users get cancer. Interestingly, antilipid drugs like lovostatin and other "statins" used to lower levels of LDL-cholesterol (the bad cholesterol) are antifungal agents. Practically all antifungal therapies will lower LDL-cholesterol and help reverse atherosclerosis. The antifungal drug *griseofulvin* has been well documented to reverse hardening of the arteries and relieve angina pain, though its developers never intended griseofulvin for this purpose.

HISTORY AND SYMPTOMS OF FUNGAL-RELATED COMPLEX

History of taking antibiotics

Persistent prostatis, vaginitis, cystitis, or other genito-urinary infections

History of taking birth control pills, female hormone-replacement therapy, or cortisone-like drugs

Reactions to perfumes, tobacco, chemicals

Development of multiple food and chemical allergies (universal reactor phenomenon)

Athlete's foot, ringworm, jock itch, chronic fungal nail or skin infections

Chronic rashes or itching, psoriasis, recurrent hives

Cravings for sugar, breads, or alcoholic beverages

Fatigue, spaciness, lethargy, poor memory, numbness, tingling, burning

Insomnia, muscle aches, weakness, paralysis, joint pain or swelling

Dry mouth or throat, rash or blisters in mouth, bad breath

Nasal congestion or postnasal drip, nasal itching, sore throat, recurrent cough

Bronchitis, laryngitis, wheezing, ear infections (otitis), or ear pain (otalgia)

Abdominal pain, bloating, gas, diarrhea/constipation

Rectal itching, heartburn, food hypersensitivity, mucus in the stools

Impotence, loss of libido, endometriosis, infertility, premenstrual syndrome

Anxiety, depression, irritability, cold extremities, drowsiness, uncoordination, mood swings

Headaches, dizziness

Foot, hair, or body odor not relieved by washing

The fungal-related complex manifests primarily in five areas of the body:

1. Digestive System

   Symptoms include bloating, gas, cramps, alternating diarrhea with constipation, or multiple food allergies. The individual may feel allergic to all foods (pan-allergic).

2. Nervous System

   Symptoms include abnormal fatigue, spaciness, anxiety, mood swings, drowsiness, memory loss, depression, insomnia, and/or mental fogginess. In extreme cases, hallucinations and violent behavior can occur. Autism, hyperactivity, and learning disabilities in children can be manifestations of fungal infestation.

3. Skin

   Symptoms include hives, psoriasis, eczema, excessive sweating, acne, and nail infections.

4. Genito-Urinary Tract

   In women, common problems include premenstrual syndrome (depression, mood swings, bloating, fluid retention, cramps, craving for sweets, and headaches prior to menstruation), recurrent bladder or vaginal infections, and a loss of interest in sex. In males, common problems include chronic rectal or anal itching, recurrent prostatitis, impotence, genital rashes, and jock itch.

5. Endocrine System

An intimate relationship exists in the body between the immune system, the nervous system, and the endocrine system. The thyroid and adrenal glands in particular may be involved. Both hypo- and hyperthyroidism, especially the autoimmune variety, are strongly linked to fungal overgrowth.

Candida/fungal toxins can travel to virtually all organs and tissues in the body. The syndrome has been associated with practically every medical condition, including cancer, heart disease, multiple sclerosis, AIDS, asthma, arthritis, chronic sinusitis, recurrent flu, middle ear infection, alcoholism, addiction, diabetes, eating disorders, hypoglycemia, and many other less common conditions. In some of these diseases fungi are secondary "opportunistic" infections. In many, the fungal mycotoxin may be the cause. In either case, a healthy immune system is the only natural defense against these microbes and their poisons.

CHICKEN OR THE EGG?

Do fungal infections occur because of altered immunity due to some other cause? Or do fungal infections cause altered immunity, which leads to immune disorders such as chronic fatigue syndrome? The answer to both questions is yes. The debate is similar to the theories on tuberculosis in the early half of this century. No matter which came first, the chicken or the egg, the microorganisms involved must be directly dealt with to reverse the disease. As with tuberculosis, the overall health of the host must be enhanced by better nutrition, reduced stress, cigarette and alcohol cessation, aerobic exercise, spiritual and psychological therapy, and a less-contaminated, less-polluted environment. Dietary changes alone do not reverse Candida/fungal syndromes. Aggressive antifungal therapy is also necessary in most cases.

Chapter 2

DO YOU HAVE CANDIDA ALBICANS?

BY DR. ZOLTAN P. RONA

THE MOST TROUBLESOME ASPECT OF THIS SYNDROME is the diagnosis. Doctors skeptical of Candida or the fungal complex frequently point out that there are no unequivocal objective tests to verify its existence. I agree completely. Over the past decade I have used virtually every imaginable laboratory test in my practice to help diagnose Candida or fungal infections. Some of these have included the use of symptom questionnaires, skin tests, RAST or ELISA blood tests, and stool analysis.

Nonmedical practitioners may use electroacupuncture techniques like Vega or Interro testing to diagnose Candida. Others use iridology, muscle testing, pendulum swinging, and radionics. Candida questionnaires of all kinds usually overdiagnose the problem. Lab tests (scratch test, serum RAST, serum antibody complexes, stool analysis, and others) used to detect the presence of Candida or fungi are associated with many false positives and negatives. Candida is normally an inhabitant of the gastrointestinal tract and skin of even the healthiest individuals, so a positive result on a lab test has little meaning. As for the long list of nonmedical Candida tests, correlation with treatment outcomes has not been documented.

Some lab tests can indirectly show the presence of fungi in our bodies. Uric acid is not manufactured by the human body, despite what some medical texts claim and what most doctors believe. Fungi, on the other hand, have been proven to be capable of manufacturing uric acid. If blood tests show elevated uric acid in the body, this is nearly always a sign of fungal overgrowth or infection. The use of antifungal therapy lowers the uric acid blood levels, further supporting the concept that high uric acid blood levels and gout are really the end result of fungal invasion. A normal or low uric acid blood level, however, is no guarantee of a negative diagnosis (no infection).

There is no universal agreement about the relative merits of any single Candida/fungal test, save direct microscopic examination of blood or biopsied tissue. A promising new test, live-cell microscopy, offers a quick, reliable means of visualizing Candida, parasites, bacteria, and other organisms and their debris in live whole blood. One drop of blood coming from a fingertip puncture clearly reveals living organisms floating freely in the bloodstream by use of a microscope attached to a high-quality color video camera connected to a color monitor and video recorder. Live-cell microscopy, pioneered by Canadian scientist Gaston Naessens, creator of the 714X alternative cancer treatment, can reveal some health and disease data not possible through conventional microscopy.

Most microscope technicians charge $50 to $100 for this test. Beware of untrained microscopists affiliated with multilevel-marketing vitamin companies who sell the products they recommend! Some insurance companies cover the test and all types of remedies if recommended by a medical doctor.

Trial therapy based on signs, symptoms, and a high "index of suspicion" is a recommended alternative. In my clinical practice, the symptom that consistently appears in an otherwise medically healthy individual as a reliable indicator for trial therapy of antifungals is debilitating fatigue accompanied by spaciness or short-term memory loss.

The cholesterol in our blood does not come from dietary sources. Eating cholesterol does not cause heart disease. Cholesterol is a fat made by the body in response to the presence of fungal mycotoxins. It is a sign that something is wrong, not a sign that we should try to lower the cholesterol in our bodies by reducing the cholesterol intake in our diet. The more fungal mycotoxins in the body, the more the liver will manufacture cholesterol to help neutralize the toxins. Studies indicate that a high sugar and yeast diet (eating lots of bread and desserts) increases the Candida or fungal population in the gastrointestinal tract, elevates cholesterol, and increases the risk of heart disease.

The real role of cholesterol in the body is to serve as a defense against mycotoxins. Cholesterol reduces the toxicity of mycotoxins by helping bind ("chelate") them. In other words, high blood fats (hyperlipidemia) are protective. For this reason, a high blood level of cholesterol is a sign of fungal overgrowth or infection. Studies support the fact that the use of antifungal therapies lowers cholesterol and reverses atherosclerosis. Every cholesterol-lowering prescription drug is also antifungal. A normal cholesterol level does not necessarily indicate no fungal infection. A cholesterol level well below the normal reference range (below 150) might also be connected to fungal infections. Severely depressed cholesterol blood levels are frequently seen in AIDS patients, who are rarely free of fungal overgrowth. In view of the confusion in both the medical and lay literature, the cholesterol-fungal connection is a concept that may take many years to accept.

Platelets are important blood-clotting factors. Another clue to the presence of fungal invasion is a low blood platelet count. Over the years I have seen several cases of thrombocytopenia (low platelets) cleared by an antifungal program of diet changes and food supplements combined with prescription antifungal drugs. A normal platelet count, however, does not necessarily mean that a fungal infection does not exist in the body.

UNSUSPECTED FUNGAL CONNECTIONS

Through authors such as Orian Truss and William Crook, we have become aware of the Candida/fungal connection to chronic fatigue syndrome, intractable allergies, fibromyalgia, premenstrual syndrome, endometriosis, recurrent vaginitis, cystitis, infertility, loss of libido, and many other debilitating conditions. Recently, the fungal-mycotoxin connection has been made with heart disease, hyperlipidemia, cancer, gout, autoimmune disease, and other age-related and degenerative diseases. The ultimate presence or absence of disease may well be related to the outcome of a lifelong race between fungi and our immune system's defenses against their toxins. If we are to survive, we will have to outwit and defeat this unsuspected impact of Candida and other fungi.

AUTISM
The cause of autism is unknown, but many published studies indicate that autistic children can be helped by the following:

1. Folic acid supplementation (particularly in autistic males with the fragile X syndrome). Folic acid is antifungal. Its effectiveness in the treatment of autism may well be due to its antifungal properties.

2. High doses of supplemental vitamin B_6 and magnesium. Numerous studies by world-renowned autism expert Dr. Bernard Rimland indicate this to be the case.

3. Amino acid analysis and balancing. Recent studies indicate that autistic children have high levels of free tryptophan and serotonin in their blood. They may be helped by supplements of glutamine, phenylalanine, and tyrosine.

4. Food allergy testing and treatment may significantly help autistic symptoms. The ELISA/ACT test may be helpful in diagnosing hidden food allergies. Several published case reports indicate that nearly 50 percent of autistic cases improve when sugar, milk, and wheat are removed from the diet.

5. Testing for heavy metal toxicity (lead, mercury, cadmium, and others) by blood, urine, and hair may reveal a previously unsuspected cause of brain chemistry imbalance.

6. Supplementation of the diet with other nutrients designed to enhance brain function, including DMG (dimethyl glycine), octacosanol, choline, B-complex vitamins, vitamin C, vitamin E, and ginkgo biloba extract.

7. Fungal metabolites have been found in the urine of a large percentage of autistic children. Antifungal therapies of all types have been reported to help reverse some cases of autistic behavior.

The guidance of a natural health-care practitioner is essential in any of these nutritional diagnoses and treatments.

BODY ODOR AND HALITOSIS

Poor hygiene, uncleanliness, and stress are the most common causes of offensive body odor. Sweat itself has no odor, but after a few hours bacteria on the skin interacts with it, producing odor. Eating foods like garlic, curry, and other spices in high amounts increases body odor in susceptible people. Excessive caffeine consumption can influence body odors. Deficiencies in zinc, silicon, selenium, magnesium, protein, vitamin A, B vitamins, and especially biotin and vitamin C are unsuspected causes of body odor in some individuals. In others, chronic illnesses or negative health conditions like diabetes, liver disease, parasites, intestinal fungal or Candida infection, chronic constipation, and other gastrointestinal diseases are indirectly responsible. Anyone suffering from an offensive body odor problem that responds poorly to the usual daily hygiene methods should get biochemical and digestive system testing done by a natural health-care practitioner. Once the source of the problem has been isolated, specific treatment (bowel detoxification, antifungal herbs, or other treatments) can be started.

Halitosis (bad breath) is a common problem that may be a sign of many different conditions. The most common causes include dental and gum disease, upper or lower respiratory tract infections (nose, sinus, throat, lungs), improper diet (too much refined food and red meat), constipation, and cigarette smoking. Other fairly common causes of halitosis are food allergies, sugar diabetes, and hypochlorhydria (low stomach acid).

Low or absent stomach acid causes poor digestion of foods, leading to excessive bacterial fermentation. The heavy intake of certain foods such as onions, garlic, alcoholic beverages, and other odoriferous foods can be a factor. Fasting causes bad breath due to the production of ketones, easily relieved when the fast is broken.

If you have ruled out these potential causes of halitosis and conventional treatment has been unsuccessful, consider a number of effective measures. First, brush your teeth and tongue after every meal. To prevent bacteria buildup, change toothbrushes every month. Use dental floss and a chlorophyll mouthwash daily (2 tablespoons to 1 glass of water). Green drinks such as liquid chlorophyll, wheatgrass, or barley juice are very effective against bad breath. Drink these liberally. Use herbal toothpastes made from myrrh, peppermint, spearmint, rosemary, and sage.

Nutritional supplements that are helpful in most cases of halitosis include vitamin A, beta-carotene, B-complex vitamins (especially folic acid), vitamin C, Coenzyme Q_{10}, and bee propolis. These are important for the healing of mouth and gum disease and control of infection. An overgrowth of harmful bacteria in the large bowel can cause bad breath. So can hidden Candida or parasitic infections. Lactobacillus acidophilus supplements are recommended to offset critters with friendly bacteria in the large intestine.

If these self-help measures fail to eliminate halitosis, see a naturopath or nutritional medical doctor in your area for more detailed investigations and specific treatments.

Breast Cancer and the Fungal Connection

When I graduated from medical school in 1977, breast cancer was said to occur in one of every eleven women. The accepted conventional treatment at the time was radical mastectomy—the complete surgical excision of the breast, the lymph nodes under the arm, and some of the underlying muscle layers.

This was then followed by radiation, chemotherapy, and, in some cases, more surgery to remove the ovaries or other organs.

In the following two decades, the good news was that radical mastectomy had slowly been replaced by the simple lumpectomy—the surgical excision of the cancerous tissue only. The bad news, however, was that by the year 2000, the incidence of breast cancer had gone up to a whopping one in every seven women.

While great strides have been made medically and surgically in the treatment of breast cancer, nothing much has been done by the forces of orthodoxy to help women prevent breast cancer in the first place. One of my concerns is that, in the past five years, I have been seeing more younger women in their thirties being stricken with the disease.

In 1998, the National Cancer Institute reported 19,300 new cases of breast cancer and 5,300 breast cancer deaths in Canada. In the past 40 years in North America, the occurrence of breast cancer has increased steadily at the rate of 1 percent each year. Conventional methods of early detection and treatment are not prevention. They have clearly failed to make a dent in these disappointing statistics. Despite these shocking statistics, groups like the American Cancer Society continue to deny that a problem exists here.

While it may be true that breast cancer is strongly connected to the genes, studies show that diet and lifestyle changes can prevent or delay the expression of unfavorable genetic programming. In other words, if you happen to have a very positive family history of breast cancer and are thus blessed with less than favorable genetics, you can do a great deal to prevent the breast cancer genes from expressing themselves in you as breast cancer.

Dr. A. V. Costantini, retired head of the World Health Organization (WHO) Collaborating Center for Mycotoxins in Food at the School of Medicine in Freiburg, Germany, (see his new book *Prevention of Breast Cancer, Hope at Last*) has also advanced a well-documented theory that eradicating fungal mycotoxins from the body is the best form of prevention against breast cancer. It is interesting to note that tamoxifen, a drug touted as effective breast cancer prevention and treatment, is antifungal. Dr. Costantini postulates that this is the reason for some of its effectiveness in breast cancer therapy. If his theory is valid, it would help explain the efficacy of vegetarian diets (red meats are a heavy source of fungal mycotoxins) and many natural cancer therapies.

Of course, there are less toxic, more effective natural and prescription antifungals that can be used in place of tamoxifen to rid the body of fungi and their mycotoxins, and this is, of course, the subject of this book. The fungal-mycotoxin connection is one of the areas that needs to be addressed for the natural prevention of breast cancer.

The fungal connection may be one of the more important reasons that women with a strong family history of breast cancer should do everything they can to avoid fungi. Sugar suppresses immunity within minutes of its consumption. It causes high circulating levels of insulin and greater deposition of fat in the body. A study (presented at the Annual Meeting of the American Society of Clinical Oncology, New Orleans, May 23, 2000) now shows that breast cancer patients with high levels of insulin are eight times more likely to die from their disease and four times more likely to have the cancer recur at a distant site. Insulin promotes cell growth and, most likely, breast cancer cell growth. The higher the insulin, the higher the breast cancer risk.

Research shows that the replacement of all refined carbohydrates (i.e., sugar, honey, white flour, fruit juice, etc.) with a whole-foods, high-fiber diet of fruits, vegetables, beans, nuts, and seeds is effective in lowering high circulating levels of insulin. The best insulin-lowering foods are:

Soybeans and other legumes—1 cup or more daily of soybeans, kidney beans, lentils, black-eyed peas, chickpeas, or lima beans retards the rate of absorption of carbohydrates into the bloodstream.

Onions and garlic—½ a clove of garlic and 1 medium-sized onion twice daily normalizes blood sugar regulation by decreasing the rate of insulin elimination by the liver.

Aloe vera gel—½ teaspoon twice daily stimulates the increased synthesis of insulin by the pancreas.

Fenugreek seeds—½ ounce twice daily reduces fasting and postprandial (after meal) blood sugar levels in both juvenile and adult-onset diabetics by improving cell sensitivity to insulin.

Blueberry leaf tea—1 cup twice daily reduces high blood sugar levels through the action of the active component, myrtillin.

Bitter melon (balsam pear)—a tropical fruit widely cultivated in Asia, Africa and South America, the juice of which (2 ounces daily) contains several compounds with strong blood sugar–lowering action.

Jerusalem artichokes and asparagus—(1 to 2 cups daily) contain inulin, a soluble fiber that stabilizes blood glucose levels, preventing both hyper- (high) and hypoglycemia (low blood sugar). Inulin can also be found in high concentrations in chicory (Chicolin), the dahlia plant, dandelion, burdock, garlic, and onions.

Incidentally, these are also the same foods that will normalize blood sugar levels in people with adult-onset diabetes, as well as those suffering from hypoglycemia (low blood sugar attacks).

The average North American consumes the equivalent of 35 teaspoons of simple sugar daily (about 150 pounds annually). At least half of this comes from hidden sources such as pickles, pasta sauces, cheese spreads, crackers, boxed cereals, peanut butter, ketchup, and so forth. Simple sugars include fructose (fruits, honey, pop, and some processed foods), sucrose (white and brown sugars), lactose (milk sugar), and maltose (rice, corn, or barley syrup). Most experts agree that too much sugar leads to tooth decay, extremes in blood sugar levels, and higher body fat. Studies at Yale University by Dr. Judith Rodin show that sugar stimulates the appetite and leads to repeated food cravings or addictions.

In *Lick the Sugar Habit* (Avery Publishing Group, 1996), Dr. Nancy Appleton recommends the following measures:

- Don't keep sugar-laden foods at home (helps prevent feeding the habit).
- Remove corn from the diet (a major sugar source in processed foods that brings on cravings).
- Eat complex carbohydrates made of multiple sugar molecules linked together in long chains called polysaccharides (whole grains, brown rice, potatoes, beans, and vegetables) to avoid the yo-yo effect of simple sugars.
- Read labels and avoid sugar equivalents like honey, maple and corn syrup, dextrose, malt, and so on.
- Eat small portions of high-protein foods (large portions might trigger cravings).
- Get help from friends (the buddy system provides needed psychological support).
- Increase exercise (vigorous exercise decreases appetite while burning calories).
- Avoid artificial sweeteners (studies show no benefit for curing sugar cravings).
- Avoid fruit, caffeine, and alcohol because all cause greater sugar cravings due to their blood sugar–lowering effects.

- Take dietary supplements that curb sugar cravings:
    Glutamic acid or L-glutamine (2,000 milligrams three or more times daily)
    GTF chromium (1 milligram three times daily)
    Zinc (30 milligrams daily)
    Multiple vitamin and mineral supplement (1 tablet daily)
- Work with a natural health-care practitioner for a personalized diet, exercise, and supplement program.

CHRONIC FATIGUE SYNDROME, FIBROMYALGIA, AND THE FUNGAL CONNECTION

In 1978, fibromyalgia and chronic fatigue syndrome were rare conditions of little to no concern to most medical practitioners. In the mid-1980s, however, this changed dramatically. Now, hardly a day goes by that I don't see a CFS or fibromyalgia patient. No one is completely sure what happened, but suddenly doctors began seeing an ever-growing number of people with multiple, non-specific complaints. Often, it was impossible to distinguish these people from those who were labeled as having "Candidiasis." The major symptoms included chronic fatigue, sleep disturbances, generalized muscle and joint pains, intermittent flu-like illnesses, depression, anxiety, general malaise, and cognitive impairment. With all these signs and symptoms occurring in the same individual at roughly the same time, doctors were baffled about both the diagnosis and how to treat the problem.

Initially, medical experts who could find no evidence of bacterial, viral, or other infection theorized that this was a psychiatric illness, a form of depression. To this day, many doctors still believe that CFS and fibromyalgia are "in your head." Evidence is now accumulating that CFS and fibromyalgia are primarily a disorder of the immune system. The type of immune system disorder involved fits the category known as autoimmune disease.

An autoimmune disease is defined as one in which the body's immune system starts making antibodies against its own tissues or organs. In a normal state of health, the immune system recognizes the body's organs as native, or a part of self: It does not attack them in any way. A healthy immune system only attacks foreign invaders (e.g., bacteria, viruses, parasites, fungi, or other potentially unfriendly particles) or tissues (cancer cells). When one's immune system attacks one's own body (normal healthy tissues and organs), this is defined as an autoimmune reaction.

An immune system reaction to joints (as in rheumatoid arthritis) is one example of an autoimmune reaction leading to an autoimmune disease. When the immune system mounts an attack against the thyroid, autoimmune thyroiditis results. When it attacks the lining of the gastrointestinal tract, autoimmune colitis (ulcerative colitis or Crohn's disease) results, and so on. Current thinking is that fibromyalgia syndrome (FMS) is the result of such an autoimmune mechanism of action.

Autoimmune diseases often respond to antifungal treatments. Evidence exists that fungi, through their production of mycotoxins, initiate many autoimmune diseases by triggering inflammation in the gastrointestinal tract, which in turn leads to the development of the "leaky gut syndrome." The major killer diseases in North America, cancer and heart disease, are intimately connected to fungal mycotoxins. Diseases of "unknown etiology" often have a fungal connection, with treatment of the fungal infection bringing about an improvement or elimination of that disease.

In treating any fungal infection, it is important to realize that many foods, even those considered to be healthful, are heavily colonized by fungi and their mycotoxins. These include corn, peanuts, cashews, and dried coconuts. To a lesser degree, fungi can also be found in barley, rye, wheat, rice, millet, and practically all cereal grains. A diet high in contaminated grains and nuts increases the likelihood of fungal colonization of the gastrointestinal tract. Worse, animals fed mycotoxin-contaminated grains end up with fungal overgrowth. This is evidenced by the fact that the fat and muscles of most grain-fed animals in North America are loaded with mycotoxins. Animal fat has been well documented to be associated with a greater risk of both heart disease and cancer. According to some researchers, it is not the animal fat that increases the cancer and heart disease risk, but the mycotoxin load found in the fat itself.

There is a fungal connection to CFS and fibromyalgia. While it cannot be said that fungi cause these diseases, numerous reports state that the use of antifungal remedies clears or improves many cases.

ECZEMA

Eczema can be caused by stress and emotional factors, nutritional deficiencies, food allergies, and digestive function abnormalities, including low stomach acidity and low pancreatic digestive enzyme levels. Chronic eczema has also been associated with fungal infections, especially in cases in which antibiotics have been used. The antibiotics kill off even the friendly bacteria that usually keep fungi like Candida albicans at bay, allowing the latter to flourish. Candida and other fungi secrete a toxin that can cause a long list of health problems, including eczema. Parasites, bacterial flora imbalances, and various toxicities (e.g., mercury) are other possible etiologies in some cases of eczema.

Eczema is usually treated by dermatologists with prescriptions for various cortisone-based creams. Dermatologists rarely prescribe remedies directed at the systemic source of a rash, preferring to suppress skin problems with assorted steroid lotions and creams. For many people, this is acceptable practice.

For those who wish to use a more natural approach in reversing eczema, their diet should be as fresh and unrefined as possible. They should avoid chemicals, chlorinated tap water (they may want to avoid chlorine in both drinking and bath water), animal products, processed foods, coffee, tea, alcohol, and sugar in any form. Even the sugar found naturally in fruit and fruit juices might aggravate eczema in some individuals because sugar feeds bacteria, parasites, or fungi that might already be present in the gastrointestinal tract in larger than acceptable numbers.

Dairy products and eggs are strongly allergenic and a trial therapy of strict avoidance of these foods and anything derived from them for several weeks is usually a very good idea. Animal products may also be loaded with drugs such as antibiotics, synthetic hormones, nitrates, nitrites, and other skin toxins. For short-term relief, an organic, plant-based diet is best. As symptoms improve, poultry and fish can be added back to the diet. Later, whole fresh fruits can be consumed on a trial basis. If the eczema returns upon reintroduction of any food, a stricter dietary approach of either complete avoidance or a four-day rotation of reactive foods can be instituted. One can avoid the food trial-and-error approach by getting food allergy testing by blood tests like the RAST or the ELISA/ACT test.

Nutrient supplements that may be very helpful for both treatment and prevention include essential fatty acids (e.g., salmon oil, evening primrose oil, flaxseed oil, black current seed oil, oil of borage, etc.), vitamin A, B-complex vitamins (including biotin), vitamin C, bioflavonoids (pycnogenol, hesperidin, catechin, quercetin), vitamin E, zinc, calendula, tea tree oil, and aloe vera. Treatment depends mainly on biochemical individuality, which is something that can be determined from professional consultation and testing. Topically, calendula cream helps healing and prevents infections. So does vitamin E cream and aloe vera gel. See a naturopath or a medical doctor familiar with the natural approach for a personalized program based on a thorough clinical evaluation and biochemical tests.

GOUT

Gout is the name given to a condition that results from too much uric acid in the blood, joints, kidneys, or other body tissues. When uric acid accumulates, it forms crystals and causes pain and swelling in the joints. If uric acid crystallizes in the kidney, stones may be produced. There are many causes of gout, including a long list of metabolic conditions: cancer, psoriasis, hemolytic anemia, specific enzyme defects such as Lesch-Nyhan syndrome and others, and several kidney diseases. Some cytotoxic drugs, chronic lead poisoning, and high fructose (sugar) consumption can also lead to gout.

The human body does not synthesize uric acid. All the uric acid present in the body comes from production and secretion by fungi. Therapy must ultimately be aimed at reducing the fungal population of the body. All anti-gout or uric acid–lowering drugs are antifungal. This fact has been documented for the drugs *colchicine* and *allopurinol*. Natural uric acid–lowering substances like vitamin C and folic acid are also antifungal.

In uncomplicated cases, diet is very important in the prevention and treatment of gout. Weight reduction in obese individuals reduces uric acid levels significantly. Drink at least eight glasses of distilled water daily. For short-term relief, vegetables and their juices (especially celery, liquid chlorophyll, carrot, spinach, and parsley) are recommended in large amounts. Avoid fruits and fruit juices, as these may be mold-contaminated or too high in sugar, albeit natural sugar, which can contribute to the uric acid load. Blueberries, blackberries, raspberries, strawberries, and hawthorn berries, all high in bioflavonoids, have the ability to neutralize uric acid however. Whole grains, seeds, and nuts can be included in a uric acid–lowering diet.

Rich foods, coffee, sugar, and white flour products aggravate gout. Avoidance of purine-rich foods and alcohol will help prevent the accumulation of uric acid. Purine-rich foods include red meats, sweetbreads, shellfish, anchovies, herring, sardines, meat gravies, consommé, mussels, all organ meats, asparagus, and yeast products. Other foods that increase uric acid are fish, poultry, dried beans, lentils, peas, spinach, cauliflower, oatmeal, and mushrooms. These latter foods may be added back to the diet in small amounts once the acute attack is under control. Vitamin B3 (niacin) in large doses may also elevate uric acid and must be avoided in anything other than a B-complex supplement. Recent studies have also speculated that vitamin A toxicity and gout may be related. Supplementation with vitamin A should be questioned.

Supplements that help in the treatment of gout include vitamin B-complex, folic acid, vitamin C, vitamin E, and magnesium chelate. Folic acid is antifungal and inhibits the enzyme *xanthine oxidase*, which is responsible for producing uric acid. The prescription anti-gout drug allopurinol works because it inhibits this same enzyme in fungi.

Omega-3 and omega-6 EPA oils (flaxseed oil and oil of evening primrose or borage) are important for their role in limiting inflammation. Another potent natural anti-inflammatory agent is bromelain. Bromelain is a proteolytic enzyme found in pineapples. The bioflavonoid quercetin is also helpful in gout because of its anti-inflammatory effect and its ability to inhibit xanthine oxidase in fungi. Studies also show that the amino acids alanine, aspartic acid, glutamic acid, and glycine lower uric acid levels. One or more of these health-food store supplements may be effective alternatives to prescription anti-inflammatory drugs.

Traditional herbal remedies for gout include devil's claw, burdock, and juniper. Devil's claw not only relieves joint pain but also reduces both serum cholesterol and uric acid levels. It can be used as a complement to other anti-gout remedies. See your health-care practitioner for advice and supervision with these and all other natural remedies.

HEMORRHOIDS

Hemorrhoids (piles) are distended or ruptured veins located within or just outside the anus. They are varicose veins that result from several factors, including heredity; pregnancy; prostate enlargement; obesity; straining at stool; constipation; improper or heavy lifting; sedentary lifestyle; standing for long periods of time; sitting on cold, hard surfaces; liver disease (cirrhosis); food allergies; alcohol or drug abuse; and anal intercourse. Hemorrhoids may itch, bleed, tear, and cause pain. They can usually be treated naturally, but severe cases may require surgery.

From a dietary standpoint, it is important to increase fluids. A high-fiber, high-complex-carbohydrate diet is recommended. Avoid animal products as much as possible, as well as coffee, spicy foods, fried foods, alcohol, hot sauces, fatty foods, rich foods, salty foods, sugar, and refined carbohydrates. Eat more cranberries, water chestnuts, buckwheat, (tangerines, figs, plums, prunes, guavas), bamboo shoots, mung beans, (melons), black sesame seeds, (persimmons, bananas), squash, cucumbers, and tofu. Avoid cigarette smoking and a lack of exercise; both habits make hemorrhoids worse. Some of these foods, the ones in parentheses, must be avoided if Candida is present.

Fresh juices that may be therapeutic include carrot, spinach, potato, turnip, watercress, celery, and parsley. Topical herbal remedies that may be soothing are aloe vera and calendula. Herbs helpful in an oral supplement form are plantago (psyllium seed husks and powder), chamomile, buckthorn, collinsonia root, and elderberry. Flaxseed oil (1 to 2 tablespoons daily) creates a natural lubricating effect by softening stools. A garlic clove or raw potato can be made into a rectal suppository for relief of rectal itching. Homeopathic rectal suppositories (BHI, HEEL) can be quite effective. Mineral (sitz) baths using the health-food store product Batherapy on a daily basis helps.

Itchiness from hemorrhoids is usually caused by yeast or Candida overgrowth and their mycotoxins. A daily supplement of a good lactobacillus acidophilus supplement helps crowd out the fungi and eventually the itching stops. Fast-relieving topical remedies that you can experiment with are: tea tree oil, aloe vera gel, garlic oil, oregano oil, olive oil, flaxseed oil, and calendula cream. Follow an antifungal Candida diet. Avoid leftovers and tobacco products. Eat more fish and fish oils, garlic, onions, olives, olive oil, green vegetables, herbs, spices, soy products like tofu, yogurt, psyllium, pectin, and milled (ground) flaxseed. An increased intake of fiber significantly reduces the impact of mycotoxins.

Daily supplemental nutrients often prescribed to shrink hemorrhoidal tissue and promote healing are:

Vitamin A	10,000 mgs.
Beta-Carotene	10,000 mgs.
Vitamin B complex	50 mgs. 3 times daily
Vitamin C	3,000 to 6,000 mgs.
Vitamin E	800 IU
Bioflavonoids (rutin*, hesperidin)	1,000 mgs.
Pycnogenol	150 to 200 mgs.
Coenzyme Q_{10}	200 mgs.

*There is no need to be concerned about the safety of rutin or other bioflavonoids; there is no known toxicity. Bioflavonoids strengthen capillaries and help lessen the effects of food allergies.

For bleeding hemorrhoids, supplementation with vitamin K may be necessary. To get adequate amounts of vitamin K from the diet, eat more dark green leafy vegetables, such as spinach, alfalfa, kale, and lettuce. Dosages for all supplements should be individualized. Supervision by a naturopath or medical doctor familiar with vitamins, minerals, and herbs is recommended.

HYPERACTIVITY

Hyperactive behavior (also known as ADD or attention deficit disorder) and learning disabilities have been linked to sugar intake; hidden or unsuspected food and chemical (especially food dye) allergies; salicylate sensitivity; lead, cadmium, and other toxic minerals; and psychological and other factors.

Many reports have claimed that hidden (masked, delayed hypersensitivity) allergies to foods and chemicals may be involved in hyperactivity. The most common allergies reported are to corn (present in almost all sweetened foods), milk, wheat, eggs, yeast, chocolate, and citrus fruits. I have found that the best way to clinically diagnose hidden allergies to foods or chemicals is with the ELISA/ACT blood test. It can reveal your immune system's reactions to over 300 foods and chemicals. In many ways, this blood test is similar to other ELISA tests that measure antibodies to viruses, bacteria, and fungi. For more information on the ELISA/ACT test and doctors in your area who can order it for you, contact:

Serammune Physicians Laboratories
1890 Preston White Drive, Suite 201, Reston, VA 22091
800-553-5472

Dr. Russell Jaffe is the person who developed this test and made it available to physicians in Canada and the United States. He can be reached for further information at SPL Ltd.

Second, serum amino acid analysis is another test that should be considered, based on the work of Dr. Jaffe and other nutritional doctors. Since amino acids are the precursors to neurotransmitters, low levels can lead to neurotransmitter deficiency. Higher than accepted levels may lead to neurotransmitter excess. Once the amino acid levels are determined, treatment can be aimed at balancing brain chemicals more accurately.

Third, it is important to look for micronutrient deficiencies or dependencies. For example, zinc deficiency can have deleterious effects on both short- and long-term memory. White spots on the nails could be a sign of zinc deficiency, even when blood tests for zinc are normal. The expression, "No zinc, no think" is not without merit. Many studies have shown that zinc supplementation is helpful for memory, thinking, and IQ. The best way of getting zinc is to optimize the diet. The most recently published RDA (Recommended Dietary Allowance) for adults is 15 milligrams per day. The richest sources of zinc are generally the high-protein foods such as organ meats, seafood (especially shellfish), oysters, whole grains, and legumes (beans and peas). Beyond ensuring zinc adequacy from the diet, see a health-care practitioner to decide whether supplementation is worth trying.

Cognitive impairment may also be associated with a deficiency in iron. Studies show that cognitive development can be impaired when iron blood levels are low. Deficiencies in B vitamins, particularly vitamin B_1 and choline may also be involved. Toxic heavy metals such as cadmium and lead can accumulate in the body and cause both hyperactive behavior and learning disabilities in some susceptible children. A hair mineral analysis can reveal whether or not these toxic heavy metals are building up in the body. The good news is that, with a natural program of vitamins and minerals, accumulations of lead and cadmium can be removed from the system.

Many scientific studies show that GBE (ginkgo biloba extract) has remarkable effects on different parts of the circulatory and nervous system. Some of its actions include enhancement of energy production, an increase in cellular glucose uptake, an increase in blood flow to the brain, and an improvement of the transmission of nerve signals. Theoretically, one might assume that GBE could have a beneficial effect on learning disabilities (LD). Unfortunately, no one has ever studied its effects in this area. Studies supporting the use of GBE were for conditions such as the major symptoms of cerebral vascular insufficiency (short-term memory loss, vertigo, headache, ringing in the ears, lack of vigilance, and depression), senility, Alzheimer's disease, peripheral vascular disorders, Raynaud's syndrome, and postphlebitis syndrome.

Since GBE is a safe herbal extract, a trial therapy for LD under the supervision of a naturopath, herbalist, or holistic doctor couldn't do any harm. There is no guarantee that it would be effective. More studies and documented clinical experience would have to be done before I could recommend it as a treatment for learning disabilities. GBE and all the nutrients mentioned here are available from most health food stores and some pharmacies.

Evidence also links this disorder to Candida or fungal infections. According to Dr. William Crook, "I now feel that sugar-sensitive, hyperactive children (especially those who have taken repeated courses of antibiotic drugs) react to sugar because the sugar promotes the proliferation of Candida."

Dr. Crook, reaffirmed by several authors, states, "In my experience, if a hyperactive, learning-disabled child gives a history of recurrent ear and other infections and his hyperactive behavior is triggered by sugar, I feel that a sugar-free special diet and anti-yeast medication should be important parts of his overall management." Work with your doctor to put together a comprehensive nutritional program designed to rebalance the system.

INFLAMMATORY BOWEL DISEASE

The general term *inflammatory bowel disease* includes two major gastrointestinal diseases: Crohn's disease and ulcerative colitis. Both involve large bowel inflammation and tissues outside the colon. There is some overlap of signs and symptoms in both conditions but the cause is poorly understood.

Common to both conditions is the fact that antifungal medications colchicine, nystatin, and ketoconazole have been documented to reverse inflammation in the gut. This and the many positive reports of disease reversal by naturopaths using natural antifungal therapies support the theory that both Crohn's disease and ulcerative colitis have a strong connection to chronic fungal infection.

Crohn's disease is primarily a disease of white adults between the ages of twenty and forty, although it can occur in both children and the elderly. Its main signs and symptoms include abdominal pain, diarrhea, weight loss, rectal bleeding, anal fissures, abscesses, and arthritis. In a minority of cases there may be inflammation of the liver, kidney, and skin. The disease process involves the small bowel only in 30 percent of patients, the colon in 15 percent, and both the small bowel and colon in 55 percent.

Ulcerative colitis is a chronic inflammatory disease that deteriorates the lining of the large bowel. It shows up primarily in the twenty-to-forty age group and effects predominantly females. Most often, the inflammation begins at the rectum and extends up through the colon. The inflammation can progress until ulcerations and abscesses develop. In some patients, the disease can be mild and localized, or excruciatingly painful with perforations of the colon. There is usually diarrhea with blood and mucus in the stool. Sudden attacks followed by periods of remission are typical.

Ulcerative colitis tends to recur in families and there is a high incidence of eczema, hay fever, arthritis, and ankylosing spondylitis. One school of thought believes that inflammatory bowel disease, especially ulcerative colitis, is the result of an allergy or hypersensitivity reaction to food by the colon. Salicylate (e.g., aspirin) sensitivity has been found in some patients with ulcerative colitis. Researchers have shown the existence of circulating antibodies against cow's milk and other foods. The most common offending foods triggering ulcerative colitis are milk, wheat, and yeast-containing foods. It is also known that a chronic Candida or fungal infection increases the incidence of food allergies and that clearing the infection improves allergic symptoms.

Conventional medical treatments for Crohn's and ulcerative colitis often ignore the value of diet, despite a large amount of published medical literature that stresses its importance. Studies and research information are well documented in the book *Breaking the Vicious Cycle: Intestinal Health Through Diet* by Elaine Gottschall (The Kirkton Press, RR1, Kirkton, Ontario, Canada N0K 1K0). Many victims of inflammatory bowel disease can control symptoms simply by eliminating lactose (milk sugar), starches, grains, yeast, and refined carbohydrates from the diet. Gottschall's book contains menus, recipes, and other self-help information for anyone suffering from inflammatory bowel disease. The salicylate-free diet and the Gottschall Specific Carbohydrate Diet have a high success rate in both Crohn's disease and ulcerative colitis, probably because the foods eliminated or reduced are the very ones that stimulate the growth of fungi in the gut. Some patients need only follow these diets for six months, while others must follow them for years before being able to eat the disallowed foods again without symptoms.

More difficult cases require help from a natural health-care practitioner for treatment of hidden food allergies, Candida/fungal infections, bacterial flora imbalances, and parasite infestations. The best currently available immunological test for determining hidden food or chemical hypersensitivities (allergies) is the ELISA/ACT test. This is a special blood test developed by Dr. Russell Jaffe that measures circulating antibody levels to as many as 300 foods and chemicals. Parasitic infections can be diagnosed by comprehensive parasitology stool analysis. Diet therapy can be tailored to account for individual food allergies or infections.

Nutritional imbalances and deficiencies arise in sufferers of Crohn's because of malabsorption. Zinc deficiency is common, as are deficiencies in B vitamins, especially B_{12}, vitamin A, and vitamin D. Most cases require periodic vitamin B_{12} injections.

Herbs that benefit inflammatory bowel disease include chamomile, ginger, comfrey, and a combination of slippery elm, Turkish rhubarb, burdock, sheep sorrel, and cress, known as Essiac. This same combination of herbs can be used in the complementary treatment of hemorrhoids, constipation, ulcers, diverticulitis, obesity, adult-onset diabetes, and hypoglycemia. Side effects are negligible.

Barley is a grain and might be a problem for Crohn's and colitis sufferers. Aloe vera juice is soothing for practically all gastrointestinal inflammations. Garlic and acidophilus (dairy- and grain-free) may be helpful. None of the natural treatments interfere with conventional medical treatments. In fact, dietetic change will help make any medical therapy work better.

Low Platelets and Thrombocytopenic Purpura

Idiopathic thrombocytopenic purpura (ITP) is an immune system disorder characterized primarily by rapid destruction of blood-clotting factors called platelets. The cause is unknown and treatment usually involves steroids (prednisone) and removal of the spleen. There are no proven effective alternative therapies; however, complementary nutritional therapies may help speed recovery.

Elimination of allergenic foods from the diet prevents the inflammatory response that manifests as flare-ups of the disease. The most common food allergy associated with ITP is milk. If you do not know your food allergies, go on a hypoallergenic diet (no animal products, processed foods, sugar, white flour products, coffee, tea, or alcohol). At your earliest opportunity, get food allergy testing done (ELISA/ACT test).

Some studies indicate that high doses of vitamin C and bioflavonoids are helpful in the treatment of ITP. Bioflavonoids such as rutin, hesperidin, catechin, quercetin, eriodictyol, and pycnogenol help strengthen the walls of capillaries, preventing bruising (purpura). They stabilize the mast cell membranes and block the series of reactions associated with almost any allergy. If your condition is associated with an allergy, vitamin C and bioflavonoids would be beneficial.

Bioflavonoids are found in many foods, including citrus fruits (the white material just beneath the peel), onions, garlic, peppers, buckwheat, and black currants. In supplemental form, they have been successfully used for many years as a treatment for pain, bumps, bruises, and more severe athletic injuries.

Bioflavonoids work together with vitamin C to protect blood vessels. They are also useful in the treatment of asthma and other allergic conditions.

Side effects of bioflavonoid supplementation, even in megadoses, are unlikely, but due to the serious nature of ITP, it is important that even this natural therapy be supervised by a doctor. In other words, do not attempt this without medical supervision.

Antifungal treatments with natural antifungals like garlic or oil of oregano or prescription drugs can help ITP. Colchicine, an anti-gout as well as antifungal prescription drug, has been documented to help reverse low platelet levels. Successful treatment may take a year or longer but is well worth attempting under medical supervision.

MULTIPLE SCLEROSIS

Multiple sclerosis (MS) is a disease that affects different parts of the nervous system through the destruction of the myelin sheaths, the structures that cover the nerves. The inflammatory response produces any number of symptoms, including blurred vision, staggering gait, numbness, dizziness, tremors, slurred speech, bowel and bladder problems, sexual impotence in men, and paralysis.

MS usually occurs in persons between the ages of twenty-five and forty. The disease may disappear for long periods of time, then return with acute symptom flare-ups. It progresses slowly and may last decades in many cases. In a minority of people, it can develop rapidly and progress unremittingly to death. There is no universally accepted treatment for multiple sclerosis. ACTH (hormone) injections are often used in acute exacerbations, as are immunosuppressive drugs. These have severe side effects. When asked about the role of nutrition in MS, most conventional medical doctors claim no benefit to diet changes. I disagree.

The definitive cause of MS is unknown, but a growing number of scientific studies suggest that nutrition may be a very important factor. Nutrition-oriented health-care practitioners have noticed that early MS can be helped by optimizing nutritional status with respect to essential fatty acids; amino acids; minerals such as zinc, selenium, and magnesium; and B vitamins, especially vitamin B_{12} and folic acid.

In my practice, I have noted tremendous subjective improvements in many MS patients after a series of vitamin B_{12} and folic acid injections. Not only did patients have greater energy, but there were objective improvements in nerve conduction studies done by neurologists. Spontaneous remission?

Not likely; both vitamins have been demonstrated to improve nerve cell function. It is indeed possible that some cases of MS are really B-vitamin deficiencies in disguise.

Most cases of MS (over 80 percent, according to one 25-year study) improve on a low saturated fat diet (Swank diet for MS). Researchers have reported that symptoms improve when food intolerances (allergies) are eliminated. In my experience the most common hidden food allergies are wheat, milk, eggs, yeast, and corn. Testing and treatment of these allergies may unlock the door to recovery for many MS sufferers.

Supplements very effective in both prevention and treatment of MS include fish oil (omega-3 EPA) and evening primrose oil capsules. Dosages depend on the severity of the illness and the patient's tolerance for these supplements. Alternatives include flaxseed oil, edible linseed oil, oil of borage, and black currant oil. Vitamin E and other antioxidants (vitamin A, beta-carotene, B-complex vitamins, vitamin C, zinc, selenium, pycnogenol, and others) are also beneficial.

The hormone DHEA has been touted as an effective remedy for helping multiple sclerosis. A recently published book on DHEA by Dr. Neecie Moore, *Bountiful Health, Boundless Energy, Brilliant Youth: The Facts About DHEA*, is well documented and easy to read. One can also get a great deal of information on DHEA from the Life Extension Foundation (1-800-544-4440).

DHEA has been used successfully in the treatment of many autoimmune disorders, including multiple sclerosis, lupus, and fibromyalgia. DHEA regulates the immune system and maintains the metabolic and structural integrity of the nervous system. DHEA has been shown to be antiviral and has benefited conditions as serious as HIV infection and AIDS.

DHEA is the most abundant androgen (male hormone) produced by the adrenal cortex of both men and women. It can be found in almost any organ, including the testes, ovaries, lungs, and brain. Testosterone is synthesized from DHEA in both men and women. One theory as to why men get lupus and other autoimmune diseases eight or more times less than women is because of their relatively higher levels of DHEA and testosterone. Nutritional doctors have used DHEA in the treatment of fatigue, obesity, loss of libido, allergies, autoimmune diseases (thyroiditis, vitiligo, alopecia areata, rheumatoid arthritis, lupus, scleroderma), stress, and hypoglycemia with varying degrees of success.

One 1990 study by Roberts indicated that MS victims had low DHEA levels, which were improved by DHEA administration. The majority of these patients had discernible improvement in quality of life, including increased energy levels, better dexterity, greater limb strength, decreased sensations of numbness, more power in the lower limbs, and an increase in libido. Another 1990 study by Calabrese concluded that DHEA helped to improve the fatigue so often associated with MS.

In the United States and Canada, DHEA is available only on a doctor's prescription. Natural precursors to DHEA can be found in wild yam, but studies do not indicate that this is equivalent to the pure hormone.

Hypersensitivity to toxic heavy metals such as mercury can produce all the symptoms of MS. So can Lyme disease. Testing for these two possibilities is certainly worthwhile. Some dentists have advocated the replacement of all mercury dental fillings with nonmetal fillings as a therapy for MS. Testimonials that support the replacement of the common mercury filling in MS patients are legion, but it is a controversial topic. In my practice I have had at least a dozen MS victims improve drastically after replacement of mercury dental fillings; an equal number had no change in health status as a result of this treatment.

Hair mineral analysis and urine tests can screen for excess body burdens of mercury, as well as other toxic heavy metals that may interfere with the immune system. High levels can usually be offset by supplementation with vitamin C, selenium, garlic, cysteine, methionine, and other high sulfur-containing compounds. If you are one of these people with a mouthful of dental hardware, get yourself a copy of *Eliminating Poison in Your Mouth* by Klaus Kaufmann and find a dentist familiar with the mercury problem.

Autoimmune diseases like MS often also respond to antifungal treatments. For more information on autoimmune diseases and antifungal treatments, see the earlier section on Chronic Fatigue Syndrome.

Diet is very important in the treatment of any fungal infection. Sugar feeds fungi and must be eliminated from the diet. This includes maple syrup, honey, molasses, and fruit juice. In severe infections, even whole fruits should be eliminated for several weeks. Milk, white flour products, foods containing yeast, peanuts, mushrooms, melons, and moldy foods (e.g., leftovers) all contribute to worsening any fungal infection.

The key elements of diet revision for MS are:

1. Avoid all dairy, grains, legumes, eggs, and yeast.

2. Avoid all allergenic foods that are identified by skin and ELISA tests.

3. Avoid all red meat and margarine.

4. Eat fish and skinless breast of chicken and turkey for protein, fruits and vegetables for carbohydrates and micro-nutrients, and extra virgin olive oil and unrefined sunflower oil for fats.

This diet is essentially a "Paleolithic Diet" (Eaton and Konner, 1985) and is the one that our genetic structure evolved in concert with over 2 million years. Thus, it is very compatible with our genetic makeup and results in few, if any, biochemical failures.

The treatment approach taken to MS or any autoimmune disease depends on many different factors and is best individualized for the patient by a natural health-care practitioner.

Web sites with MS treatment and testing info:

http://www.2cowherd.net/q

http://www.helsinki.fi/~ahalko/ms.html

http://aspin.asu.edu/msnews

http://www.nutramed.com/

http://www.allergy.co.uk/

http://www.srvitamins.com

http://www.thbot.com/

http://www.greatsmokies-lab.com/

Tests

1. Blood Allergy Test by ELISA/ACT or RAST for IgG4
   Available from:

Meridan Valley Clinical Laboratory
515 W. Harrison St.
Kent, Washington 98032
Tel.: (206) 859-8700
Fax: (206) 859-1135

Serammune Physicians Laboratories (ELISA/ACT test)
1890 Preston White Dr., Suite 201
Reston, VA 22091
Tel.: (800) 553-5472

Immuno Diagnostics Labs (RAST for IgG4)
1620 West Oakland Park Blvd.
Ft. Lauderdale, Florida 33311
Tel.: (954) 486-4500

York Nutritional Laboratory (RAST for IgG4)
Murton Way, Osbaldwick
York
YO19 5US, United Kingdom
Tel.: 44 1904 410410
Fax: 44 1904 422000
E-mail: info@allergy.co.uk

2. Intestinal Permeability Test and CDSA
   Available from:

Great Smokies Diagnostic Laboratory
63 Zillicoa Street
Asheville, North Carolina, 28801
Tel.:(800) 522-4762
Fax: (828) 285-9293
http://www.greatsmokies-lab.com/

3. Candida Analysis
   Available from:

Antibody Assay Laboratories
1715 E Wilshire #715
Santa Ana, California 92705
Tel.: (714) 972-9979

4. Whole Blood Elements
   Available from:

Doctor's Data Laboratories
170 W. Roosevelt Rd.
West Chicago, Illinois
Toll free: (800) 323-2784
Fax: (708) 231-9190
(Hair Multi-element Analysis also available.)

5. Amino Acid Analysis, Food Allergy Testing
   Available from:

METAMETRIX
5000 Peachtree Ind. Blvd.
Norcross, GA 30071
Tel.: (800) 221-4640
Fax: (770) 441-2237
E-Mail nutrition@metametrix.com

If you have trouble finding a doctor who will do the test for you, phone or fax one of the laboratories and they will likely be able to give you the name of a physician in your area who will arrange the test.

NAIL DISEASE

Fungal nail problems may be associated with internal disorders such as diabetes, liver disease, low hydrochloric acid production by the stomach, respiratory disease, nutritional deficiencies, and problems with the lymphatic system. A fungus rarely grows on a healthy person's nails but even seemingly healthy people can be plagued by chronic fungal infestations of their hair, skin, and nails.

The use of prescription antifungal drugs often requires a year or longer for a complete cure. Aside from prescription drugs like Lamisil, Diflucan, Nizoral, Sporanox, and Fulvicin, fungi can be killed on contact with selenium-containing shampoos. Soak your toes and feet in a full-strength selenium-containing shampoo every night for at least half an hour. Use it as your shampoo and hand and body soap on a regular basis. Avoid using commercial soaps, which can clog skin pores and aggravate any skin and nail condition. Another effective topical treatment is calendula cream in a flaxseed oil base. This can be applied to the nails and surrounding skin at least twice a day.

Consider using tea tree oil both topically and internally. Tea tree oil is derived from the Australian native tree *Melaleucea alternifolia*. It has a variety of antimicrobial activities and has been used successfully in the treatment of many different skin conditions, especially those associated with fungi or Candida. Despite what you might read on the bottle label, tea tree oil is effective as a systemic antifungal remedy when swallowed with some water. The usual effective dose is about 15 drops in water swallowed three times daily. Other effective antifungal oils taken internally are flaxseed oil, oregano oil, olive oil, borage oil, castor bean oil, evening primrose oil, and fish oils.

Fungi can be difficult to eradicate from toenails, and natural remedies can take months to fully clear them from the body. Oil of oregano is a stronger antifungal than tea tree oil and would work faster for toenail fungus. It does give off a strong odor, but wearing shoes would cut that off considerably. Comments like "Who ordered the pizza?" rarely occur with people who use topical oregano oil. It's worth trying for three months, applied twice daily. Applying some 3 percent hydrogen peroxide to the nails a few minutes before using either tea tree oil or oil of oregano would speed the healing. Taking 2 drops of the oregano oil under the tongue twice daily is also helpful to accelerate fungal eradication.

If enough "friendly" bacteria reside in your body, fungi are less likely to grow on your nails. Take a regular supplement of lactobacillus acidophilus to help your immune system. Other natural antifungal remedies are garlic, caprylic acid, echinacea, colloidal silver, and whole-leaf aloe vera juice. Taken internally, these can kill most harmful bacteria and fungi without significant side effects.

Healthy nails are dependent on adequate intake of protein; vitamin A; B-complex vitamins, especially biotin; vitamin C; vitamin E; selenium; calcium; magnesium; silicon; zinc; and iron. Low stomach hydrochloric acid secretion, as well as a low output of digestive enzymes by the pancreas, may also contribute to nail problems and should be corrected by appropriate digestive aids like betaine and pepsin and/or pancreatin. Get a nutrition evaluation done to determine your specific needs. Optimizing your nutritional status will make a tremendous difference for prevention of further nail problems.

Polycythemia

Polycythemia is a condition in which there is an increase in the total red cell mass of the blood. On lab tests this is manifested by an elevation of the packed cell volume (PCV), the hematocrit, or the hemoglobin level. Symptoms include either those associated with poor cardiovascular function (chest pain, shortness of breath, high blood pressure) or with abnormal nervous system function (fatigue, dizziness, vague aches and pains, numbness, and tingling). The increase in red cell mass may develop in response to a tissue lack of oxygen (hypoxia) or rare disorders causing an elevation in the hormone erythropoietin, produced by the kidney. Polycythemia may also arise from an autonomous overproduction of red cells unrelated to hypoxia or altered erythropoietin levels.

Treatment of polycythemia depends on the cause but usually involves phlebotomy (bloodletting) several times each month, advice on cessation of smoking, a weight-loss program if necessary, management of high blood fats, and control of high blood pressure.

One plausible theory is that some cases of polycythemia are a manifestation of a chronic systemic fungal/Candida infection. If this is true, victims are likely to respond positively to a sugar-free, yeast-free diet and antifungal supplements like garlic, olive oil, oregano oil, ozone, hydrogen peroxide, tea tree oil, taheebo tea, Essiac herbal tea, caprylic acid, acidophilus, betaine and pepsin, pancreatic digestive enzymes, psyllium, and/or prescription antifungal drugs. Certainly, a trial therapy of anti-Candida/antifungal therapy is safe and likely to improve general health status.

Increasing oxygen intake, either via aerobic exercise or oxygen therapies like ozone and hydrogen peroxide, certainly improves cardiovascular health, while decreasing the stimulus to manufacture more red cells. Antioxidants like Coenzyme Q_{10}; beta-carotene; vitamin C; bioflavonoids, especially pycnogenol; vitamin E; selenium; and zinc might also be helpful in improving the health of the cardiovascular system. A naturopath or holistic medical doctor can prescribe and monitor the treatment, depending on individual biochemistry.

PROSTATE CANCER

About a decade ago I became aware of the connection between cancer of the prostate and unsuspected fungal infections. Research made use of the antifungal drug ketoconazole, and I prescribed this to a patient with cancer of the prostate who had refused the conventional cut, slash, and burn medical and surgical interventions. I was more than amazed to discover that the cancer all but disappeared within six months of high-dose antifungal drug therapy. Since then, five other cases of cancer of the prostate were treated with the antifungal approach, and all are doing extremely well, as evidenced by normal PSA (prostate-specific antigen) blood tests, without other conventional therapy.

Prostate cancer is very rarely seen in males under fifty years old and is rated third in cancer deaths in male patients over the age of sixty-five (behind lung and colon). Most are adenocarcinomas. They are associated with benign prostatic hypertrophy (BPH), but there is no specific causative link. Men with prostate cancer may be asymptomatic but often complain of urinary frequency, urgency, and nocturia (a need to wake up to urinate at night).

The diagnosis is usually made by a positive prostate biopsy, but blood tests may show an increased serum acid phosphatase as well as an increased prostate-specific antigen (PSA). Prostate cancer spreads or metastases to the bone, and this can be monitored by other types of tests.

Conventional treatment is prostatectomy and/or radiation, or female hormone therapy. In nonmetastatic disease, the 10-year survival rate is 65 percent, although the male almost always becomes impotent and urinary incontinence can develop (5 to 15 percent of patients) following surgical removal of the prostate. Hormone therapy with estrogen can provide excellent results. Once bony metastasis has occurred, the survival rate declines to two to three years.

From the alternative cancer treatment point of view, many doctors have become aware of the connection between cancer and fungal infections. Many people, including those advocating the antifungal herb taheebo, have observed the shrinkage or disappearance of prostate and bladder cancers when individuals go on a program of diet and supplements designed to control Candida or other fungi. Cancer has also been associated with the presence of parasites. Live-cell (darkfield) microscopy and comprehensive stool and digestive analyses can be done to confirm their presence. Specific parasite cleansing therapies, as well as antifungal treatments, can then be done using herbs, enzymes, probiotics, and other natural approaches.

Aside from the antifungal drugs like ketoconazole (Nizoral) or nystatin, cancer of the prostate responds very well to high doses of vitamin C. It just so happens that vitamin C has powerful antifungal effects. High doses pushed to bowel tolerance levels (the dose that causes diarrhea or very loose bowel movements) are recommended.

Natural antifungal therapy includes a low-carbohydrate diet, garlic, folic acid, lactobacillus acidophilus, pau d'arco (taheebo), Essiac (a combination of burdock, slippery elm, Turkish rhubarb and sheep sorrel), caprylic acid, psyllium seed powder, digestive enzymes, essential fatty acids like flaxseed oil and evening primrose oil, gentian, berberine, grapefruit seed extract, and artemisia annua. Ozone, hydrogen peroxide, tea tree oil, oregano oil, and olive oil are other natural antifungals.

People who have cancer of the prostate should consume more of the following therapeutic foods and juices as often as possible in unlimited amounts:

- garlic, walnut, mulberries, burdock, dandelion greens, taro roots, pearl barley, grains, fresh fruits, and vegetables (avoid leftovers that are likely fungal contaminated)
- pumpkin seeds (raw), beet tops, papaya, mung beans, licorice, sea cucumbers
- anise, tangerine, cherries, figs, lychee, sunflower seeds, mangoes, and seaweeds

- foods rich in zinc and vitamin E like squash seeds, almonds, sesame seeds, tahini, and kelp
- fresh juices made from carrot, beet, spinach, celery, asparagus, lettuce, lemon, and cucumber

Recommendations for all cancers:

Cancer victims, in general, are best off avoiding:

- sugar; white flour products; dairy products; fatty foods; coffee; caffeine; alcohol; meat; chicken; tobacco smoke, which is contaminated with both sugar and yeast; refined foods

Supplements

- Vitamin A (antioxidant with cancer-fighting properties)
- Vitamin C (antioxidant with cancer-fighting properties)
- Vitamin E (antioxidant with cancer-fighting properties)
- Proanthocyanidins (bioflavonoids also known as grape seed extract, pine bark extract, pycnogenol, and so on, are very strong antioxidants)
- Saturated potassium iodide solution (has antimicrobial and cancer-fighting properties)
- Selenium (antioxidant with cancer-fighting properties)
- Germanium (antioxidant with cancer-fighting properties)
- Zinc (antioxidant with cancer-fighting properties)
- Coenzyme Q_{10} (antioxidant with cancer-fighting properties)
- Green foods (e.g., Green Life or Greens Plus for antioxidants like the carotenes and immune enhancement)
- Aloe vera juice (improves digestion and has cancer-fighting properties)
- Immunocal (a special extract of whey protein that elevates glutathione, one of the body's strongest antioxidants and cancer-fighters)
- Lactobacillus acidophilus and bifidus (friendly bowel bacteria that boost immunity against cancer)
- Ecogen (a very high-potency soy isoflavone concentrate that blocks the spread of cancer of the prostate, breast and several others)
- Pectasol (modified citrus pectin that has been demonstrated to prevent the spread of many different cancers)

- Essiac (Flor-Essence, Can-Aid, and Native Legend Tea all contain the cancer-fighting herbs burdock, slippery elm, Turkish rhubarb, and sheep sorrel)
- Taheebo (Pau d'arco is a strongly antifungal herb with documented anti-cancer effects)
- *Avena sativa* (oats are nourishing and soothing for urinary tract problems)
- *Baptisia tinctoria* (wild indigo has anti-cancer effects)
- *Berberis* (Oregon grape fights cancerous cachexia)
- Echinacea (increases interferon production, purifies blood, and boosts immunity)
- *Gentiana lutea* (gentian promotes appetite and improves digestion in chronic debility associated with cancer)
- *Larrea divaricata* (chaparral, creosote bush, or greasewood has long been acknowledged as a natural cancer fighter)
- *Rumex crispus* (yellow dock is especially helpful in the early stages of cancer to prevent its spread)
- *Taraxacum officinale* (dandelion is effective for loss of appetite, liver problems, and weak digestion)
- Curcumin (an extract of tumeric that is anti-inflammatory as well as anti-cancer)
- *Trifolium pratense* (red clover is an alterative that is thought to purify blood, fight cancer, and boost immunity)
- *Viola odorata* (sweet violet is safe and effective in malignant disease, especially after tumor resection, to protect against metastases)
- *Viscum album* (mistletoe: parts of this herb can be toxic and supervision of a knowledgeable herbalist or naturopath is important; tumor-inhibiting effects are reported; its main use is as follow-up therapy after surgery or radiation)
- Hoxsey-like formula is a constitutional cleansing and cancer support formula made up of
  Glycyrrhiza glabra (licorice root)
  Trifolium pratense (red clover)
  Arctium lappa (burdock)
  Berberis (Oregon grape)
  Rhamnus purshiana (buckthorn)
  Xanthoxylum americanum (prickly ash)

Some or all of these treatments can be combined in different ways under the supervision of a natural health-care practitioner. They are, for the most part, compatible with conventional cancer therapies. For more information, see your naturopath or holistic medical doctor.

PSORIASIS

Psoriasis is a common skin condition that results in red, scaly plaques on the arms, legs, and trunk. It affects the scalp but rarely the face. The most common sites include the points of the elbows and knees. Toes and fingernails become dull and develop ridges and pits. It is most commonly seen in people between the ages of fifteen and twenty-five. The cause is unknown and sufferers respond to a variety of medical treatments, including coal tar, steroid creams, and ultraviolet light. Stress, anxiety, surgery, cuts, other illnesses, infections, and drugs such as lithium, chloroquine, and beta-blockers may all trigger attacks. Some studies have demonstrated that psoriasis benefits from fasting and gluten-free, elimination, and complete vegetarian diets. Food allergy detection and control may be very important in some cases. The disease lessens in severity in the summer. It may go into remission from time to time, but it can always return.

Researchers have reported that most psoriasis sufferers have abnormal serum levels of free fatty acids. Long-term dietary changes with respect to fat intake may produce improvement. Animal fat, especially from red meat and dairy products, must be reduced or eliminated. Fresh fruits and vegetables should be increased. Get fats from fish, sesame seeds, flaxseed, or soybeans. Supplementation of the diet with flaxseed oil or edible linseed oil is recommended.

Fish oils (omega-3 EPA oils) are especially helpful. Greenland Eskimos, who consume a high amount of these oils, have a very low incidence of psoriasis despite limited exposure to the sun. Many recent double-blind studies have shown that supplementation of the diet with 10 to 12 grams of EPA oils daily results in significant improvement in psoriasis. This is roughly equivalent to a daily intake of 150 grams of mackerel or herring. Cod liver oil or salmon oil capsules may be more palatable for those with less than a love for fish. The essential oils in these fish, flaxseeds, and soybeans interfere with the body's production of inflammatory chemicals that cause psoriasis lesions to swell and turn red. Red meats and dairy products do the opposite and are best eliminated from the diet. It may take three to six months to see the full benefit of supplementation with essential fatty acids. The diet changes are not expensive and may actually reduce your total grocery bill.

Other supplements reported to be helpful include daily vitamin A, folic acid, vitamin B_{12}, selenium, zinc, evening primrose oil, digestive enzymes, and vitamin E. Supervision by a naturopath or medical doctor familiar with potential side effects from such high doses is advisable. Herbal remedies that may be of help to psoriasis sufferers include silymarin, dandelion, goldenseal, sarsaparilla, yellow dock, lavender, and chaparral. Poultices made from these herbs may be helpful for topical application.

Some cases of psoriasis benefit from antifungal treatment. All the natural anti-psoriasis remedies are also antifungal. Prescription antifungal drugs documented to improve or eliminate psoriasis are colchicine and Nystatin.

Psychiatrists at McGill University have recently reported that stress-reduction techniques such as meditation produce significant improvements in psoriasis symptoms.

RHEUMATOID ARTHRITIS

Rheumatoid arthritis is a chronic joint disease affecting one or more joints, usually those of the hands and feet, particularly the knuckle and toe joints. The synovium and other parts of the joint may gradually become inflamed and swollen with tissue destruction and deformities occurring in the most severe cases. Rheumatoid arthritis, unlike osteoarthritis, is a condition that waxes and wanes, occurring as a single attack or as several episodes that leave the victim increasingly disabled. The disease may also be associated with damage to the lungs, heart, nerves, and eyes. Although this form of arthritis predominantly affects those between the ages of forty and sixty, it can also affect children and teenagers (juvenile rheumatoid arthritis). The cause of the disease is unknown, but is considered to be an autoimmune process (components of the immune system attacking the joints). As with all autoimmune diseases, a fungal connection should be suspected and trial therapy instituted, especially in those cases where both conventional and natural treatments have met with limited success.

Conventional medicine treats arthritis with anti-inflammatory drugs (most commonly aspirin) and physiotherapy. In severe cases of rheumatoid arthritis, more potent anti-inflammatory drugs are used: nonsteroidal anti-inflammatory drugs such as indomethacin, cortisone-like drugs, antimalarials, gold salts, penicillamine, and even experimental cytotoxic drugs.

This approach may produce pain relief, but it does little, if anything, to alter the arthritic process itself. Surgical removal of badly inflamed joint synovium may be required (synovectomy), arthroplasty (joint realignment and reconstruction), tendon repair, arthrodesis (joint fusion), and even artificial joint replacement.

NSAIDS (nonsteroidal anti-inflammatory drugs) are the most common therapy for arthritis. They are big business for the pharmaceutical companies. They cause bleeding from the gastrointestinal tract in close to 25,000 people a year. There is evidence that these drugs accelerate the destructive nature of the disease. Are there safer, more effective alternatives?

Nutritional approaches to arthritis emphasize a diet aimed at eliminating refined carbohydrates (sugar and white flour products) and animal fats (especially those found in red meats). Certain types of fats, however, may, in higher than average intake amounts, act in the same way as standard anti-inflammatory drugs. Examples of this include cold-pressed linseed oil (flaxseed oil), gamma linolenic acid (GLA, found in evening primrose oil), and EPA (found in cod, halibut, mackerel, salmon, shark, herring, and other seafood). Increasing these in the diet or taking them in encapsulated supplement form, while decreasing the intake of saturated animal fats, can have a remarkably good anti-inflammatory effect. These essential fatty acids are also antifungal.

All forms of arthritis benefit from an optimal balance of important trace minerals like zinc, copper, manganese, calcium, magnesium, silicon, boron, and selenium. Vitamins such as A, B-complex, C, beta-carotene, bioflavonoids, and E can be supplemented in higher than RDA doses because of their antioxidant properties. The recommended doses for all these nutrients should be determined by a qualified health-care practitioner, based on appropriate biochemical tests.

Many arthritis sufferers have reported benefits from the use of herbs: alfalfa, devil's claw, Essiac (a combination of burdock, slippery elm, Turkish rhubarb, and sheep sorrel), licorice root, yucca, white oak, comfrey, and sassafras.

A growing number of studies demonstrate the relationship between food allergies (hypersensitivity) and arthritis. The purported benefits of juice or water fasting for all types of arthritis may simply occur because the fast eliminates the food or foods to which the person is allergic. For years, testimonial reports have suggested that some individuals are adversely affected by plants from the *Solanaceae* group (the nightshades). These include tomatoes, potatoes, eggplants, peppers, paprika, and tobacco. It can do no harm for an arthritis sufferer to exclude these foods from the diet for at least two months to see whether avoidance has an impact on the disease process. For those who find the rigors of fasting and food elimination diets too inconvenient or risky, the RAST or ELISA/ACT blood tests can pick up allergies to the nightshades and other hidden food hypersensitivities.

In people who react adversely to all foods (pan-allergic), the probability of an intestinal tract parasitic or fungal (Candida) infection is high. Although one cannot say that parasites or Candida cause arthritis, many nutrition-oriented physicians and clinical ecologists have reported success in the treatment of arthritis when the Candida or parasitic infection was cleared first. Mainstream medical literature documents the fact that colchicine, a drug with antifungal properties, has a beneficial effect on some cases of rheumatoid arthritis.

The ecology of your gastrointestinal tract is intimately connected to the health of the immune system. The intestine is involved with nutrient uptake but also serves as a barrier to toxic substances. Nutrition-oriented doctors and naturopaths have noticed that a large number of people suffering from varying degrees of environmental illness and autoimmune diseases (rheumatoid arthritis, lupus, thyroiditis, scleroderma, and others) have "leaky gut" syndrome. In this syndrome, the intestinal barrier is porous or more permeable to microbial toxins, including fungal mycotoxins, food allergens, polysaccharides, and polypeptides. When these materials penetrate the intestinal mucosa, they induce inflammation and stimulate the immune system to manufacture antibodies that cross-react with your own tissues. Systemic immune complexes are formed, and these lead to many of the symptoms of autoimmune disorders or environmental illnesses: total allergy syndrome, 20th-century disease, chronic fatigue syndrome, and so on.

What causes this condition? The list of potential etiologies is a long one, the most common being undiagnosed infections with parasites, fungi, Candida albicans, and pathogenic bacteria. Leaky gut syndrome can be caused by excessive use of alcohol, NSAIDS (nonsteroidal anti-inflammatory drugs like aspirin and ibuprofen), steroids, broad spectrum antibiotics, a deficiency of pancreatic digestive enzymes, inadequate stomach acidity, a highly refined diet, and food allergies.

The gut becomes leaky in the sense that substances (undigested proteins, toxins) normally not absorbed in the healthy state pass through a damaged or "leaky" gut. The microorganisms secrete various toxins that damage intestinal mucosa and various organ systems, including the joints. Intractable arthritis cases have been documented to respond to therapy aimed at clearing a chronic, unsuspected bowel infection with parasites, fungi, or pathogenic bacteria. Herbs, antioxidant vitamins and minerals, glutamine, glucosamine, essential fatty acids, soluble fiber like psyllium and fruit pectin, digestive enzyme supplements, and lactobacillus acidophilus might all be considered as part of the leaky bowel healing program.

Special lab tests (intestinal permeability test, comprehensive parasitology, and comprehensive stool and digestive analysis) can be ordered to diagnose leaky gut syndrome and lead to effective treatment. At present, one of the best labs offering these services is Great Smokies Diagnostic Laboratory. Any doctor can request test kits, written information on leaky gut syndrome, and other information. Contact:

Great Smokies Diagnostic Laboratory (CDSA, Parasite testing, etc.)
63 Zillicoa Street, Asheville, NC 28801
800-522-4762

Autoimmune diseases like rheumatoid arthritis often respond to antifungal treatments. Evidence now exists that fungi, through their production of mycotoxins, initiate many autoimmune diseases by triggering inflammation in the gastrointestinal tract, leading to the development of the leaky gut syndrome. (See Multiple Sclerosis for more information regarding this; also, diet and animal fat.)

Seborrhea, Folliculitis, and Scalp Problems

Scalp problems such as seborrhea and folliculitis are most often external expressions of internal imbalances and toxemia. Mild cases of seborrhea, folliculitis, and dandruff have been found to respond well to antifungal or selenium-containing shampoos. Using prescription antifungals for six weeks or more can also resolve the problem in mild to moderate cases. In severe cases, the whole body has to be addressed to achieve healing. This can best be accomplished by taking a natural approach.

Stress, emotional factors, nutritional deficiencies, food allergies, and digestive function abnormalities like low stomach acid, low pancreatic enzyme levels, or a severe intestinal flora imbalance may all be related to scalp inflammation and hair loss. Bacterial, fungal, or parasitic infections in the bowel create toxic overloads. Some toxins produced by these microbes have androgenic or estrogenic hormonal effects. Some cause the immune system to overreact to foods or the environment; some cause skin rashes: eczema, seborrhea, and psoriasis. If the body cannot eliminate toxins from these imbalances through the urine or feces, it tries to get rid of them through the skin. Along the way, skin diseases like acne, seborrhea, and folliculitis result. No identifiable fungi may be present in the hair or scalp, but this does not mean they are not in the colon or elsewhere in the body manufacturing toxins. Prescription antibiotics and steroids in pill or lotion form offer temporary relief but set the stage for a chronic fungal infection that just keeps getting worse.

Eradicating the problem usually requires a good bowel-cleansing program, as well as a complete revision of the diet: the elimination of food allergens, reimplantation of a friendly bacterial culture (lactobacillus acidophilus and bididus), and the use of several digestive enzymes and other nutritional supplements. A bowel-cleansing program might involve ozone or hydrogen peroxide therapy, magnesium oxide, aloe vera juice, psyllium seed powder, pectin, bentonite, senna, buckthorn, cascara sagrada, ground flaxseed, and a series of colonic irrigations. Juice fasting is helpful in most cases.

The diet should be as natural as possible. You may have food allergies; until you know exactly which foods are harmful to you, avoid foods high in sugar, fruit, and fruit juice; fermented foods such as beer, wine, cheese, and bread; stored grains; grain-fed animal products (red meats, especially beef and pork, animal fats, butter, whole milk, and other high-fat dairy products); nuts (especially peanuts, cashews, pistachios, and dried coconuts); seeds and refined foods; leftovers; and tobacco products. Eat more fish and fish oils, garlic, onions, olives, olive oil, green vegetables, herbs, spices, soy products like tofu, yogurt, psyllium, pectin and milled (ground) flaxseed. An increased intake of fiber significantly reduces the impact of fungal and other microbe toxins.

Nutrient supplements helpful for treatment and prevention include: essential fatty acids (evening primrose oil, flaxseed oil, black currant seed oil, oil of borage, and others); vitamin A; B-complex vitamins, including biotin; vitamin C; bioflavonoids (pycnogenol, hesperidin, catechin, quercetin); vitamin E; zinc; silica; selenium; calendula; echinacea; goldenseal; chaparral; cayenne; propolis; hypericum; lomatium; and aloe vera juice.

Topically, the use of tea tree oil and calendula cream is beneficial. So is topical vitamin E, silica gel, and aloe vera. Colloidal silver is a natural antimicrobial that can be taken internally and/or applied topically to skin lesions. If possible, see a natural health-care practitioner for biochemical individuality testing (blood, urine, hair analysis, food allergy testing, comprehensive digestive and stool analysis, and so on). A personalized nutritional program can reverse scalp problems and restore general health.

STROKE, TIA, ATHEROSCLEROSIS, AND HEART DISEASE

Stroke (CVA or cerebrovascular disease) is defined as an injury to the brain caused by a lack of oxygen, due either to a blockage of a cerebral artery or a hemorrhage. A transient ischemic attack (TIA) is a type of minor stroke that can cause sudden and brief neurological abnormalities. TIAs are usually the result of pathology in the internal carotid-middle cerebral, or vertebral-basilar arterial system of the brain. The attacks are often recurrent and are premonitions of a full stroke in the future. Most TIAs stem from atherosclerosis (hardening of the arteries) and emboli. Emboli are tiny fragments that may break off the vessel walls of atherosclerotic arteries and lodge in smaller arteries in the brain, causing an interruption or blockage of the blood supply. TIAs are more common in those suffering from high blood pressure, heart disease, atherosclerosis, diabetes mellitus, and polycythemia. Conventional treatment addresses lowering cholesterol or stabilizing high blood pressure. Other conventional treatments are anticoagulants, platelet inhibitors, and, if possible, surgical resection of the diseased artery.

The natural treatment of strokes is similar to that used for the reversal of atherosclerosis and heart disease. The more severe the case, the more strictly one has to adhere to an atherosclerosis-reversing nutrition program. For the most serious cases I usually recommend a complete vegetarian diet, such as those described in books by Dr. Dean Ornish and Dr. John McDougall. There must be complete avoidance of saturated animal fats, sugar, refined carbohydrates, white flour products, and refined and processed foods. Also avoid trans-fatty acids and hydrogenated oils found in commercial margarine, vegetable shortenings, imitation butter spreads, and most commercial peanut butters. Avoid oxidized fats (deep-fried foods, fast food, ghee, and barbecued or smoked foods). All these may increase the levels of free radicals in the bloodstream and lead to hardening of the arteries.

Evidence suggests that many forms of heart disease, including strokes, could be related to fungal infections. Taheebo tea, a natural antifungal, has often been reported to help in recovery from heart disease and stroke. Other natural antifungals include garlic, onion, most soya products, olive oil, tea tree oil, fish oils, oregano oil, caprylic acid, flaxseed oil, psyllium, lactobacillus acidophilus, colloidal silver, whole-leaf aloe vera juice, and digestive enzymes of all types. Just about any natural antifungal remedy is effective in the promotion of sound cardiovascular health.

Interestingly, antilipid drugs such as lovostatin and other "statins" used to bring LDL (the bad cholesterol) levels down are all antifungal agents. Practically all prescription antifungal therapies lower LDL-cholesterol and help reverse atherosclerosis. The antifungal drug griseofulvin has been well documented to reverse hardening of the arteries and relieve angina pain, despite the fact that its developers never intended griseofulvin to reverse coronary artery disease.

Foods that may have a therapeutic effect in the reversal of atherosclerosis include garlic, wheat germ, liquid chlorophyll, alfalfa sprouts, buckwheat, carrots, watercress, rice polishings, apple, and celery. Water-soluble fiber added to the diet can assist in further lowering blood cholesterol levels and cleansing the body of toxins: flaxseed, pectin, guar gum, and oat bran. Other foods with therapeutic benefits include onions, beans, legumes, soy products like tofu, and ginger. A great deal of evidence also indicates that one can prevent cardiovascular and cerebrovascular disease by increasing the intake of omega-3 and omega-6-EPA oils. I recommend vegetarian sources for these oils such as walnuts, flaxseed oil, borage oil, evening primrose oil, or black currant oil.

Fresh vegetable juices are an important part of the nutritional program. The best juices include combinations of carrot, liquid chlorophyll, beet, asparagus, lettuce, parsley, alfalfa, spinach, and celery.

Supplemental Nutrients

Dosages vary from individual to individual; consult a medical doctor or naturopath for supervision.

Chromium can decrease both cholesterol and triglycerides while improving glucose tolerance. A good source of chromium is brewer's yeast (not torula yeast, which is chromium-poor). The best supplemental forms are chromium picolinate and polynicotinate.

Copper in optimal doses controls cholesterol and is vital in the prevention of aortic aneurysms. The zinc-to-copper ratio must be balanced in the body (8:1 zinc to copper is ideal); the best ratio for you can be determined through a combination of blood, urine, and hair tests.

Magnesium can do virtually anything that prescription heart medications can do. Doctors frequently prescribe "calcium channel blockers" to treat heart problems; magnesium has been referred to as "nature's calcium channel blocker." To correct an arrhythmia, magnesium usually has to be given at dosages far above those that can safely be tolerated in oral supplement form. In practice it is always wise to balance magnesium intake with both calcium and potassium. Evaluation of blood and tissue levels can be done with the help of a health-care practitioner.

If one takes high amounts of magnesium (2,000 to 5,000 milligrams per day), the effect after a day or so is diarrhea and loss of magnesium and other minerals from the body, known as "magnesium-induced magnesium deficiency." To avoid this, many people learn to give themselves intramuscular injections of magnesium.

Potassium is a mineral like magnesium and calcium and is very important in control of blood pressure and heart rhythm. Balance with calcium and magnesium is crucial. Best food sources include bananas, oranges, cantaloupe, kiwi, baked potato, spinach, lentils, split peas, and all beans.

Omega-3-EPA oils reduce cholesterol and prevent platelet stickiness. Good dietary sources include flaxseed oil, rice bran oil, trout, mackerel, salmon, herring, sardines, cod, halibut, and shark. Controversy exists about the cholesterol-lowering effects of fish oils; some studies report an elevation of blood fats.

Selenium is an antioxidant that works in conjunction with vitamin E to protect vascular tissue from damage by toxins. Low selenium levels are associated with an increased risk of atherosclerosis.

Vitamin E is otherwise known as alpha-tocopherol. Studies indicate that supplementation of as little as 200 IU daily in men can reduce the risk of a heart attack by 46 percent; in women the risk is reduced by 26 percent. Whether from a natural or synthetic source, all forms supply the body with at least some vitamin E activity. The natural forms of vitamin E are d-alpha-tocopherol, d-alpha-tocopheryl acetate, d-alpha-tocopheryl succinate, and mixed tocopherols. The synthetic forms are dl-alpha-tocopherol, dl-alpha-tocopheryl acetate, or dl-alpha-tocopheryl succinate.

Studies indicate that the most biologically active are the esterified natural forms: d-alpha-tocopheryl acetate and d-alpha-tocopheryl succinate. Both have been found to provide full antioxidant activity in the body and are recommended by the top authorities on vitamin E at the Shute Institute and Medical Clinic in London, Ontario.

Recent studies indicate that high levels of stored iron in the body (ferritin) are associated with a greater risk of heart disease and diabetes. High-dose vitamin E supplements can interfere with iron absorption. If you have been prescribed iron to correct iron deficiency, take the iron supplement about twelve hours apart from vitamin E. Iron absorption is enhanced by sufficient acid in the stomach. Iron destroys vitamin E in the body. A supplement of vitamin C (500 to 1,000 milligrams) can increase iron absorption by up to 30 percent. Other good absorption aids include Swedish bitters, betaine or glutamic acid hydrochloride, apple cider vinegar, and lemon juice.

Vitamin C lowers high blood cholesterol levels and helps prevent atherosclerosis. It directly promotes the breakdown of triglycerides and regulates arterial wall integrity via its essential role in collagen formation. Vitamin C regenerates and reactivates the vitamin E used to block oxidation of LDL-cholesterol. It is also antifungal.

Beta-carotene, a precursor to vitamin A, is a fat-soluble antioxidant that protects LDL-cholesterol from oxidation. Supplementation has been shown to raise HDL-cholesterol levels. Beta-carotene has also been shown to protect smokers from coronary artery disease.

Vitamin B$_6$ prevents accumulation of high levels of the amino acid homocysteine, implicated as one of the tissue-injuring substances initiating atherosclerosis. Other supplements shown to lower homocysteine levels include vitamin B$_{12}$ and folic acid. B$_6$ deficiency has been associated with a greater risk of coronary artery disease, elevated serum cholesterol, and atherosclerosis. Vitamin B$_6$, B$_{12}$, and folic acid are best taken together in the form of a B-complex vitamin supplement to fully balance all the B vitamins.

Folic acid has recently been heralded as a potent preventive remedy against heart disease. Aside from its ability to lower dangerously high homocysteine blood levels, folic acid appears to be antifungal. Folic acid lowers uric acid levels in the body. Gout results from a fungal production of uric acid; folic acid may be an effective gout remedy simply because it is antifungal.

Carnitine is therapeutically effective in the treatment of coronary heart disease. Normal cardiac function is dependent on adequate concentrations of carnitine in heart muscle. Carnitine helps increase muscle strength and stamina. In the body, carnitine is manufactured from the amino acids lysine and methionine with the help of vitamins B$_3$, B$_6$, and C. Linus Pauling advocated the use of high doses of L-lysine and vitamin C in patients with angina. His studies indicate a significant improvement, possibly because of greater manufacture of carnitine in the body from the lysine and vitamin C.

L-carnitine transports fatty acids into cells where they can be burned as fuel. In fact, some types of metabolic obesity are caused by a deficiency of carnitine. L-carnitine can dramatically lower blood levels of triglycerides. D-carnitine and D, L-carnitine can be toxic and should not be used. Use only the L-carnitine, an amino acid supplement only available in the United States.

N-acetyl-cysteine (NAC) is a sulfur-containing amino acid and is a strong antioxidant. It is a constituent of glutathione peroxidase, one of the most important antioxidants in the body. NAC is important in the treatment of angina because it can make patients more sensitive to the beneficial effects of nitroglycerine. NAC must be used with caution in diabetics and should be supervised by a physician.

Choline lowers blood levels of triglycerides and cholesterol. Lecithin is a source of choline, but some brands of lecithin may have 20 percent or less choline content, the remainder being saturated fat. Unfortunately, no study confirms the benefits of lecithin in lowering cholesterol. Much of the lecithin sold commercially in pill or loose powder form may be nothing more than rancid fat. Look for pure choline capsules.

Chondroitin sulfate is a component of collagen and lowers cholesterol and triglycerides while preventing thrombus (vessel blockage) formation.

DHEA (dehydroepiandrosterone) is a steroid hormone produced in the adrenal gland. It has been found in significantly lower levels in men with documented coronary artery disease and men who die of heart attack. DHEA supplementation (a natural source is the Mexican wild yam) has benefits not only for heart disease but also for obesity, diabetes, arthritis, cancer, immune system problems, memory loss, and osteoporosis.

Niacin has long been known as a potent cholesterol-lowering agent. Severe side effects (flushing, gastrointestinal distress, ulcers, glucose intolerance, and liver irritation) make it an unpopular remedy. Those wishing to take it should be under the care of a physician. There are time-release forms as well as forms combining niacin with inositol, which are not associated with any significant flushing reaction. Inositol hexaniacinate is the safest form of niacin and produces virtually no flushing effects. Niacin can lower total cholesterol blood levels by as much as 18 percent, raise HDL-cholesterol by 32 percent, and lower triglycerides by 26 percent at dosages ranging from 600 to 1,800 milligrams daily.

Coenzyme Q_{10} (CoQ_{10}) is an antioxidant supplement successful in the prevention and treatment of coronary artery disease. It has been found particularly effective in the treatment of chest pain and heartbeat irregularities. It improves cardiac function in cardiomyopathies (diseases of weak heart muscle), reduces angina attacks and pain, and works synergistically with other antioxidants like vitamin E, beta-carotene, and vitamin C. CoQ_{10} can significantly lower high blood pressure, and lower LDL-cholesterol while raising HDL-cholesterol.

Bioflavonoids are special antioxidant compounds found in many fruits, especially berries, vegetables, green tea, and wine. Some better-known bioflavonoids include catechin, hesperidin, rutin, quercetin, pycnogenol, pronogenol, and polyphenols. Bioflavonoids can lower LDL-cholesterol levels and inhibit platelet stickiness. Together with vitamin C in large doses, bioflavonoids are effective in the treatment of allergies.

Ginkgo biloba increases the blood supply to the brain, prevents platelet aggregation, and controls angina pectoris (chest pain from coronary heart disease). It is a potent antioxidant much like vitamin E.

Garlic is probably the best-known herb that lowers cholesterol (by up to 10 percent) and triglycerides (by up to 13 percent), while raising HDL-cholesterol (by up to 31 percent). Garlic prevents thrombus formation and lowers blood pressure.

Gugulipid is a standardized extract of the mukul myrrh tree native to India. Gugulipid can lower cholesterol by 27 percent and triglyceride levels by up to 30 percent. It has no side effects and is even considered safe for use during pregnancy.

Hawthorn is best known for its use in cardiac weakness, valvular murmurs, shortness of breath, mitral valve regurgitation, chest/angina pain, anemia associated with heart irregularity, and nervous exhaustion. Hawthorn has traditionally been used in the complementary medical treatment of coronary artery disease, angina pectoris, arrhythmias, arteriosclerosis, and other circulatory weaknesses. Hawthorn reduces cholesterol, dilates coronary blood vessels, and thereby increases blood flow to the heart muscle. It prevents and reverses plaque formation. It has a potent synergistic effect with the digitalis cardiac glycosides and should be used with caution in people taking prescription cardiac drugs.

Onions have effects on lowering blood pressure and cholesterol as well as on preventing platelet aggregation.

Alfalfa lowers cholesterol because of its content of saponins.

Ginger has a tonic effect on the heart, lowers cholesterol, and inhibits platelet aggregation.

Cayenne lowers cholesterol and inhibits platelet aggregation. Cayenne is an excellent natural remedy for the chest pain seen in angina pectoris.

Bromelain is a proteolytic enzyme found in pineapples that can break down atherosclerotic plaques.

Many of these nutrients are sold in combination form at health food stores; it may, therefore, not be necessary to take large numbers of capsules or tablets.

A naturopath or medical doctor familiar with herbal remedies can recommend dosages. The world's leading medical journals increasingly report that diet and lifestyle changes by themselves can reverse hardening of the arteries and its complications. Drugs and surgery are not always a fact of life. Discuss all this with your health-care practitioner and use his or her experience and expertise to guide you with an individualized holistic health program aimed at reversing circulatory disease.

CHRONIC VAGINITIS

Chronic fungal or Candida vaginitis does not always show up on cultures. In fact, cultures are a poor way of making the diagnosis. The problem is usually systemic and requires more than just the dietary approach of a yeast-free, sugar-free diet and natural antifungals. Such cases usually require fairly long-term prescription antifungal medication. Ketoconazole (Nizoral) would be my first choice. Other options include fluconazole (Diflucan), itraconazole (Sporanox), and nystatin (Nilstat). All these drugs have a high degree of safety and efficacy, both short- and long-term.

Women with chronic fungal vaginitis should be assessed for hormonal imbalances, especially for a deficiency in progesterone and thyroid hormone. Using natural progesterone cream (3 percent or 6 percent) might help soothe vaginal pain and burning, irrespective of special hormone tests. Calendula cream, flaxseed oil cream, aloe vera gel, and vitamin E oil are all soothing for genital area irritation and could be tried if progesterone cream does not provide immediate relief. Food and chemical allergies are common in chronic inflammatory conditions.

Natural remedies applicable in chronic fungal vaginitis are: dong quai, ginseng, black cohosh, aloe vera juice, flaxseed oil, evening primrose oil, borage oil, tea tree oil, lactobacillus acidophilus and bifidus, silicon (silica gel), boron, zinc, selenium, copper, vitamin A, vitamin B_6, and vitamin E. Soy products contain phytochemicals that can help normalize estrogen levels. If estrogen is too high, soy products help lower it; if it is too low, they help raise it. Yams and mistletoe are good sources of natural progesterone. A naturopath or holistic medical doctor can prescribe and supervise a personalized program.

Vitiligo

Vitiligo is a skin condition marked by areas of depigmentation (white spots) and is considered an autoimmune disease associated with a lack or insufficiency of hydrochloric acid production by the stomach. It may also be associated with an endocrine (adrenal or thyroid) imbalance as well as a chronic systemic fungal infection.

Achlorhydria (no acid) or hypochlorhydria (low acid) leads to dozens of nutrient deficiencies. Most high-protein foods need acid for digestion. If acid is low or absent, amino acids, vitamins, and minerals are poorly absorbed. The best-recognized nutrient deficiency caused by low or deficient stomach acid is vitamin B_{12} deficiency. This deficiency leads to pernicious anemia and can usually only be rectified by regular vitamin B_{12} injections.

Low stomach acid may be the result of heredity, extended use of drugs such as antacids and anti-ulcer medications (cimetidine, ranitidine, and others), infection in the gut, or food allergies (especially to milk, dairy, and wheat products). Doctors specializing in nutritional medicine can do several tests to determine the etiology. One is the comprehensive digestive and stool analysis. The CDSA is a battery of 24 screening tests of gastrointestinal status. The main value of the test is in assessing how well a person digests and assimilates food; the existence of a bacterial bowel flora imbalance; hidden infections with fungi, Candida, or parasites; possible food allergies; or digestive enzyme insufficiencies. Once the specific functional problem is determined by the CDSA, further investigations and treatment can be carried out as indicated by the results of the test.

If the cause of low stomach acid is heredity, a variety of things can be tried. These include supplements of glutamic acid hydrochloride, betaine hydrochloride, pepsin, apple cider vinegar, lemon juice, stomach bitters, pantothenic acid (vitamin B5), vitamin C, PABA, and pyridoxine hydrochloride (vitamin B_6). These supplements are usually safe but may, on occasion, lead to too much acidity and intolerance. All are best taken in the middle of each meal or directly afterward.

Aside from acid supplementation, autoimmune diseases like vitiligo might also respond to antifungal treatments.

Natural antifungal remedies may include lactobacillus acidophilus, garlic, caprylic acid, echinacea, tea tree oil, colloidal silver, or whole-leaf aloe vera juice. Taken internally, these can kill most harmful bacteria and fungi without significant side effects. Some individuals respond poorly to the natural approach and are only helped by prescription antifungal drugs (such as Sporanox, Lamisil, Diflucan, and others).

Autoimmune diseases like vitiligo have also been reported to respond to the hormone DHEA (dehydroepiandrosterone). DHEA is the most abundant androgen (male hormone) produced by the adrenal cortex of both men and women. It can be found in almost any organ, including the testes, ovaries, lungs, and brain. Testosterone is synthesized from DHEA in both men and women. One theory as to why men get lupus and other autoimmune diseases eight or more times less than women is because of their relatively higher levels of DHEA and testosterone. Nutritional doctors have used DHEA in the treatment of fatigue, obesity, loss of libido, allergies, autoimmune diseases (thyroiditis, vitiligo, alopecia areata, rheumatoid arthritis, lupus, scleroderma), stress, and hypoglycemia with varying degrees of success.

In low doses (under 1,200 IU per day), vitamin E may have little or no effect on autoimmune disease. In doses well above 2,000 IU, vitamin E weakens autoimmune disease. Herbs such as aloe vera, comfrey, licorice root, white willow bark, feverfew, devil's claw, yarrow, yucca, and marshmallow may also be helpful. Doses of supplemental nutrients have to be carefully individualized. Supervision by a nutritional medical doctor or naturopath is highly desirable.

The transplantation of pigment cells is a promising new treatment for vitiligo. For more information on this type of treatment, ask your family doctor or dermatologist to refer you to a plastic surgeon.

WEIGHT CONTROL AND CANDIDA

A long-term (more than three months) diet in which less than 10 percent of the calories comes from fat is unhealthy because certain essential fats are vital to cell membranes, the synthesis of hormones, and the health of various tissues and organs. Fatigue, memory loss, confusion, eczema, cancer, and heart disease are just a few of the many diseases related to a deficiency of essential fats. It is possible to lower one's fat intake to as low as 10 percent of the diet (e.g., Pritikin Diet) for extended periods of time, but deficiencies in essential fatty acids will eventually occur. Thankfully, it is next to impossible to create a totally fat-free diet from natural foods alone. For a better understanding of the role of protein, carbohydrates, and fat on metabolic rate and weight loss, see *Enter the Zone* by Dr. Barry Sears.

One's metabolism and ability to lose weight on a low-calorie diet depend on many factors, including heredity, blood type, and the status of the endocrine system, especially thyroid hormones, adrenal hormones, gonadal hormones, growth hormone, insulin, and glucagon levels. For example, people who are blood type O are able to lose weight easier on a high protein diet but will gain weight if they eat too many carbohydrates (breads, pastas, cereals, etc.). People who are blood type A will do better on a high carbohydrate, low protein vegetarian diet. For more information on the association between blood types and diet, see *Eat Right for Your Type* by Dr. Peter D'Adamo.

Women who have been on the birth control pill, multiple antibiotic prescriptions, or steroid hormones of other types (e.g., fertility-enhancing drugs) and who follow a high carbohydrate diet, drink alcohol, or smoke cigarettes might well be suffering from a chronic, low-grade Candida (yeast) infection. These prescription drugs and chemicals stimulate the growth of fungi normally present in the gastrointestinal tract. Candida secretes toxins that are sometimes responsible for chronic health problems, including slow metabolism; obesity; cravings for sweets, breads, or yeast-filled foods; fatigue; and a long list of other health problems. Controlling Candida/fungal overgrowth may well be crucial in reversing some chronic cases of slow metabolism of unknown etiology.

Other important factors in weight loss are the adequacy of digestive enzymes, the rate of waste elimination, the health of the liver and kidneys, the levels of B-complex vitamins, mineral levels and the levels of brain neurotransmitters like serotonin and dopamine. Naturally, severe life stresses can contribute to abnormal levels of any of these hormones and micronutrients, making weight loss difficult on practically any diet. Before beginning any weight loss regime, it is best to get a thorough nutritional and biochemical evaluation done by a natural health-care practitioner.

CONCLUSION

If you suffer from one of the many autoimmune diseases like lupus, rheumatoid arthritis, thyroiditis, multiple sclerosis, colitis, or Crohn's disease, your treatment may be incomplete without attention to hidden fungal infections. In cases of chronic illness, especially in allergic conditions like hay fever, asthma, psoriasis, and eczema, Candidal or fungal infestation may well be the culprits causing the seemingly never-ending symptoms. A trial therapy with antifungal remedies might make all the difference to a complete recovery. Since the majority of these treatments are quite harmless, victims of chronic immune system impairment can only win by complementing their medical or naturopathic treatments with an antifungal program.

Chapter 3

TYPES OF TREATMENT

BY DR. ZOLTAN P. RONA

THE RECOMMENDED TREATMENT OF CANDIDA AND other fungal infections is highly variable from author to author and from one health-care practitioner to another. The most important thing is to improve digestive competence and immune defense functions. The goal should never be just to kill all the Candida and fungi in the body. By improving digestion and the general health of the immune system, Candida and other fungi will not find a hospitable environment that allows them to do damage.

Most mild and moderate cases can be treated without prescription drugs. Persistent or severe fungal infections, although responsive to the natural approach of diet changes and food supplements, often require antifungal drugs. The decision about drugs should be made after considerable discussion with one or more doctors.

The most common natural and drug treatments used by naturopaths and holistic medical doctors are described here. Most of these recommendations can be easily implemented, but it is never a good idea to self-diagnose or self-prescribe. Arm yourself with knowledge, then see a health-care practitioner for an assessment and a personalized treatment regimen.

DIET

Food allergies can make fungal infections worse—and vice versa. A natural health-care practitioner can help pinpoint unsuspected food allergies that should be eliminated from the diet. Whenever we speak of diet, we are referring to organically grown foods.

Fungi thrive on sugar, especially the milk sugar lactose. Whether or not you have allergies, avoid foods high in sugar; fruit; fruit juice; fermented foods such as beer, wine, and cheese; bread; stored grains; grain-fed animal products (red meats, especially beef and pork, animal fats, butter, milk, and other high-fat dairy products); nuts (especially peanuts, cashews, pistachios, and dried coconuts); seeds; and refined foods. Avoid leftovers and tobacco products. Eliminate mushrooms from your diet because they feed the fungal population in the gut.

Eat more fish and fish oils, garlic, onions, olives, olive oil, green vegetables, herbs, spices, soy products like tofu, yogurt, psyllium, pectin, and milled (ground) flaxseed—provided you can tolerate them without symptoms. Raw sauerkraut is a rich source of D-lactic acid, an inhibitor of fungal growth. Eating six to eight ounces daily of sauerkraut or high D-lactic acid juices sold at health food stores is a good natural way of controlling fungal infections. Increased intake of fiber significantly reduces the impact of mycotoxins.

Brush your teeth only with buffered vitamin C powder or baking soda. The sweetener found in almost any type of commercial toothpaste encourages the growth of Candida or other fungi. At any sign of Candida in the mouth, gargle with 0.5 percent peroxide solution.

For more information on healthy eating to help prevent and treat Candida and other fungal infections, see Part II: Diet Plans, Menus, and Recipes.

HYPOTHYROIDISM

An undiagnosed low thyroid condition (subclinical hypothyroidism) can make it difficult to eradicate a fungal infection. Standard blood tests for thyroid disease will tell a doctor if the thyroid gland is diseased, but not whether thyroid hormones are functioning at optimal levels. According to alternative health-care doctors, regular underarm temperatures of 97.6°F or below (or average oral temperatures below 98.6°F), combined with symptoms of low metabolism are likely due to a hidden hypothyroid (low thyroid) condition.

Classically, low-functioning thyroid symptoms include depression, fatigue, cold extremities, fluid retention, trouble losing weight, higher-than-average body fat composition, "hypoglycemia," gastrointestinal symptoms such as multiple food sensitivities or allergies, and poor response to exercise (for example, getting weaker after months of aerobic exercising).

Checking your temperature for low thyroid is best done using an old-fashioned shake-down thermometer. Take daily readings for a few weeks; this will show an accurate trend. Not all cases of low temperatures are caused by a functionally low thyroid. Aspects of low thyroid are clearly explained in Broda Barnes's book *Hypothyroidism: The Unsuspected Illness.*

Hair loss may be a symptom of hypothyroidism or other hormonal imbalances (such as adrenal, gonadal, or others). Nutritional factors include deficiencies in protein, zinc, selenium, silicon, iodine (sea kelp), vitamin A, B-complex vitamins (particularly biotin and inositol), essential fatty acids, vitamin C, and vitamin E. Low temperatures may reflect suboptimal nutrient levels in the body.

Routine blood tests (T3, T4, T7, TSH) for thyroid may show normal results in unsuspected ("subclinical") hypothyroidism. Or you may find higher-than-normal cholesterol, low vitamin A, and a high carotene level. Active thyroid hormone is required to convert carotene from the diet into vitamin A (retinol), and to help keep cholesterol blood levels low.

In most hypothyroidism, especially in vegetarians, vitamin A will be low and carotene will be high on the blood tests. Evidence is a carrot-orange color on the palms and soles. Many people who have normal thyroid function tests with multiple hypothyroid symptoms will occasionally show high levels of antithyroid antibodies and antimicrosomal antibodies (Hashimoto's thyroiditis). The B vitamin PABA, high doses of primrose oil or other essential fatty acids, and vitamin E in high doses may help reverse the condition. If not, low doses of prescribed thyroid hormone (such as desiccated thyroid), slow-release liothyronine (T3), glandular thyroid extract, or homeopathic thyroid drops may relieve symptoms.

In some cases there may be a goiter (enlarged thyroid gland) in the neck. A goiter is a definite indication of weak thyroid function. Supplements with thyroid extract and/or iodine eliminate the signs and symptoms within six weeks. Suddenly, a depression of many years, unresponsive to antidepressant drugs, disappears. Food sensitivities, inability to lose weight on very low-calorie diets, lack of positive results from exercise, and general malaise improve dramatically.

Treatment with desiccated thyroid is safe when supervised. Alternatives are supplementation with zinc, vitamin B_6, tyrosine, and iodine, but these do not always work; thyroid hormone (L-thyroxin) supplementation may be necessary. Some companies make a glandular thyroid extract without L-thyroxin, although there are trace amounts of this active hormone. These may work as well as the hormone tablet. A homeopathic doctor should assess suitability for this remedy.

Another alternative treatment for subclinical hypothyroidism is time-release liothyronine (T3). For more information on T3, see *Wilson's Syndrome: The Miracle of Feeling Well* by Dr. Denis Wilson. Wilson's syndrome treatment can get complicated. Regular supervision by a medical doctor is required, mainly to decide on dosages and monitor for side effects. T3 has a very low toxicity potential; side effects can be controlled entirely by drinking much more water and reducing the two daily doses by 7.5 micrograms or more. Make sure you are taking compounded, slow-release liothyronine capsules, not the Cytomel tablets. There is a world of difference between the two prescription forms of T3.

Endocrinologists often object to the use of thyroid medication in a person with normal thyroid blood tests. This is understandable, given the rigidity of medical education—but illogical. In insulin-dependent diabetics with high blood sugar levels, insulin blood levels are usually normal or higher than normal. Despite this, doctors give insulin. Diabetes is an endocrine disease; the real problem is not blood levels of insulin but tissue receptivity to insulin. To get around lack of receptivity, the person is given more insulin, forcing the tissues to use the excess insulin. Megadoses of insulin are used; standard diabetes therapy is an orthomolecular therapy.

In the orthomolecular treatment of hypothyroidism, the levels of thyroxin are increased despite normal thyroxin levels. If blood levels of insulin or thyroxin alone are used to make a diagnosis of diabetes or hypothyroidism, few patients would get proper treatment for either of these conditions. It is unwise to rely only on biochemical tests, which are guides and must be considered together with individual history and a complete physical examination. Ask your natural health-care practitioner for a comprehensive assessment.

MERCURY DENTAL AMALGAMS

The mercury contained in dental restorations is hazardous to the human body. If you have mercury in your mouth, embedded deeply in your teeth or not, you certainly have Candida or fungi there as well. Conventional dental authorities in North America and Britain have attempted to defuse the toxicity issue by ignoring voluminous amounts of scientific research. Persistent denial of the dangers of mercury in dental fillings comes in the form of written pronouncements and attacks on the media by heads of dental associations. But concern about mercury amalgams refuses to die.

Over 100 published scientific papers directly implicate mercury released from amalgam restorations as a major contributing factor in chronic illness. No government or professional agency has ever shown that mercury in dental amalgams is safe. This includes the American Dental Association (ADA), the Canadian Dental Association (CDA), the Food and Drug Association (FDA), and the Canadian Health Protection Branch (HPB). The ADA has published literature claiming that any dentist who removes amalgam restorations due to mercury toxicity is unethical.

One American dental group, the American Academy of Head, Neck, and Facial Pain, has taken a stand against the ADA and its outdated policy. In recent literature this group states, "The evidence is too overwhelming to continue to practice in ignorance and avoidance of the facts. The Board of Directors, under the name of our Academy, has written a petition to several agencies (the FDA, OSHA, NIH, NIDR, U.S. Public Health Service, and the National Institute of Environmental Health Services) asking that all past and current scientific literature concerning mercury and dental amalgams be reevaluated."

What evidence incriminates mercury dental fillings?

1. Mercury damages DNA, alters the structure of proteins, disrupts communication between cells, induces free-radical tissue damage, and inhibits antioxidant enzymes like glutathione peroxidase. Mercury from a single dental filling (nanogram amounts) is enough to inhibit the activity of white blood cells. Mercury can indirectly increase antibiotic-resistant oral and intestinal bacteria, impair kidney function, and induce autoimmune diseases like multiple sclerosis, systemic lupus erythematosus, and chronic fatigue syndrome. Several neurological diseases are linked to mercury hypersensitivity or toxicity, including Lou Gehrig's disease (amyotrophic lateral sclerosis or ALS), Parkinson's disease, and Alzheimer's.

   Eight of the eleven-symptom criteria set by the Centers for Disease Control for chronic fatigue syndrome are well-known symptoms of mercury poisoning. The World Health Organization (WHO) has recently stated: "It is not scientifically possible to set a level for mercury in blood or urine below which mercury-related symptoms will not occur." The medical literature reports a long list of signs and symptoms alleviated by replacement of mercury dental fillings: allergies, gastrointestinal problems of all types, tension headaches, migraine headaches, unexplained hair loss in women, eczema, asthma, multiple sclerosis, lupus, Parkinson's disease, and urinary tract problems.

2. Mercury is continually released in the mouth from amalgam restorations. Those with amalgam fillings have an average mercury vapor concentration ten times higher than people without such fillings. Chewing gum, brushing teeth, and drinking hot beverages all increase mercury release.

3. Mercury vapors from dental amalgams absorb directly into the blood and practically all body tissues, including the oral cavity, lungs, and gastrointestinal tract. Mercury fillings in pregnant women affect the growing fetus: Within three days of placing amalgam fillings in pregnant sheep, mercury shows up in the placenta of their babies. One study showed that around the time of birth, most fetal tissue had higher levels of mercury than that of the mothers. Mercury amalgams may affect fertility. Autopsies done on aborted human babies found that mercury levels in the brain, liver, and kidney correlated significantly with the number of amalgam fillings in their mothers.

4. Mercury levels in the blood, urine, brain, nerves, endocrine glands, and kidneys increase in direct proportion to the number of amalgam restorations present in the mouth. Studies indicate that 80 percent of inhaled mercury vapor is absorbed into the bloodstream. There is a direct transport of mercury through peripheral nerves into the central nervous system. Autopsy studies reveal statistically significant correlations between measured mercury tissue concentrations and the number of amalgam fillings.

5. Dentists who use mercury amalgam restorations have detectable tissue levels of mercury in their bodies and measurable biological dysfunction in the form of polyneuropathies. They have double the number of brain tumors and perform less well on neurological function tests than dentists not using mercury. Several studies have indicated the higher the exposure to mercury, the worse the performance on the neurological tests. Subtle losses of manual dexterity and concentration have been documented, as have abnormal psychiatric behaviors. The saying often associated with mercury poisoning —"mad as a hatter"—is not without merit. It is unfortunate that it is increasingly being associated with dentists.

6. Based on extensive scientific documentation, several world governments (Germany, Austria, Sweden, and Norway) have either banned the use of

mercury dental amalgams outright or severely curtailed the use, especially in pregnant women or those with kidney problems.

The safety of mercury-containing dental amalgams has never been proven in long-term clinical trials with control groups receiving different treatment. Where are the double-blind, placebo-controlled studies on dental amalgam safety? Mercury dental amalgams are unsafe and unproved therapy. Mainstream dental dogma dictates that any unproved treatment be labeled quackery, yet supposedly scientific groups like the ADA and CDA declare that amalgams are safe for all but 3 percent of the population (who have an allergy or sensitivity to mercury).

A growing number of dentists work without mercury for the health protection of themselves and their patients. Mercury is a toxic substance in any amount. It does not belong in your mouth. Find a dentist who works without mercury. Ugly black fillings can be replaced by inert, nonmetal composite or porcelain fillings that are safer and look better.

The removal and replacement of amalgam fillings will release mercury vapors and can temporarily worsen symptoms, especially in sensitive individuals suffering from chronic fatigue syndrome or severe environmental hypersensitivity syndromes (such as 20th-century disease). Some individuals should not replace mercury fillings at all or should do so carefully on the advice of their natural health-care practitioner or medical specialist.

To prevent or offset damage from the replacement of dental amalgams, follow a high-fiber diet, eat more garlic and onions, drink distilled water, and supplement with high doses of beta-carotene; vitamin A; vitamin C; selenium; vitamin E; aloe vera juice; green drinks like barley green, chlorella, spirulina, and blue green algae; and high sulfur-containing amino acids like cysteine, methionine, N-acetyl-cysteine, and glutathione. This regimen prevents free-radical damage to the body by any toxic heavy metal, including mercury. To find a dentist in your area who knows about mercury alternatives, contact one of these organizations for a referral:

Consumer Health Organization of Canada
280 Sheppard Ave. E., #207, P.O. Box 248, Willowdale, Ontario, CANADA M2N 5S9
416-222-6517

Environmental Dental Association
9974 Scripps Ranch Blvd., Suite #36, San Diego, CA 92131
Call 619-586-1208 or fax 619-693-0724 for educational materials, research, referrals, and other resources for nontoxic dentistry.

PARASITES

One reason for the failure of antifungal therapies is the presence of an undiagnosed infection with parasites (*blastocystis hominis, giardia lamblia, entamoeba coli*, or others). According to Dr. Leo Galland, an expert in the treatment of Candida and parasitic infections, "Every patient with disorders of immune function, including multiple allergies, patients with unexplained fatigue, or with chronic bowel symptoms, should be evaluated for the presence of intestinal parasites." In a study reported in the *Journal of Nutritional Medicine* in 1990, Dr. Galland found that one symptom of hidden giardia infection may be constipation. In the United States, it is estimated that about 50 percent of the water supplied to communities is contaminated with the parasite giardia lamblia. This parasite and several others (especially blastocystis hominis and entamoeba histolytica) have been implicated in a large number of physical and emotional illnesses.

People can easily pick up these infestations from salad bars, day-care centers, and household pets. Natural herbal remedies are available to treat the growing epidemic of these parasites in the North American population. Remedies include artemisia annua, berberine, grapefruit seed extract, cloves, black walnut, pumpkin seeds, chinchona, and garlic. Goldenseal, ginger root, vitamin B_6, stomach bitters, plant enzymes, and pancreatic digestive enzymes (pancreatin) may also be helpful and are free of side effects.

THE PARASITE CLEANSE

Naturopaths have for centuries advocated colon cleansing as a way of detoxifying the entire body. In early cases of parasite infections (before the parasites have reached the liver, bloodstream, and other internal organs) it may be enough just to detoxify the GI tract. Some have relied on the use of high colonic irrigation as a way of cleansing all bowel toxins, including parasites, but this does little, if anything, to rid the bloodstream or organs of parasites.

In any case of diagnosed parasitic infection, the first thing to do is to cleanse the gastrointestinal tract, the usual source of parasites for the rest of the body. No drug or herb by itself can reach parasites that have become embedded in the intestinal wall, sometimes for years. The mucus-encrusted waste matter surrounding worms, amoebae, or flukes has to be softened and exposed first. This is something that can be accomplished by using what is usually called a "colon cleanser," made up of a combination of soluble fibers like ground flaxseeds, psyllium husks, sodium alginate, agar-agar, comfrey root, beet root, citrus pectin, apple pectin, bentonite, and dried fruit extracts from figs, prunes, dates and papayas. These water-soluble fibers all have a de-sludging effect, ridding the intestinal walls of encrusted debris and mucus materials for better waste elimination. Water intake has to be increased whenever one uses a bowel cleanser to enhance toxin elimination. If constipation results from using a colon cleanser, one of the reasons for this may well be inadequate pure water intake.

Colonic irrigation and enemas can also be used to clear the colon, but these are not necessary if one improves the diet to include more high-fiber foods and uses a colon cleanser. Many very good ones are on the market, several of which are sold by network marketing distributors.

THE ANTIPARASITE DIET

No matter what you may have been told about parasite programs, no colon cleanser or herbal remedy works all that well unless the diet is modified to make it difficult for parasites to take a foothold in the first place.

This means that it's very important to eliminate all foods in one's diet that stimulate or feed parasites. It's generally better at the beginning of a cleansing program to cook most of your fruits and vegetables to encourage easier digestion. Later, with symptom improvement, more raw foods can be reintroduced. Avoid cold or iced foods or leftovers that may be contaminated with molds. Work with a natural health-care practitioner to develop a personalized dietary regime suitable for your unique biochemical makeup. The Phase II and III diets in this book work perfectly for parasite cleanses.

Parasite Growth-Inhibiting Foods
fresh pineapple and papayas—contain high amounts of bromelain and papain, two protein-digesting enzymes capable of dissolving many parasites
papaya, pumpkin, and lemon seeds
garlic, onions, carrot tops, radish roots, kelp, raw cabbage, ground almonds, blackberries, sauerkraut, and fig extract

SUPPLEMENTS

Digestive Enzymes

A lack (achlorhydria) or insufficiency (hypochlohydria) of hydrochloric acid production by the stomach predisposes an individual to parasites. In normal, healthy individuals, the high acid content of the gastric juices will help kill off most of the harmful microorganisms found in food. Parasites exposed to hydrochloric acid are killed and basically converted into a good protein supplement.

As one grows older (after age forty, and especially after age sixty) and the stomach's ability to produce hydrochloric acid diminishes, parasites can get past the stomach acid barrier and overpopulate the gut. One of the major inhibitors of hydrochloric acid production is unsuspected food allergies, especially to wheat, milk, and other dairy products. The problem can be reversed by eliminating the offending allergenic foods and by supplementing the diet with acidifying nutritional supplements. Examples of acid supplements include glutamic acid, betaine hydrochloride, pepsin, apple cider vinegar, and Swedish or stomach bitters.

Strict vegetarian diets also decrease the body's ability to produce hydrochloric acid. In addition, people who are born with Type A blood do not secrete enough hydrochloric acid.

Pancreatic enzyme insufficiency is another reason why parasites can flourish in the gastrointestinal tract. Like hydrochloric acid, pancreatic enzymes (protease, lipase, amylase, and others) help digest and inactivate parasites that enter the body with food.

Both low stomach acid production and pancreatic enzyme insufficiency can be diagnosed through a comprehensive stool and digestive analysis ordered by a natural health-care practitioner. Acid or pancreatic digestive enzyme supplements can be taken to improve the situation. Plant enzymes derived from aspergillus, a friendly mold used in fermenting miso and soy sauce, can help digest food in both the stomach and the small intestine, while the animal-based pancreatin will usually only work in the more alkaline small intestinal tract. Other good parasite-dissolving enzymes are bromelain from pineapple and papain from papayas.

Herbs

garlic
pink root
black walnut
green or black walnut
  hulls
ground cloves
grapefruit seed extract
butternut
artemisia annua
mugwort
wormwood
slippery elm
senna
black seed
bitter sophora
gentian
peppermint leaves
psyllium

rhubarb
fennel
corn silk
King Solomon seed
kelp
cramp bark
thyme
fennel seed
ginger root
capsicum
olive leaf extract
colloidal silver—while
  not a herbal remedy,
  this natural anti-
  microbial has been
  reported to be effec-
  tive against many
  parasites

Oxygen

Ozone therapy can be given by a health-care practitioner or self-administered into the rectum on a daily basis. Medical ozone is probably the most effective of any natural anti-parasitic therapy. Once it has killed the parasites, ozone converts to oxygen and water, and, provided the right amounts are used, toxicity potential is extremely low. To get information on ozone generators, ask your naturopath or holistic medical doctor where you could buy an ozone generator for home use. Alternatives to ozone are hydrogen peroxide (35 percent food grade combined with aloe vera juice) and liquid, stabilized oxygen drops.

Probiotics

Effective products that support a healthy bacterial flora include:

Inulin (a.k.a. fructo-oligosaccharides or FOS) from Jerusalem artichoke, burdock, chicory or the dahlia plant—FOS stimulates the growth of friendly bifidobacteria in the gastrointestinal tract.

Lactobacillus acidophilus and bifidus, lactobacillus sporogenes, and *sachromyces boulardii* are all friendly bacteria that can be used in either powdered or capsule form.

Colostrum from bovine sources is another powerful immune system modulator that stimulates a sluggish immune system or dampens an overactive immune response as occurs with autoimmune diseases. For more information on colostrum, see Colostrum/Bovine Colostrum under Natural Antifungal Treatments later in this chapter.

Not everyone suffering from the effects of parasites needs to take all these food supplements and herbal remedies. Each individual is different, and personalized diet and supplement programs used to fight parasites should ideally be prescribed and supervised by a qualified natural health-care practitioner.

Even if you do not travel outside of Canada and the United States, you are still at risk for getting parasites at any age and any profession. Here are some simple and effective guidelines that you can use to protect yourself and your family from parasite infestations:

1. Wash your hands often, using tea tree oil skin washes, if possible, especially before meals, after going to the bathroom, after changing diapers, after handling pets, and after physical contact with any sick individuals. Tea tree oil is a natural antimicrobial that can inhibit most bacteria, fungi, and parasites. It can be used for shampooing as well as for disinfecting just about every body orifice. For example, it can be used as a mouth rinse or used to gargle with for sore throats. Most doctors do not recommend swallowing it, but some who advocate oral use find it extremely effective against Candida.

2. Drink only filtered water. A fine pore filter of not more than one micron diameter is necessary to filter small parasites like cryptosporidium. Ideally, ozonate the filtered water or add some hydrogen peroxide or stabilized oxygen drops to help disinfect your drinking water from parasites. Reverse osmosis filtration systems, distilled water, or other types of at-source filtration, combined with ozonation or stabilized oxygen, are all acceptable drinking waters for parasite prevention. You can take stabilized oxygen drops with you to add to food or water when you travel out of the country.

3. Meat, fish, fruits, and vegetables can all be treated with a cleansing bath of 1 teaspoon of peroxide (35 percent) to 1 gallon of water. This not only rids foods of parasites but also of bacteria, fungi, and chemical sprays. All cooking utensils can also be cleaned the same way or with Chlorox bleach.

4. Use condoms during sexual intercourse.

5. Women should wipe from front to back after urinating to avoid introducing microbes from the rectum into the vagina.

6. Get tested for toxoplasmosis if you are pregnant or trying to get pregnant. Cats are carriers of toxoplasmosis, so it's best to avoid exposure to cats as much as possible.

7. Use herbal-based antiparasite combination products as well as digestive enzymes while traveling. Discuss brands with your natural health-care provider or product distributor.

8. An old expression basically says that a fungus never grows on a healthy tree. If your body is well balanced with respect to vitamins, minerals, amino acids, enzymes, antioxidants, pH, and waste elimination, it is very hard for parasites to become invasive. Boost your immunity to parasites by taking a broad spectrum antioxidant combination product containing beta-carotene, vitamin A, zinc, selenium, and vitamins C and E. Other herbs that can be taken to boost the body's ability to resist parasites are echinacea; astragalus; thymus gland extract; ginseng; whey powder; whole leaf aloe vera juice; boneset; chlorophyll; green food supplements like spirulina, chlorella or blue green algae; and Coenzyme Q_{10}. Along with a sugar-free, organic food, high-fiber diet, all these safe and effective natural supplements can be taken to increase your resistance to parasites.

The famous scientist Max Planck once said, "Science progresses, funeral by funeral." This statement may well be applicable to the subject of parasites. It is estimated by some scientists that, by the year 2025, over 8 billion people worldwide will be harboring at least one parasite in their bodies. This rapid escalation of the parasite problem is largely fueled by ignorance as well as denial. The more we pretend that parasites are not a problem, the more we will see illness and epidemics in our society.

Anyone ignoring the hidden or silent parasite epidemic in the United States and Canada, whether a doctor or a patient being treated for cancer, is ignoring a potentially devastating yet curable or reversible condition. If you have been suffering from a chronic illness and especially if that illness has "no known cause" (which, by the way, is a common phrase used by doctors and medical textbooks), consider yourself infested with parasites until proven otherwise by objective tests. Whatever you do, do not allow yourself to be brainwashed by anybody into believing that your chronic health problem, whatever it may be, is just in your head. It may well be directly related to a hidden parasitic infection.

I urge you to spread the word about what parasites can do to your health and how easily they can be prevented or eradicated from the body without drugs. If you need more information about parasites, pick up a copy of Ann Louise Gittlemann's book called *Guess What Came to Dinner: Parasites and Your Health* (also *Parasites: The Enemy Within* by Hanna Kroeger).

NATURAL ANTIFUNGAL TREATMENTS

Candida and fungal overgrowth signs and symptoms can often be treated successfully with the natural approach alone. In more severe or resistant cases, prescription medications are necessary. The decision to use either the natural, the drug, or a combination of the two approaches should be made in consultation with the patient's health-care provider and depends very much on the severity of the problem and the patient's response to treatment.

The major disadvantage of drug therapy is the cost, but significant side effects can also be a problem with any non-natural treatments. Natural therapies, for the most part, are safe. They involve diet changes and the use of one or a combination of the following supplement options.

Aerobic exercise is an effective antifungal therapy because Candida and fungi do not thrive in a high-oxygen environment. A higher oxygen level can be created in the body by regular aerobic exercise. Many people who suffer from the more serious effects of fungal infections, however, are physically incapable of exercise without aggravating the symptoms. For those who can, aerobic exercise is beneficial.

Aloe vera juice has long been known for its antimicrobial properties. It is loaded with antioxidants, enzymes, and a long list of phytochemicals with immune system-boosting properties to help keep fungi under control. In choosing an effective aloe vera juice, check its MPS (methanol-precipitated solids) units. A good aloe juice has at least 10,000 MPS per liter.

Larch arabinogalactan has very potent immune-enhancing properties and has been approved by the FDA as an excellent source of dietary fiber. Supplementation will lower the generation and subsequent absorption of ammonia, a potent neurotoxin. It also protects colon cells against cancer-promoting agents.

Larch arabinogalactan is found in a wide range of plants, including carrots, radishes, black beans, pears, wheat, and tomatoes, but most abundantly in the Larch tree. Immune-enhancing herbs like echinacea also contain significant amounts.

Like colostrum and probiotics, larch arabinogalactan has an array of clinical uses, in both the prevention and the treatment of numerous conditions associated with lowered immune function.

As a food supplement, larch arabinogalactan is available in powdered form. It has a very slight pinelike odor and a sweet taste. It mixes very well with any beverage. The usual adult dose is one to three tablespoons daily. Children under age four can easily take ½ teaspoon daily. Both children and adults can take much higher amounts for various medical conditions. It has no significant side effects except for occasional bloating and flatulence. While not yet well documented or studied for its clinical applications, larch arabinogalactan shows a great deal of promise as a natural immunizing agent against viruses, Candida, parasites, and bacteria.

Berberine is an alkaloid found in herbs such as goldenseal, barberry, and Oregon grape. It fights Candida and parasite overgrowth (especially amoebae) and normalizes intestinal flora. Berberine stimulates the immune system, soothes inflamed mucous membranes, and helps diarrhea and other gastrointestinal symptoms. It is very well tolerated and generally associated with no side effects.

Betaine and pepsin hydrochloride, as well as other stomach acidifiers like glutamic acid and stomach bitters, dissolve Candida and fungi in the stomach. Antacids and acid-suppressing drugs like cimetidine and ranitidine lead to fungal infections because they eliminate the fungal-protective effect of hydrochloric acid. Excess acid, however, can cause severe heartburn and lead to gastritis or peptic ulcer disease. The need for acid supplementation should be determined by tests ordered by a natural health-care practitioner. One of these tests is the CSDA (comprehensive stool and digestive analysis).

To correct low stomach acidity, most naturopaths recommend starting the treatment by taking one capsule of betaine and pepsin hydrochloride (10 grains) with the first large meal. If this is tolerated, then increase to two capsules at the next large meal and keep increasing to a maximum of six capsules per large meal or to the point where a warm sensation is felt in the stomach. Smaller meals require proportionately lower doses of the betaine and pepsin. A warm sensation means that you have taken more than the amount of acid required to digest your protein completely. At the next large meal take less than the dose that produced the warmth and stay at that dosage until the warm feeling returns. Then, lower the dosage of betaine and pepsin again. This treatment is continued until one capsule per large meal produces the warm feeling, then the treatment is stopped. At this point, the stomach has healed enough to secrete adequate amounts of acid on its own. Smaller meals (a sandwich, for example) require less betaine, and a warm feeling in the stomach will alert you to an excessive dose. When taking more than two capsules per meal, it's best to take the capsules during the meal at five-minute intervals. In most young adults, the entire treatment will take an average of three months. During this time it is best to avoid dairy products and foods containing gluten (all grains except rice) since a sensitivity to these two food categories is often the reason for the low stomach acidity in the first place.

Biotin is one of the B-complex vitamins. It is important particularly for the health of the hair, skin, and nails. It inhibits the conversion of the benign yeast form of Candida to the invasive mycelial form. The usual effective therapeutic dose in adults is 1 milligram or more daily.

Caprylic acid is a naturally occurring antifungal fatty acid (from coconut oil) and works primarily at the level of the gastrointestinal tract. It is comparable in its antifungal activity to the prescription drug nystatin. It has only weak systemic antifungal properties.

Citrus seed extracts (paracan 144, paramicrocidin, Citricidal) are advocated by several well-known holistic doctors such as Dr. Leo Galland. His experience is that these products are as effective as nystatin and caprylic acid in the treatment of gut fungal overgrowth. Parasites like giardia and blastocystis hominis are effectively treated by citrus seed extracts. Mix with warm water, one hour or more before or after meals or starches to avoid stomach upset.

Cloves and clove tea have a similar effect to pau d'arco and can be used effectively against any fungal or parasitic infestation.

Coenzyme Q_{10} is an antioxidant normally found in the body that is involved in optimizing the effects of oxygen in the body. CoQ_{10} (ubiquinone) has been well documented in helping the many symptoms of chronic fatigue syndrome, angina pectoris, and high blood pressure. It has no side effects or significant toxicity.

Colloidal silver is both an immune system stimulant and a natural antimicrobial agent. The popularity of colloidal silver is on the rise, especially because of growing concerns over the many hazards of commonly prescribed antibiotic drugs.

Colloidal silver has been documented to contain broad-spectrum germicidal properties and was used as an antibiotic by doctors before the development of modern antibiotics. The dosages of silver used in the pre-antibiotic era were far in excess of the dosages now recommended. Recent studies suggest that the relatively dilute colloidal silver products sold without a prescription lack effective germicidal activity or immune-stimulating effects. Despite these drawbacks, hundreds of anecdotal reports recount the effectiveness of colloidal silver for a long list of infectious diseases.

Colloidal silver is said to work by disabling the enzyme that all one-celled pathogens (microorganisms in their reproductive stage) use for their oxygen metabolism, thus causing the microorganisms to suffocate in six minutes or less upon contact.

Any mineral, including iron, zinc, chromium, copper, and calcium, can become toxic to the human body if the dosage is high enough. The same can be said for silver. Silver can accumulate in the body and lead to toxicity. Critics of colloidal silver claim that accumulated silver causes kidney damage, pulmonary edema, arteriosclerosis, and death. While this may be true with high doses of silver, it does not apply to the typical doses of colloidal silver recommended by natural health-care practitioners.

One should be aware that the long-term use of colloidal silver increases the risk of developing a condition called argyria, whereby excess silver is deposited in the skin and tissues, causing discoloration and skin damage. Colloidal silver could conceivably work well as a homeopathic remedy for a broad range of infectious diseases on a short-term basis.

Colostrum/bovine colostrum Since the first edition of this book was published, many practitioners have started recommending bovine colostrum as a treatment for Candida infections as well as for a host of immune system problems.

Colostrum is the first mammary secretion nourishment that any mammal, including man, provides for its newborn for the first 24 to 48 hours of life. It contains numerous immune system and growth factors that trigger at least 50 processes in a newborn, ranging from the development of the immune system to the growth of all body cells. Laboratory analysis of immune and growth factors from bovine colostrum are identical to those found in human colostrum except for the fact that the levels of these factors are significantly higher in the bovine version.

Conventional medical doctors were, at one time, enthusiastic about using colostrum for antibiotic purposes. This occurred prior to the introduction of sulfa drugs and penicillin. In the 1950s, prior to the widescale use of corticosteroids as anti-inflammatory agents, colostrum was used for the treatment of rheumatoid arthritis. Polio vaccine developer Dr. Albert Sabin discovered that colostrum contained antibodies against polio and recommended it for children susceptible to catching the disease. Bovine colostrum has been used therapeutically in India for thousands of years by Ayurvedic physicians.

In the past five years, North American scientists and health-care practitioners have rediscovered this natural, whole-food supplement. Bovine colostrum is gaining prominence because of its myriad clinical and preventive applications in humans, a fact that has not escaped the notice of drug manufacturers who have tried to copy (genetically engineer), patent, and market several of the individual components of colostrum.

Well-known colostrum components like interferon, gamma globulin, growth hormone, IgF-1, and protease inhibitors are all used by conventional medical specialists in the treatment of cancer, chronic viral infections, including HIV and autoimmune disease. Now over 4,000 clinical studies from around the world detail research that has been done using colostrum in the treatment of dozens of different diseases.

Genetically engineered versions of IgF-1 and GH are presently marketed as anti-aging and AIDS drugs, which are sold by prescription for between $800 to $1,200 dollars per month. They are found naturally in high concentrations in colostrum but at a fraction of the cost of the genetically engineered versions.

Components
The two major components of colostrum are immune factors and
  growth factors:

Immune Factors
- Immunoglobulins (A, D, E, G, and M)—neutralize toxins, viruses, and bacteria in the lymph and circulatory systems.
- Lactoferrin—antiviral, antibacterial, anti-inflammatory, iron-binding protein with therapeutic effects on cancer, HIV, cytomegalovirus, herpes, chronic fatigue syndrome, Candida albicans, and other infections.

- Proline-Rich Polypeptide (PRP)—a hormone that regulates the thymus gland, stimulating an underactive immune system or dampening an overactive immune system as seen in autoimmune disease (MS, rheumatoid arthritis, lupus, scleroderma, chronic fatigue syndrome, allergies, etc.).
- Leukocytes—white blood cells that stimulate the production of interferon, which slows viral reproduction and the penetration of cell walls.
- Enzymes—lactoperoxidase-thiocyanate, peroxidase, and xanthine oxidase destroy bacteria through their ability to release hydrogen peroxide.
- Lysozyme—a hydrolyzing agent and immune system booster capable of destroying bacteria and viruses on contact.
- Cytokines—interleukins, which regulate the duration and intensity of the immune response, are responsible for cell to cell communication and boost T-cell activity and the production of immunoglobulins. Interleukin-10 is strongly anti-inflammatory, especially in arthritic joints.
- Trypsin Inhibitors and Protease Inhibitors—prevent the destruction of immune and growth factors in colostrum from being broken down in the GI tract; they also prevent *H. pylori* from attaching to the walls of the stomach and can have a beneficial role in the treatment of peptic ulcers.
- Lymphokines—hormone-like peptides produced by activated lymphocytes, which mediate the immune response.
- Oligo Polysaccharides and Glycoconjugates—attract and bind to pathogens (*Streptococcus, E. coli, salmonella, cryptosporidium, giardia lamblia, entamoeba, shigella, clostridium* Difficile Toxins A and B, and cholera), preventing them from attaching or entering the mucous membranes.
- Other Immune Factors—some of the documented immune factors include orotic acid, secretory IgA, IgA Specific Helper, B lactoglobulin, lactalbumin, albumin, prealbumin, alpha 1-antitripsin, alpha 1-fetoprotein, alpha 2-macroglobulin, alpha 2-AP glycoprotein, C3, C4, and orosomucoids.
- Vitamins—A, B_{12}, and E are found in small amounts, while traces of all other vitamins are also present in colostrum.

- Sulfur—a mineral with multiple uses in metabolism and as part of many structural body proteins.

Growth Factors

The growth factors found in bovine colostrum all boost cell and tissue growth by stimulating DNA and RNA formation. Studies show that these growth factors are capable of increasing T cells, accelerating healing, balancing blood glucose, reducing insulin need, and increasing muscle and bone growth while metabolizing fat. Colostrum growth factors include:

- Epithelial growth factor (EgF)
- Insulin-like growth factor-I and II (IgF-1 and IgF-II)
- Fibroblast growth factor (FgF)
- Platelet-derived growth factor (PDGF)
- Transforming growth factors A and B (TgA and B)
- Growth hormone (GH)

Important Uses

Completely healthy individuals can supplement with colostrum just to maintain their vitality and good health. Colostrum stimulates lean muscle growth and increases endurance, while encouraging the burning of excessive body fat. It helps to reverse this and many other signs of aging.

IgF-1 is required by the body to metabolize fat for energy through the Krebs cycle. With aging, less IgF-1 is produced in the body. Inadequate levels are associated with an increased incidence of Type II diabetes and difficulty in losing weight despite a proper nutritional intake and adequate exercise. Colostrum provides a good source of IgF-1 as a complementary therapy for successful weight loss.

Colostrum is an ideal supplement for athletes. Exhaustive workouts and athletic competition can temporarily depress the immune system, decreasing the number of T-lymphocytes and NK cells. Athletes are therefore more prone to develop infections, including chronic fatigue syndrome. Many of colostrum's immune factors can help significantly reduce the number and severity of infections caused by both physical and emotional stress.

Fighting viruses with the use of conventional medical approaches is, at best, problematic. Standard vaccinations and antiviral drugs can all cause significant side effects, including death. On the other hand, hundreds of studies indicate that colostrum is a safe and effective agent for both the prevention and treatment of common viral illnesses.

Heart disease of all kinds can be helped by colostrum's ability to regenerate heart muscle via its growth factors. The interferon and lymphokine components of colostrum fight cancer, while diabetics can benefit from colostrum's growth factors.

Colostrum benefits over 60 known immune and autoimmune diseases, including the following:

AIDS	Candidiasis
Allergies	Crohn's disease
Arthritis	Depression
Asthma	Fibromyalgia
Attention deficit disorder (ADD)	Multiple sclerosis
Bacterial infections	Parasites
Chronic fatigue syndrome	Rheumatoid arthritis

Product Quality

The number of supplement manufacturers offering bovine colostrum to the public is growing with each passing day. At present, bovine colostrum is available at health food stores, through health-care practitioners, or from multilevel marketing distributors without prescription. Unfortunately, several poor quality colostrum products are on the market, which are biologically inactive due to improper processing through the use of high temperatures and pasteurization. The formation of colostrum into tablets is a method that requires high pressure and generates heat, thereby destroying activity.

Colostrum in liquid form is also less than ideal. It is not as concentrated as the powdered versions of the product, must be kept refrigerated due to its short shelf life, and preservatives must be added, which further dilute and destroy its biological capabilities. Further, some sensitive individuals can react adversely to these chemical preservatives.

To get optimal health results from colostrum supplementation, make sure that the brand you purchase is either in powdered or encapsulated powder form and produced organically—free of pesticides, herbicides, and anabolic hormones. Purchase a product that originates only from USDA-certified plants that follow strict quality control procedures and that, by law, must test all the colostrum they produce.

Low heat processing and the removal of fat, whey, and lactose, as well as laboratory testing to ensure biological integrity and safety, are the rigid standards that must be met by high-quality supplements. The supplement manufacturer must be able to supply the consumer with independent assays demonstrating that the product contains the active immune and growth factors.

Dosages

In the treatment of adults with serious immune system diseases, clinicians usually prescribe 1,000 to 2,000 milligrams twice daily of the dried, encapsulated form of colostrum, best taken on an empty stomach with 8 to12 ounces of water. Preventive doses have not been established, but several authors recommend continuous dosing at levels decided upon primarily by the consumer/patient. For those who show no clinical response to colostrum, the dosage can safely be doubled or even tripled as needed until the desired results are obtained.

Children can also take colostrum but require proportionately less. Herxheimer reactions (mainly flulike symptoms) can occur as part of the healing response in up to 40 percent of the cases but are usually mild and disappear with continued supplementation at the same dosage level. Through hundreds of years of use and over 1,000 clinical studies, colostrum has been demonstrated to be completely safe without drug interactions or side effects at any level of ingestion.

The Healing Crisis

In *Colostrum: Life's First Food, the White Gold Discovery*, Dr. Bernard Jensen describes a process of healing that can be triggered by colostrum in at least 40 percent of the cases. It involves what he refers to as a "healing crisis," which may be signaled by symptoms such as nausea, vomiting, diarrhea, headaches, fever, chills, rashes, muscle aches, itching, cough, and various body discharges. Critics contend that "healing crises" are just another term to describe side effects. It is, however, fairly well established that detoxification programs (e.g., fasting, the master cleanser, parasite cleansing, etc.) and nutritional supplements (e.g., vitamin C taken to bowel tolerance) can trigger such reactions as a prelude to healing. The end result of such a crisis, according to Jensen, is "a restoration of tissue integrity."

The healing crisis is most severe on the first day, then progressively less severe each day thereafter. The usual length of time for such a crisis is from three to five days. This is markedly different from an allergic reaction, which does not dissipate with continued intake of the given food or supplement.

Although not reported in the scientific literature or by health-care practitioners, some individuals will likely not be able to tolerate colostrum. To avoid severe healing crisis reactions, it is recommended that one starts supplementing with the lowest possible dose (500 milligrams or 1 capsule) on the first day and, if symptoms develop, then stay on that dose until the healing reaction abates. The dosage can then be increased gradually to 2,000 mg. twice daily or higher, depending on tolerance and the therapeutic goals.

One thirty-six-year-old patient in my practice noted that she was unable to experience any weight loss with colostrum until she boosted the dosage to 10 capsules (5,000 milligrams) twice daily, at which time she had a healing crisis and started to lose weight steadily. After several months she has been maintaining her weight successfully by supplementing with 4 capsules (2,000 milligrams) twice daily. Given the biochemical uniqueness of each individual, the right dosage and impact on health may be quite variable. A natural health-care practitioner's supervision may be of value in certain cases.

Colostrum may well be the only practical protection on the planet against autoimmune disease, cancer, and other incurable diseases. It is completely natural, free of side effects, and an excellent alternative to hundreds of drugs. If you are worried about vaccinations, AIDS, hepatitis, biological warfare, herpes, allergies, and chronic fatigue syndrome, colostrum is definitely worth your consideration.

Desensitization injections against Candida are used by alternative health-care physicians and may help selected patients. The Candida syndrome is linked to perhaps thousands of different fungi or strains of Candida, and injections may not be specific enough for many victims of fungal infection or hypersensitivity. Scientific documentation to date is scanty, but patient testimonials are encouraging.

Dioxychlor, aerobic oxygen, Bioxy Cleanse, and other oral forms of oxygen work based on the ability to harm fungi by increasing oxygen in the body. They may not be as effective as intravenous ozone or hydrogen peroxide therapy, but case histories indicate a substantial benefit and symptom reversal in many cases.

Fish and fish oils (omega-3- and omega-6-EPA fatty acids) have been demonstrated to substantially reduce the mortality rate from atherosclerosis. Fish oils and other fatty acids have strong antifungal properties. Controversy exists in the medical literature about the cholesterol-lowering effects of fish oil capsules. It is clear that at least some individuals benefit a great deal from supplementing the diet with fish like trout, salmon, cod, halibut, sardines, mackerel, swordfish, and tuna.

Flaxseed oil is a good source of omega-3- and omega-6-EPA fatty acids. Evening primrose oil, borage oil, and black currant seed oil are excellent sources of omega-6-EPA fatty acids. All are antifungal.

Hempseed oil is one of the best sources of essential fats. It contains roughly double the amount of omega-3 and omega-6 fatty acids as flaxseed oil. If your skin is on the dry side, use more. If your skin turns oily with this supplement, reduce the dose. A combination of fish oils and flaxseed oil is an alternative to hempseed oil. Raw sunflower and pumpkin seeds are also good sources of these fats. Avoid peanuts, peanut butter, and peanut oil at all costs. They contain mold and aflatoxin, a known immune suppressor. According to experts in mycology (the study of fungi), no peanut sold in North America is free of aflatoxin, even organic ones.

Fructo-oligosaccharides (FOS) are sucrose molecules linked in sequence with fructose. They are widely found occurring naturally in vegetables, grains, and fruits. FOS promote the growth of beneficial gut bacteria (lactobacillus acidophilus and bifidus). In Japan FOS is used as a sweetener. It is not broadly available in North America yet; its use is inhibited by its currently high price. A good natural source of FOS is Jerusalem artichoke flour. Some documented beneficial effects of FOS are reduction of bowel toxins, prevention of diarrhea and constipation, reduction in serum cholesterol, protection of liver function, anticancer effects, and improvement of chronic inflammatory bowel disease symptoms.

Garlic and onions have been used for thousands of years as antibiotic, antifungal, and health-enhancing foods. They have a significant role to play in the prevention and treatment of heart disease and cancer. Garlic and onions are mainstays of any effective natural antifungal program. Both are potent in lowering cholesterol and triglycerides. For those who cannot tolerate the taste or odor caused by garlic, deodorized forms (garlic oil capsules or combinations of garlic and parsley) are good substitutes.

Gentian formula (Biocidin, available from Bio-Botanical Research) is a unique antifungal, antiparasitic formula made up of gentiana, chlorophyll, impatiens, hydrastis, sanguinaria, allicin, and other natural antibiotic herbs. Many health-care practitioners find it helpful in very resistant cases.

Germanium is a trace mineral that enhances the effects of oxygen in the body. The inorganic form is potentially toxic to kidneys and best avoided. Organic forms of germanium have not been proven harmful in any way. Many practitioners use this trace mineral for the treatment of chronic fatigue, allergies, infections, and cancer. A good source of naturally occurring germanium is Korean ginseng. Other good sources include: aloe vera, shiitake mushrooms, garlic, and onions. One's levels of germanium can be determined through hair mineral analysis. If levels are low, supplementation is warranted.

Ginger tea is the hot beverage of choice to soothe inflammation in the gastrointestinal tract caused by Candida or fungal overgrowth, as well as to help repair inflamed tissues. Quick nausea relief can frequently be obtained by using capsules of ginger root powder at a dose of 250 milligrams four times a day. It is a carminative and intestinal antispasmodic. Recent double-blind studies show ginger to be effective in preventing the symptoms of motion sickness and morning sickness during pregnancy (hyperemesis gravidarum) without harmful side effects. Some studies show that ginger is superior to Dramamine in its antinauseant properties. Ginger also has potent anti-inflammatory effects and has been successfully used in treating rheumatoid arthritis and other inflammatory conditions.

Goldenseal (hydrastis) is an herbal remedy that helps fungal infections by encouraging the growth of friendly intestinal bacteria. Goldenseal and lactobacillus acidophilus are valuable supplements to prevent fungal overgrowth if one has been prescribed antibiotics in the treatment of a bacterial infection. Goldenseal is often combined with echinacea.

Green food supplements are effective against Candida and fungi primarily because of their immune system–boosting properties. High chlorophyll content prevents the spread of fungal or bacterial infection and promotes the growth of friendly colonic bacteria. Some of the best-known, well-documented beneficial green foods are barley green, chlorella, spirulina, blue green algae, and green kamut. High-quality popular brands blended with synergistic herbs and plant enzymes are Greens Plus (Supplements Plus) and Green Life (Bioquest). Both are available in powdered, tablet, and capsule forms and are often prescribed for boosting energy and immunity.

Homeopathic remedies (aquaflora, candex, and others) contain very dilute, almost imperceptible amounts of Candida albicans and other fungi. Unlike herbal, vitamin, mineral, enzyme, and prescription medicine antifungals, homeopathic remedies for fungi have little scientific documentation to support their use. It is unknown how many people suffering from fungal infections clear the infection or hypersensitivity with these products. The Candida syndrome is linked to perhaps thousands of different fungi or strains of Candida; the Candida albicans homeopathic dilutions might not be specific enough for many victims of fungal infection or hypersensitivity.

Thousands of patients and homeopathic doctors, however, have claimed excellent results in reversing signs and symptoms of chronic fungal problems with homeopathic remedies. These products are harmless and, under supervision of a qualified homeopathic doctor, may make a big difference for select individuals.

Interferon Boosters Interferon is a substance produced naturally by the body's white cells to fight and prevent viral and other infections, including those by fungi, as well as cancer, allergies, and toxic poisoning of the body. A fever stimulates the body to make more interferon, one of the reasons why naturopaths recommend against the use of drugs to suppress fevers. Interferon can stimulate the immune system to produce more of the disease-fighting T cells that can keep fungi like Candida under control. In therapy, interferon is given as an injection by medical doctors for the treatment of hepatitis C and certain types of bone marrow–related cancers. The cost of these injections runs into the thousands of dollars, and many people who wish to boost their immunity against Candida cannot afford such expensive treatment.

The good news is that you can inexpensively boost your own production of interferon through the use of several herbs and other nutritional supplements. Some of the best-known and documented ones are listed here (in alphabetical order):

Astragalus This Chinese herb enhances antibody reaction to antigens, increases T-lymphocyte activity, improves symptoms of many HIV-related problems, and increases the body's production of interferon. In traditional Chinese medicine, astragalus enjoys a long history of use as an immune system booster and potent tonic for increasing energy levels. Astragalus has been proven to enhance immunity in cancer patients and offsets bone marrow suppression and gastrointestinal toxicity caused by chemotherapy and radiation. No side effects have been reported.

Boneset Native American Indians use this herb successfully for the treatment of colds, flu, coughs, fevers, indigestion, and pain. It has antiseptic properties, promotes sweating, is antiviral, and boosts the immune system by enhancing the body's own secretion of interferon.

Echinacea (*Echinacea angustifolia*) North American Indians have used echinacea as a treatment for toothaches, snake bites, insect bites or stings, and all types of infections. It has a reputation as a blood purifier and also has interferon-like properties. It fights both strep and staph infections, kills Candida (yeast infections), and can kill fungi. It has been used successfully for blood poisoning, ulcers, tuberculosis, childhood infections of every kind, and a long list of skin, digestive, and immune system disorders. Most herbalists recommend that echinacea be used on an intermittent basis (three weeks on, two weeks off) because its immune-boosting effects wane if used continuously. I do not agree with this. According to a growing number of herbalists like Canada's Dr. Terry Willard, the on-off use of echinacea is unnecessary since studies indicate that continued usage is best.

Germanium (See previous listing of Germanium for information.)

Licorice Many of the world's cultures have used licorice as a tonic and energy booster, as well as for the treatment of infections and female disorders. Licorice has anti-inflammatory and antiallergenic properties. The two licorice components, glycyrrhizin and glycyrrhetinic acid, stimulate the production of interferon by the body. Licorice is very helpful for coughs, colds, and flu and heals inflamed mucous membranes in the respiratory tract.

Medicinal mushrooms Reishi, maitake, shiitake, and kombucha, among others, stimulate many aspects of the immune system, including the production of interferon. These are controversial for those individuals who are highly sensitive to mold, yeast, or fungi. In such people, these are best avoided, regardless of their immune-potentiating properties.

Pau d'arco This herb is well known for its antifungal properties and its stimulating effect on the immune system. Several anecdotal reports have indicated that it could help fight cancer. (See the Beverage chapter for the recipe for preparation.)

Vitamin A and beta-carotene Both nutrients boost interferon production.

Vitamin C and bioflavonoids Vitamin C boosts interferon production. Especially beneficial are pycnogenols like grape seed extract, pine bark extract, and bilberry, as well as quercetin, hesperidin, and catechin.

Wheat grass This "superfood" is rich in vitamins, minerals, amino acids, and enzymes. It also enhances interferon production. It is particularly used for cancer treatments and is best taken in juice form. (Avoid it if you are wheat allergic.)

Kelp, dulse, and seaweeds are exceptionally good antifungal whole foods. They are rich in iodine and selenium, two minerals known for their ability to inactivate fungi. Before antifungal drugs, iodine was the main effective remedy against Candida and fungi.

Lactobacillus acidophilus and bifidus are friendly bacteria, and normal inhabitants of the gastrointestinal tract. Their presence is one of the body's natural defenses against fungal invasion. Yogurt and other cultured dairy products are good dietary sources; these bacteria can also be obtained from nondairy sources, in powder or encapsulated forms. They are highly recommended if prescription antibiotics are used to treat bacterial infections.

Over 400 species of bacteria weighing almost 4 pounds (1.5 kilos) inhabit the digestive tracts of healthy humans. Live bacteria (a.k.a. the intestinal flora) make up 30 percent of the fecal mass. Some of these thousands of billions of bacteria are hostile and can cause disease, while many are friendly and have established a symbiotic, mutually beneficial relationship with us over the millennia. These friendly bacteria have also been referred to as "probiotics" and are being used increasingly by mainstream clinicians for both preventive and therapeutic reasons. The literal translation of the word probiotic is "for life."

Probiotics offset other intestinal bacteria that produce putrefactive and carcinogenic toxins. If harmful bacteria dominate the intestines, essential vitamins and enzymes are not produced and the level of harmful substances rises, leading to cancer, liver and kidney disease, hypertension, arteriosclerosis, and abnormal immunity. Harmful bacteria proliferate under many different circumstances, including peristalsis disorders, surgical operations of the stomach or small intestine, liver or kidney diseases, pernicious anemia, cancer, radiation or antibiotic therapies, immune disorders, emotional stress, poor diets, and aging.

The best known of the probiotics are the *lactobacilli*, a number of species of which (acidophilus, bulgaricus, casei, and sporogenes) reside in the human intestine in a symbiotic relationship with each other and with other microorganisms (the friendly *streptococci* and *bifidobacteria*). *Lactobacilli* are essential for maintaining gut microfloral health, but the overall balance of the various microorganisms in the gut is what is most important.

Another probiotic that has recently generated a great deal of interest is the friendly yeast known as *saccharomyces boulardii,* an organism that belongs to the brewer's yeast family, not the Candida albicans group. *S. boulardii* is not a permanent resident of the intestine but, taken orally, it produces lactic acid and some B vitamins, and has an overall immune-enhancing effect.

Benefits of Probiotics

The following are the best documented benefits of probiotics:

- Weaken antibiotic-resistant bacterial strains, attack new types of pathogens (supergerms) and infections in immuno-compromised people requiring treatment (i.e., resist opportunistic infections);
- Manufacture B vitamins (biotin, B_3, B_5, B_6, folic acid, B_{12}) and vitamin K;
- Secrete lactase, an enzyme required to break down lactose in milk;
- Act as anticancer factors (especially for bladder and bowel) by inhibiting bacteria that convert nitrates into nitrites and secrete carcinogens;
- Function as natural antibiotics against unfriendly bacteria, viruses, and yeast such as Candida albicans;
- Enhance bowel function and elimination;
- Reverse diarrhea conditions (Crohn's disease, AIDS, traveler's);
- Prevent skin problems, especially acne and other skin infections;
- Protect against the adverse effects of radiation and pollutants;
- Reduce the blood levels of cholesterol and triglycerides;
- Fight stress and food cravings;
- Help eliminate bad breath;
- Optimize sex hormone levels, enhance fertility, and prevent osteoporosis;
- Produce lactic acid, improve the digestibility of foods;
- Oppose putrefactive bacteria such as bacteroides, associated with a meat-rich diet; and
- Treat allergies, eczema, psoriasis, colitis, irritable bowel syndrome, gastritis, duodenitis, diverticulitis, urinary tract infections, vaginitis, other chronic infections, and autoimmune diseases (e.g., rheumatoid arthritis, ankylosing spondylitis, lupus, alopecia areata, scleroderma, etc.)

Probiotics and Pregnancy

The use of probiotics to balance the bacterial ecology of the vagina and intestine favorably influences the course of pregnancy, labor, and the postpartum period. Far safer than prescription antibiotics, *lactobacilli* and other probiotics have been documented to reduce the incidence of postpartum complications.

How They Work

Probiotics work in many different ways by their production of antimicrobial substances (organic acids, hydrogen peroxide, and bacteriocins) that inhibit pathogen adhesion and degrade toxins produced by microbial invaders. Probiotics resist colonization by competing for binding sites as well as for nutrients with pathogens. They secrete various proteins that stimulate the immune system both locally and throughout the body, boost intestinal brush border enzyme activity, and increase secretory-IgA (a family of antibodies lining the mucous membranes). Enzymes like lactase, sucrase, maltase, alpha-glucosidase, and alkaline phosphatase are enhanced by probiotics. Cholesterol and triglyceride blood levels are metabolized and lowered by healthy probiotic populations. Probiotics are able to resist translocation, defined as the passage of pathogens from the GI tract to extraintestinal sites such as the mesenteric lymph node (MLN), spleen, liver, kidneys, and blood.

"Prebiotics"

A high complex carbohydrate diet (vegetables, fruits, whole grains, legumes) encourages the proliferation of most probiotics, especially bifidobacteria. Indigestible food factors that selectively stimulate the growth and activity of probiotics in the gut are referred to as "prebiotics." Prebiotics are plant cell-wall polysaccharides, hemicellulose, pectins, gums, and indigestible oligosaccharides. The best example of a prebiotic is fructo-oligosaccharides (FOS), sucrose molecules linked in sequence with fructose. FOS are widely found naturally occurring in many vegetables, grains, and fruits, including Jerusalem artichokes, chicory, burdock, garlic, onions, and the dahlia plant. In Japan, FOS are widely used as a sweetener. Some companies that market probiotics add FOS to enhance the potency of their product. FOS are selectively fermented by most strains of bifidobacteria, which will then grow at the expense of pathogenic bacteria such as clostridia and *E. coli*.

Adverse Effects

Probiotics are considered generally to be very safe and well tolerated in the usual dosages prescribed. Highly sensitive individuals have reported the occasional occurrence of indigestion (nausea, heartburn), which disappeared when the supplement was discontinued or the brand of probiotic was changed. Very rare cases of liver abscesses due to *L. acidophilus* have been reported in cases of chronic pancreatitis undergoing surgery.

The safe and effective dosage for most people is 1 to 10 billion viable *L. acidophilus, L. casei GG,* or *B. bifidum* organisms daily. Dosages in excess of 10 billion viable organisms can produce gut disturbances. Smaller amounts of viable organisms are usually sufficient for therapeutic effect. For example, studies indicate that a daily supplement of 1.5 billion colony-forming units of *L. sporogenes* are adequate for all purposes. For *S. boulardii,* dosages up to 3 grams per day are substantiated in the literature.

Probiotic Inhibitors

Probiotics are inhibited by high simple sugar intake, a refined diet, caffeine, alcohol, chlorine, tobacco, prescription antibiotics, steroids, vaccinations, and x rays. Some evidence exists that casein, a milk protein found in most commercially available dairy products, also inhibits probiotic growth. The antibiotics found in dairy products are also a factor in suppressing probiotics.

Probiotic Sources

Cultured dairy products like yogurt, acidophilus milk, buttermilk, sour cream, cottage cheese, and kefir are the best known sources of friendly bacteria. Equally effective probiotic sources include cultured/fermented soy products like soymilk, tofu, tempeh, and miso. Other lesser-known or lesser-used food sources of probiotics are sauerkraut and sourdough breads. Ideally, one could get a good supply of probiotics from one or more of these diverse foodstuffs. If dietary sources are not easily available, supplemental probiotic powders and capsules are good alternatives. Given the large number of brands on the market, there is a probiotic for everyone (lactose-free, dairy-free, yeast-free, etc.).

Best Supplement Brands

No legitimate published research exists comparing the clinical efficacy of one brand of probiotics over others. Since the intestinal micro-ecosystem typically carries up to 400 strains of bacteria, it makes sense to use a product that provides a broad spectrum of viable organisms combined with FOS. Some suppliers claim that the probiotic strains can only work if given one at a time. No evidence suggests that this is true. Single-strain probiotics are indeed effective but in some individuals a brand with multiple strains works best. Certain single strains do not have the near-magical properties the advertising hype would lead one to believe. The best advice here is to consult the knowledge and experience of health-care practitioners familiar with probiotics.

L-cysteine is an amino acid with a detoxifying effect. It can chelate many toxins related to fungal/Candida overgrowth.

Natural progesterone Many women who suffer from fibrocystic breast disease, high breast cancer risk due to family history, PMS, migraine headaches related to their periods, menopausal problems like hot flashes, and osteoporosis are increasingly using natural progesterone cream rather than conventional hormone replacement therapy. This is fine, provided the woman is not one of those very rare individuals who is sensitive to progesterone, even the natural form.

A minority of women (perhaps 1 to 2 percent) who either have a genetic predisposition or severe immune system imbalances (e.g., allergic to most foods, mold, chemicals, and numerous other environmental pollutants) can react adversely to natural progesterone. The main reaction appears to be a worsening of a Candida or fungal infection. For the majority of women (98 to 99 percent) at risk for breast cancer, the opposite is true. Progesterone usually prevents or offsets Candida or fungal infections.

Studies suggest that many forms of breast cancer are caused by a deficiency of progesterone. Abnormal breast cancer cell proliferation can be inhibited by topical progesterone cream. The following are some of the many benefits of the use of natural progesterone cream:

1. Helps use fat for energy
2. Facilitates thyroid hormone action
3. Is a natural antidepressant
4. Is a natural diuretic
5. Normalizes blood sugar levels
6. Restores proper cell oxygen levels
7. Restores libido
8. Normalizes zinc and copper levels
9. Normalizes blood clotting
10. Protects against breast fibrocysts
11. Helps prevent breast cancer
12. Helps prevent endometrial cancer
13. Necessary for survival of embryo
14. Maintains secretory endometrium
15. Stimulates osteoblasts (bone building)
16. Precursor for cortisone production (arthritis)

Progesterone is very well absorbed transdermally (the lower abdomen, hips, buttocks, thighs, and breasts on a rotational basis), where it is stored in the fatty tissues for use as needed and, unlike progesterone taken orally, it is not subject to being intercepted by the liver. For those women who are especially deficient in progesterone, it may take two to three months to restore optimal levels. No reports exist of any significant side effects, but a few women may experience temporary incidental spotting and/or swelling of the breasts. This stops within one to three months with the normalizing of hormone levels. You can obtain natural progesterone cream in Canada by asking your doctor for a prescription, which can be filled by a compounding pharmacist (one who makes up the cream from the basic raw ingredients).

Before supplementing with any hormonal remedies, it's important to obtain lab testing to verify low hormone levels.

Research shows that saliva testing is more accurate than blood tests for assessing hormone levels. This is because steroid hormones like DHEA are carried around the bloodstream, complexed with a carrier protein. The active hormone is "free," meaning that it does not have a protein carrier. Blood tests do not distinguish between the free and the bound form of the hormone, while the saliva test only measures the free (active) hormone. It is therefore a more accurate reflection of that hormone's activity.

Some labs in the United States offer saliva testing directly to the public, thereby avoiding the necessity of consulting a doctor. One such lab offering this service is ZRT, located in Beaverton, Oregon. You can reach it at:

Phone: (503) 466-2445
Fax: (503) 466-1636
E-mail: info@salivatest.com
http://www.salivatest.com

If you feel more comfortable working with your doctor, he or she can order and interpret saliva testing for you. In addition to ZRT, the test is available from Great Smokies Diagnostic Laboratory, but it only accepts tests ordered by a doctor. Doctors can contact Great Smokies in Asheville, North Carolina, at:

Phone: (800) 522-4762
Fax: (828) 285-9293
http://www.gsdl.com

Costs vary between $50 and $100 Canadian for each test.

Unlike American consumers, Canadians need a prescription to obtain DHEA, natural progesterone, and other natural hormones. The tests, however, are available to anyone without a doctor's approval and are a good first step in optimizing your hormone levels.

Nicotinic acid (niacin or vitamin B3) in high dosages has strong antifungal properties. Medical doctors use niacin in high doses primarily as a cholesterol-lowering agent. High cholesterol blood levels are the result of fungal mycotoxins, so it makes sense that one of niacin's mechanisms of action is to inhibit fungi and their toxins. Niacin causes flushing, severe itching, nausea, and other gastrointestinal complaints in the majority of users; with continued use the body gets accustomed to the side effects and tolerates it well. Regular liver function tests should be done on anyone who takes megadoses of niacin. Do not use time-release forms; their use has been linked to liver toxicity and failure. The non-time-release forms have nearly a 50-year record of safety.

Olive leaf extract The olive leaf has long been used for fevers and the treatment of infections caused by viruses, fungi, and bacteria. In the 1850s, medical reports described olive leaves curing malaria. In this century, a bitter compound from the leaf, called oleuropein, was discovered and said to be part of the olive tree's powerful disease-resistant properties. Some of the other health conditions found to respond positively included high blood pressure, coronary artery disease, arrhythmias, and intestinal muscle spasms. Elenolic acid, a substance derived from oleuropein, has been found to have a powerful antibacterial effect.

Around 1970, research by the Upjohn Company showed that elenolic acid also inhibited the growth of viruses. In fact, it stopped every virus tested. A number of in vitro experiments with calcium elenolate, a salt of elenolic acid, demonstrated a killer effect against viruses, bacteria, fungi, and parasitic protozoans.

The usual effective adult dose for most fungal infections is two of the 500 milligram capsules taken four times daily. Like many antifungal treatments, olive leaf extract can result in temporary die-off (Herxheimer-type reactions) caused by rapid microorganism deaths and liberation of their toxins.

Olive leaf extracts contain a strong complement of flavonoids that possess antioxidant and antithrombotic (blood clotting preventing) properties useful in both the treatment and the prevention of coronary artery disease.

Olive oil, castor bean oil, and oregano oil are antifungal and have no known side effects, except diarrhea if used in excessively large amounts. Some supplement companies manufacture capsules containing these extracts.

Oil of oregano is one natural remedy that I have found quite effective for Candida. Oil of oregano is antiviral, antibacterial, antifungal, and antiparasitic. It also has strong antioxidant and anti-inflammatory effects and is an ideal product for people who suffer from CFS and/or fibromyalgia. This is not regular oregano but a wild form (wild mountain oregano, *Origanum vulgare* species) of the spice that has, until recently, not been available in Canada. Do not use a substitute or oregano from a grocery store because it will have no effect.

Oregano oil (*Origanum vulgare*) is well known in the Mediterranean world (Greece and Crete) for its ability to slow down food spoilage through its antibacterial, antifungal, antiparasitic, and antioxidant activity. The related herbs thyme and marjoram, sold in most North American supermarkets, are labeled incorrectly as oregano, and possess little of wild oregano's miraculous healing properties.

Wild mountain oregano oil contains someric phenols, primarily carvacrol. Dilutions as low as 1/50,000 destroy Candida albicans, the *aspergillus mold*, *staphylococcus*, *campylobacter*, *klebsiella*, *E. coli*, *giardia lamblia*, *pseudomonas*, and *proteus*. Another phenol constituent, thymol, boosts the immune system. These compounds also act as free radical scavengers (shield against toxins), thus preventing further tissue damage while encouraging healing.

Taking 2 or 3 drops under the tongue with some olive oil to improve palatability several times daily or applied topically is a nontoxic and effective treatment for:

acne	colds/flu	psoriasis
asthma	croup	ringworm
allergies	dandruff	rosacea
arthritis	earaches	seborrhea
athlete's foot	fatigue	sinusitis
bronchitis	gum disease	toenail problems
canker sores	insect bites	varicose veins
cold sores	muscle pain	warts

Other applications and further information on wild oregano can be found in *The Cure Is in the Cupboard: How to Use Oregano for Better Health* by Dr. Cass Ingram.

The brand of oregano oil I recommend is manufactured by a Canadian company (Phyotogenics). It should be taken in drops under the tongue.

For children with croup or respiratory tract infections, any dose is safe, but I would start by using 1 drop mixed with ½ teaspoon olive oil placed under the tongue. If your child feels okay with taking it full strength under the tongue, you don't have to add olive oil. If the taste is too strong, increase the olive oil and/or add some honey to make it more palatable. Gradually increase the oregano oil dose to 2 drops 4 times daily. You can also add a few drops of the oil to the vaporizer, hot soups, and salads. The bottle's vapors can also be sniffed or inhaled. In addition, a few drops of the oil can be mixed with calendula cream or tea tree oil cream and rubbed on the chest before bedtime. Since there is no toxicity, use as much as you feel your child needs to overcome the illness. If your child starts to smell a bit too much like an all-dressed pizza, eucalyptus and peppermint oils can be mixed with oregano oil to disguise the distinctive odor.

Oil of oregano can be used topically for itches or infections of the skin, gums, teeth, and just about any orifice in the body. Exercise care if you use it in the genital region, where it is best mixed with olive oil or coconut oil before application (1 drop per teaspoon of olive oil or coconut oil/butter).

These are adult doses. There are no side effects and oregano is compatible with any other natural remedy or prescription drug. Also, it's a good idea to complement oregano oil with a good acidophilus supplement (3 capsules or 1 teaspoon of the powdered version daily).

Other immune system–boosters reported to benefit the treatment of fungal infections include ashwaganda, astragalus, barley sprouts, chaparral, licorice root, myrrh, thymus gland extract, safflower oil, and eucalyptus oil. Blends of antifungals are found in easily tolerated Candida-zyme and Candida Cleanse.

Oxygen therapies (ozone, hydrogen peroxide, dioxychlor, and Coenzyme Q_{10}) are extremely effective natural antifungal treatments, the treatment of choice in chronic, intractable cases of systemic fungal infections and, in my opinion, superior to all prescription antifungal drugs.

In the past decade, oxygen therapies like ozone, hydrogen peroxide, Coenzyme Q_{10}, liquid-stabilized oxygen, and other oral supplements have gained prominence and credibility. The escalating demand for oxygen therapies is linked to increased incidences of allergies, chronic fatigue syndrome, AIDS, Candida, and cancer. Oxygen therapies are extremely controversial. Many physicians and clinics offering them in the United States and Canada have been forced out of practice by government agencies. For the most part, ozone and hydrogen peroxide therapies are only available in Mexico; some Caribbean countries like the Bahamas, Cuba, and the Dominican Republic; as well as in Europe, especially Germany and eastern Europe. The reasons are political, not medical or scientific. If you want ozone or hydrogen peroxide therapies in the United States or Canada, don't call your medical doctor, who cannot legally use ozone therapy. Instead, call a naturopathic physician and ask him or her to name the rare few who use ozone therapy; then call your travel agent.

Hydrogen peroxide and ozone are naturally occurring gases capable of providing more oxygen to cells, tissues, and organs. For nearly a century, both therapies have been used around the world by conventional and alternative medical doctors, in oral, rectal, vaginal, intramuscular, and intravenous forms. As with all therapies, toxicity may be encountered.

If ozone is inhaled in large quantities, it can be toxic. Overdoses (beyond the usual therapeutic doses) of either hydrogen peroxide or ozone can cause inflammation, nausea, indigestion, diarrhea, coughing, chest pain, asthma, dizziness, and headaches. Combined with environmental pollutants like petrochemical hydrocarbons, ozone can irreversibly damage lung and other body tissues. The same is true of hydrogen peroxide, oxygen, water, and any other nutrient. To categorically say "ozone is toxic" or "hydrogen peroxide is toxic" is almost as ridiculous as saying "water is toxic." Toxicity is a matter of degree. It is a biochemical fact that the body manufactures its own hydrogen peroxide under certain conditions. For ozone, hydrogen peroxide, oxygen, and water to become toxic, huge amounts—far more than the recommended levels used in therapy—would have to be consumed.

Safety of oxygen therapies is ensured when they are part of a comprehensive health-promoting program that takes into account optimal diet and antioxidant nutritional supplements such as beta-carotene, vitamin C, vitamin E, and selenium. By and large, the medical use of oxidative therapies is safe and effective for a broad range of conditions. Beware of ozone and hydrogen peroxide promoters who claim that oxygen therapies are all you need to treat cancer or AIDS. Using these therapies alone can lead to problems.

Hydrogen peroxide is found in the waters of famous healing spas around the world and in the human body, including mother's milk. Natural, friendly bacterial flora, lactobacillus acidophilus, manufactures hydrogen peroxide as a defense against Candida albicans and potential pathogens. A high vitamin C intake stimulates production of hydrogen peroxide. In the blood, white blood cells (lymphocytes) produce hydrogen peroxide to combat invasive organisms. Hydrogen peroxide transports sugar throughout the body. It has the ability to reverse plaque formation in atherosclerotic disease, thereby preventing a host of heart conditions.

Medical ozone is more bactericidal, fungicidal, and viricidal than any other natural substance, including hydrogen peroxide. Studies prove that ozone infused into donated blood samples can kill viruses 100 percent of the time. It does not do any damage to healthy cells. Blood bank centers around the world are seriously considering using medical ozone in all donated samples rather than just testing blood samples for the presence of viruses. Herpes, Epstein-Barr, influenza, mumps, measles, HIV, cytomegalovirus, hepatitis, and other viruses have been documented to be destroyed by ozone. Atherosclerotic plaque has also been reduced by intravenous ozone therapy.

Ozone is used to purify water in many European countries instead of chlorine because it does not produce carcinogenic byproducts, as chlorine does. Chlorine and other chemicals from gasoline and diesel-powered vehicles are linked to countless chronic diseases, including cancer. The city of Los

Angeles has replaced chlorination for drinking water by the largest ozone water purification system in the world. Other major North American cities will soon follow suit.

Both ozone and hydrogen peroxide break down in the body into extra oxygen. They destroy viruses, bacteria, fungi, parasites, pyrogens, and, according to some, cancer cells. No bacteria, virus, fungus, or spore can survive in the presence of ozone or peroxide. This explains the benefit in chronic viral conditions and Candidiasis.

Cancer cells are killed by ozone or peroxide, yet healthy cells are unaffected. The theory is that cancer is a plant cell that can be killed by its waste product oxygen; noncancerous cells are resistant to this type of destruction. An increasing volume of scientific research supports the fact that ozone or peroxide therapy can help in the successful treatment of a long list of infectious and degenerative diseases.

Diseases Benefitting from Oxygen Therapies

AIDS	periodontal disease
arthritis	circulatory diseases
athletic injuries of all types	cardiovascular disease
fractures	diabetes
chronic fatigue syndrome	sickle cell anemia
Candidiasis and all fungal infections	skin ulcers
cancer	infected wounds
herpes and other venereal diseases	gangrene
hepatitis	burns
mononucleosis	colitis
psoriasis and almost all skin disorders	

The availability of oxidative therapies in the United States and Canada will hinge more on increasing public demand and grassroots political action than on further scientific community acceptance. The legal status of ozone and hydrogen peroxide therapy in Canada and most parts of the United States is on shaky ground, but there are safe, effective, legal ways of getting the benefits of oxygen in both liquid and capsule form. A number of American and Canadian companies market and sell nutritional supplements that liberate oxygen to internal organs and tissues when swallowed and combined with the normally present hydrochloric acid in the stomach (Dioxychlor, Bioxy Cleanse, and others). The natural antioxidant supplement Coenzyme Q_{10} can optimize oxygen in the body. Research indicates that these products are effective, but it is unclear exactly how they compare with direct ozone and hydrogen peroxide treatments. Visit your natural health-care practitioner for personalized advice on oxygen treatments.

Pancreatic digestive enzymes are a line of protection normally found in the body. These enzymes (amylase, lipase, protease, and others) can be supplemented to increase the control of fungal growth in the gastrointestinal tract. Plant- and animal-source (beef, pork, lamb) digestive enzymes are available without prescription from any health food store or pharmacy. Some brands are combined with bile salts (to help emulsify fats) and lactobacillus acidophilus (to help crowd out fungi). Since no significant side effects occur with any of these, a trial therapy, especially in victims with symptoms such as gas, bloating, diarrhea, or constipation, is worth a try. The need for pancreatic enzyme supplementation can be determined by the CSDA (comprehensive stool and digestive analysis).

Natural health-care practitioners have found that plant-source digestive enzymes work better than the animal-source variety. Animal-based enzymes only work well at a high pH (alkaline) level. The pH in the intestine is alkaline; that of the stomach is much more acidic. Animal-based enzymes do not work in the low pH, highly acid stomach. Plant-based enzymes work well in both an acidic and alkaline environment.

PABA (para-aminobenzoic acid) is an integral part of the vitamin B complex. It is water soluble and exists in a wide range of foods, including whole grains and wheat germ. PABA is synthesized by friendly bacteria in healthy intestines. In cases of Candida overgrowth, it may become deficient and contribute to the worsening of infections. PABA is essential for the breakdown and utilization of proteins, as well for as the formation of red blood cells. It stimulates intestinal bacteria to produce folic acid, which has a strong antifungal effect. PABA is popularly known as an anti-aging supplement that prevents sun damage and helps maintain skin health, pigmentation, and intestinal health.

Therapeutically, PABA can be successfully used in the treatment of anemia, autoimmune diseases like thyroiditis and alopecia areata, constipation, burns and sunburns, and schizophrenia. It is antagonized by sulfa drugs. Generally regarded as safe, megadosing with PABA for long periods can result in nausea and vomiting—symptoms that are evidence of liver irritation.

Pau d'arco (la pacho or taheebo) is an effective antifungal remedy, available in loose tea form or as a tincture. Claims in Canada that it cures cancer have led to government raids on health food stores and its disappearance from the shelves. The quirky nature of the laws in Canada, however, allows citizens to import this antifungal remedy from the United States for personal use.

Peppermint oil (enteric-coated) is used as an antispasmodic remedy in the treatment of irritable bowel syndrome; it happens to be anti-Candidal and antifungal as well.

Psyllium husk powder is a water-soluble, high-fiber substance with a particularly beneficial effect in clearing toxic debris accumulating in the large intestine. It flushes the gastrointestinal tract of fungi and their mycotoxins. Take 1 tablespoon powder with at least 16 ounces of water to prevent constipation and optimize its use.

Selenium, a common ingredient in fungicidal shampoos and lotions, is antifungal in high doses. Over 600 micrograms daily can be toxic to the liver; care must be exercised in oral supplementation.

Tanalbit is a broad-spectrum intestinal antiseptic made up of natural tannins and zinc. It is preferred by some practitioners over nystatin and caprylic acid. Tanalbit is a formula made up of natural tannates and Chitin (N-acetyl-glucosamine derivatives) extract and Lotus rhizome extract, which provide powerful synergistic antifungal as well as antibacterial action. Tannates act through their agglutinating/astringent effects. In other words, they bind irreversibly to lipoproteins and lectins on the surface of the fungal membranes. By so doing, the fungi lose their ability to adhere to the host's epithelial membrane and to colonize. Fungal metabolism is blocked and the fungi end up sticking together and dying. The Chitin extracts and Lotus rhizome extract also protect against gastrointestinal colonization by Candida and other fungi. Tanalbit is usually effective as an anti-diarrheal agent and has not been reported to have any side effects. It is just one more natural therapy that can be used to keep fungi under control. Tanalbit is manufactured and distributed by SCS Intensive Nutrition Products. It can be found in health practitioner offices as well as in most large health food stores.

Tea tree oil (*Melaleucea alternifolia*) is a broad-spectrum antiseptic (fungi, bacteria, parasites) traditionally used as an effective remedy against acne, blisters, athlete's foot, bronchitis, cold sores, wounds, warts, boils, burns, insect bites, sore throats, and all types of Candida infections. Tea tree oil works topically as a local anesthetic (for muscle pain); it penetrates below the skin surface and does not burn skin (unlike water-soluble antiseptics). Despite warnings on the label, some holistic health practitioners recommend the oral use of tea tree oil as an antifungal (15 drops in some water two or more times daily). Tea tree oil appears to be safe when taken internally at this dose.

Thymic Protein A The thymus gland makes several proteins or hormones that stimulate white blood cells and their production of antibodies. With age, the production of these proteins gradually diminishes, making one more susceptible to both infections and cancer.

Thymic Protein A was originally discovered by Dr. Terry Beardsley while conducting cancer research. It is synthesized in a lab from a live cell line of calf thymus and is basically used therapeutically as a general immune system–enhancing supplement. It primarily boosts cell–mediated immunity, the part of the immune system particularly suppressed by fungal mycotoxins.

Health food stores have been selling thymus glandulars or drugs like thymosin, containing fractions of an entire protein, for many years. Unfortunately, these glandular extracts are only moderately effective in enhancing immune function. Thymic protein A is much more potent because it fits the receptor site of the white blood cell (T-4 lymphocyte) more easily. Thus, Thymic Protein A is more bioavailable than thymic glandulars.

Thymic Protein A supplement is available as a freeze-dried powder, contained in individually dosed packets, and is administered under the tongue. Allow it to dissolve for two to three minutes before swallowing. Dosage ranges from one packet every other day for maintenance and longevity to as many as three a day for serious illnesses. For optimal use, people over the age of forty should take the supplement on a fairly continual basis.

No known harmful effects result from using Thymic Protein A, and the only known contraindication is for people taking large doses of steroid hormones. Thymic Protein A can be used in the treatment of any illness that may be the result of a deficiency of immune system function. Commercially, Thymic Protein A is marketed by Longevity Science and should be available through most natural health-care practitioners. The product is also marketed by EcoNegenics, as well, which markets it as Thymic Longevity.

Vitamin B$_6$ is a water-soluble vitamin consisting of three related compounds: pyridoxine, pyridoxal, and pyridoxamine. It is an important adjunctive therapy for Candida problems, especially in women with a history of birth control pill usage. Vitamin B_6 is found in a large number of healthful foods, including legumes, seeds, green leafy vegetables, avocados, soybeans, and walnuts. Vitamin B_6 assists in red blood cell regeneration and helps regulate protein, fat, and carbohydrate utilization. It is needed as a cofactor for neurotransmitters like dopamine, serotonin, norepinephrine, and GABA.

Vitamin B_6 is probably best known for its role in the female reproductive system. Therapeutically, it can be used successfully in the treatment of premenstrual syndrome, the nausea of pregnancy, fluid retention, and dysmenorrhea. Neurological/psychological problems like carpal tunnel syndrome, seizure disorders, rheumatism, tardive dyskinesia, depression, dementia, hyperactivity, and schizophrenia are helped by B_6 supplementation.

Several metabolic and immune system conditions are helped by B_6 supplementation, including seborrheic dermatitis, acne, anemia, atherosclerosis, asthma, monosodium glutamate sensitivity, kidney stones, and diabetes. Many common drugs, including the birth control pill, corticosteroids, and estrogens, destroy vitamin B_6. Vitamin B_6 is required to convert tryptophan into niacinamide. Depletion may result in depression, neuropathies, and other nervous system disorders. When taken as a supplement, it must be balanced by an intake of the other B-complex vitamins to avoid the side effect of peripheral neuropathy.

Vitamin C in high doses is antifungal. Some people have bad reactions to vitamin C, including headaches, gas, nausea, and lightheadedness. Often these symptoms can be overcome by using buffered forms of vitamin C: sodium ascorbate, calcium ascorbate, Ester C, and other mineral ascorbates.

Vitamin C is important for the following reasons:
- helps with the formation of collagen and the health of bones, teeth, gums, nails, muscles, ligaments, and all other connective tissue
- strengthens blood vessels and prevents bleeding and plaque formation in the arteries
- promotes healing of all body cells
- increases resistance to infection
- aids iron absorption and utilization
- is an antioxidant that helps prevent cancer and heart disease
- is a natural antihistamine in high doses

It is best to get your vitamin C from food sources. If you do not tolerate citrus, try eating more peppers, garlic, onions, kale, parsley, turnip greens, broccoli, rose hips, black currants, strawberries, apples, acerola cherries, cabbage, and tomatoes. All fresh fruits and vegetables contain vitamin C and variable amounts of bioflavonoids.

In general, vitamin C is a weak acid. Candida, bacteria, fungi, and parasites are often killed off by high-dose vitamin C; this releases toxins into the system. Gas, headache, nausea, and lightheadedness sometimes result—a sign of a temporary cleansing or detoxification reaction. The problem can be eliminated by a vitamin C flush, done by increasing the dose of vitamin C to the point of clear, watery diarrhea, which usually results in a purge of the majority of these toxins. The vitamin C flush is best done with buffered vitamin C powder. Take 1 teaspoon in juice every half hour until watery diarrhea is reached. After this bowel tolerance level is reached, adjust the dose to where the bowels feel comfortable. Gas and other detoxification reactions should disappear.

If you do not wish to do a vitamin C flush, consider adding sodium bicarbonate to your ester C, sodium, or calcium ascorbate supplement. This is available in powdered form and can be taken immediately after taking the vitamin C. Start with low doses and increase gradually as tolerated. In addition, use a good lactobacillus acidophilus and bifidus supplement to help control bowel flora, reduce gastrointestinal toxins, and improve digestion.

Worsening hay fever and bleeding gums are signs of vitamin C deficiency. They are also a sign of a greater need for bioflavonoids, such as pycnogenol, quercetin, hesperidin, catechin, and rutin. These can be taken in high doses without side effects and might also help you tolerate vitamin C supplements better.

If you are having trouble tolerating even the buffered forms of vitamin C, consider getting yourself checked out for chronic gastrointestinal dysbiosis. It is possible that you are suffering from a bacterial flora imbalance, Candida overgrowth, bacterial infection, or parasites. A natural health-care practitioner can order a comprehensive stool and digestive analysis with a comprehensive parasitology evaluation.

DRUGS

Some fungal or Candida infections do not respond to the natural approach. This could either be because (1) the individual finds it difficult or impossible to make the diet changes or tolerate the supplements or (2) the infection is too long-standing and entrenched in many different organs and tissues in the body. Some patients who have treated their Candida overgrowth for a year or longer without much benefit could certainly give the drug approach some consideration. Careful use of antifungal drugs might be a very effective option for selected individuals. Of course, since all these drugs require a medical doctor's prescription, they must be monitored for potential side effects on a regular basis. Drugs such as ketoconazole for example, although generally well tolerated, can occasionally adversely affect liver function. Regular lab tests should be done in order to observe any abnormalities and thereby prevent organ damage. The following drugs are the most commonly prescribed ones for Candida/fungal infections.

Amphotericin B (Fungizone) in an oral form is only available in Europe and some parts of the United States. In Canada it is used intravenously to treat deep-seated fungal infections and is unavailable for oral use. At one time a combination of amphotericin B, tetracycline, and vitamin C was available in North America but was discontinued for some reason. The oral form of amphotericin B is nontoxic and an excellent alternative to nystatin; the intravenous form is reported to have a high incidence of kidney toxicity.

Aspirin is an antifungal drug, a chemical derived from natural sources (white willow bark). If you can tolerate it without it upsetting your gastrointestinal system, one aspirin each day with a meal can go a long way toward offsetting the negative effects of fungi and mycotoxins. The antifungal activity of aspirin may be a reason why this drug has been reported to prevent heart disease, stroke, and cancer—diseases all suspected to have a fungal mycotoxin etiology.

Colchicine is an antifungal plant-derived drug, most frequently used as an anti-gout remedy. It lowers uric acid and cholesterol and has an anti-inflammatory effect in gouty arthritis and some cases of rheumatoid arthritis. Several authors have documented its beneficial effects in the treatment of degenerative disc disease and herniated discs. In many individuals colchicine causes upset stomach and diarrhea, but the drug has a high safety record. Lowering the dose helps people tolerate it better.

Fluconazole (Diflucan) is a broad-spectrum antifungal drug with a similar mechanism of action to ketoconazole. Unlike ketoconazole, this drug does not inhibit steroidogenesis. It seems to be better tolerated by chronic fatigue syndrome victims, with fewer side effects than ketoconazole.

Flucytosine was originally synthesized as an anticancer drug and was found to be effective for most fungal infections as well. All anticancer drugs have some degree of antifungal activity. Although very effective, flucytosine has numerous side effects, including potentially lethal, dose-related bone marrow suppression. The availability of fluconazole has largely replaced the use of flucytosine for the treatment of stubborn fungal infections.

Griseofulvin (Fulvicin) is an antifungal drug first discovered in 1939 and has been reported an effective antiangina agent as early as the 1960s. It is used by conventional doctors as an antifungal drug, primarily in toenail and skin infections. It works by inhibiting nucleic acid synthesis and fungal cell division. It is not effective against most Candida species. It must be used for periods of up to a year; side effects include headaches, gastrointestinal symptoms, and fatigue.

Itraconazole (Sporanox) is a newer antifungal with supposedly stronger tissue penetration than either ketoconazole or fluconazole. It is the most broad spectrum of all the antifungals. Unlike ketoconazole, this drug does not inhibit steroidogenesis. It needs adequate stomach acidity for absorption and might be problematic for those with gastric hypochlorhydria. Supplemental acidifiers are sometimes necessary. Side effects are rare, even in those suffering from multiple food and chemical hypersensitivities; some degree of liver irritation (nausea and abdominal discomfort) has been reported in susceptible individuals.

Ketoconazole (Nizoral) is a broad-spectrum antifungal drug that also has a cholesterol-lowering effect. It works systemically by interrupting the conversion of lanosterol to ergosterol in fungal cells and is especially effective in chronic fungal conditions associated with chronic fatigue syndrome. Side effects include liver irritation, most commonly experienced as nausea, and inhibition of the production of steroid hormones (steroidogenesis). Ketoconazole in high doses can reversibly inhibit the synthesis of testosterone and cortisol, thereby causing enlarged breasts in males as well as deficient sperm production, loss of libido, impotence, menstrual irregularities in females and, very rarely, adrenal insufficiency. Ketoconazole combined with antihistamines may produce heart toxicity. It needs adequate stomach acidity for absorption and might be problematic for those with gastric hypochlorhydria. Supplemental acidifiers are sometimes necessary. The clear advantage of ketoconazole over the newer antifungals fluconazole and itraconazole is price. Ketoconazole is significantly less expensive.

Nystatin (Nilstat) is a broad-spectrum antifungal drug that has been on the market for over 40 years. It has been advocated for the treatment of Candida infections and is effective against many other fungi. The pure oral powdered form is preferable to oral tablets because of its better dispersal in the oral cavity and the gastrointestinal tract; it is also free of chemical additives. It is completely nontoxic when taken orally but can produce "die-off" reactions like diarrhea, indigestion, headaches, dizziness, spaciness, and flulike symptoms as a result of the drug's impact on fungi in the gut. If these reactions occur, this is proof of the existence of fungi in the body.

Since very little, if any, nystatin is absorbed into the bloodstream, there have been no reports of severe toxicity or deaths due to its use. The die-off reactions caused by oral nystatin, however, can often be quite debilitating. Adjusting the dose can reduce the severity of these temporary symptoms. According to some authors, the die-off reactions from nystatin can be more quickly eliminated by increasing the dose. Long-term use creates fungal resistance and, according to some, spread of the infection. Use this drug only under the supervision of a medical doctor.

Terbinafine (Lamisil) is a new antifungal drug that can be used both topically and orally. It is especially effective in the treatment of fungal skin and toenail infections. It may help some cases of Candida but is infrequently prescribed for it. Terbinafine interferes with fungal membrane synthesis and growth. It inhibits squalene epoxidase, an enzyme in sterol biosynthesis in fungi, resulting in a deficiency in ergosterol and a corresponding increase in squalene within the fungal cell. This leads to fungal cell death and a clearing of the rash or abnormal toenail appearance. Terbinafine is usually well tolerated (except in the pocketbook), with rarely reported side effects of gastrointestinal upset, taste disturbances, skin reactions, and headache.

ROTATING TREATMENTS

One problem associated with Candida treatments of any kind is the eventual resistance to the therapy in use. Fungi adapt to natural as well as drug remedies if these are used for extended periods of time. There is even evidence that fungi can grow and spread more rapidly on antifungal drugs after exposure for extended periods of time. Patients on prescription drugs such as nystatin often develop sensitivity to the drug, if used in high doses for months at a time. One patient of mine with a severe case of generalized eczema did well on an antifungal drug for four days, then developed a hypersensitivity to it and was forced to rotate seven different antifungal remedies to get any benefit whatsoever. If one rotates an antifungal remedy, Candida and other fungi are less likely to develop resistance and the patient is less likely to develop an allergy/hypersensitivity to that remedy.

The advice here, especially in more severely ill or environmentally hypersensitive patients, is to use a combination of four or more natural antifungals on a rotation basis, with or without prescription drugs. Here is one example of a seven-day antifungal rotation therapy that has worked well in my practice in extremely difficult cases:

Mondays: garlic capsules and lactobacillus acidophilus
Tuesdays: berberine capsules and bifidobacteria
Wednesdays: taheebo tincture and vegetable enzymes
Thursdays: nystatin oral powder and nonalcoholic Swedish bitters
Fridays: caprylic acid capsules and aloe vera juice
Saturdays: fluconazole tablets and betaine and pepsin hydrochloride
Sundays: grapefruit seed extract and a green drink

This regime is not cast in stone and can be altered to suit individual needs or financial situations (for example, nystatin and garlic are relatively cheap; fluconazole and itarconazole may be unaffordable for individuals on fixed incomes or without private health insurance).

ALLERGY INFORMATION

1. Some people have a weakened immunity as a direct result of repetitively eating foods their immune systems have come to regard as "foreign" allergens. Elimination of these foods can make a big difference in clearing Candida or fungal infections.
2. Undetected food allergies are extremely common and can be the root cause of any symptom or illness. Basically, there are two kinds of adverse reactions to foods: delayed and immediate. Wheezing, hives, and swelling are examples of immediate reac-

tions, occurring moments to a few hours after consuming the offending food. These kinds of reactions, however, only make up 10 percent of all food allergies. The vast majority occurs on a delayed basis—even as much as four days later.

DETECTING FOOD ALLERGIES

Most authorities agree that the elimination-provocation technique is the most accurate way to detect food allergies. This involves following a hypoallergenic diet for three weeks, eliminating the most common food allergens (wheat, corn, dairy, citrus, eggs, chocolate). Thereafter, the body is challenged with the eliminated foods one by one, and reactions are noted.

During the elimination diet, most people's symptoms improve (wheezing, runny nose, etc.). If symptoms return when a food is reintroduced, you're probably allergic to that food. This diet works only if all the foods to be discontinued are done so abruptly or "cold turkey." It's far less effective to ease into this diet slowly or with some other compromise. If you have a severe illness like cancer or heart disease, this approach needs close supervision by your medical doctor.

HOME TESTING KITS

One can also identify hidden food allergies using skin tests or blood tests (e.g., the ELISA/ACT or IgG RAST blood test). The drawback to skin testing is that it's designed to detect immediate reactions to foods. Since over 90 percent of food allergies are of the delayed-onset type, skin tests cannot identify the vast majority of food allergies.

Blood tests measure antibodies in the blood directed at specific foods. Results can be misleading, however, if you're taking cortisone, acetylsalicylic acid, antihistamines, or other drugs.

To do this test, all that's needed is a single drop of blood. Food allergy home testing kits allow you to test for up to 100 foods through a drop of blood taken from the fingertip. You can obtain this in the privacy of your home without consulting a doctor.

York Laboratories in England accepts such blood samples from all over the world. The lab then processes the blood to determine the level of antibodies against specific foods. Positive test results are close to 100 percent accurate, but there may be false negatives (i.e., the test may miss up to 20 percent of allergies).

To order an allergy testing kit, contact:

York Nutritional Laboratory
Murton Way
Osbaldwick, York
United Kingdom YO19 5US
Phone: 44 1904 410410
Fax: 44 1904 422000
E-mail: info@allergy.co.uk
http://www.allergy.co.uk/

You'll receive a report back from the lab within a few weeks. It will provide a list of the reactive foods and a book advising on rotation diets and alternatives to common food allergies. Testing costs vary from $200 to $500, depending on the number of foods being tested.

DIGESTIVE AIDS

It used to be said, "You are what you eat." I think it is probably much more accurate to say, "You are what you absorb." One can have the best diet in the world and take the best nutritional supplements yet not feel well because of maldigestion and malabsorption caused by deficiencies in enzymes and low stomach acidity.

Maldigestion due to insufficient digestive enzymes and hydrochloric acid is much more common than most conventional doctors believe. Adequate digestive juices can prevent or control almost all types of gastrointestinal disease, inflammatory conditions like arthritis, as well as infections with bacteria, Candida, other fungi, and parasites. High-dose supplementation with most of these digestive aids are often beneficial for victims of cancer, colitis, tendinitis, allergies, autoimmune diseases, and a long list of other metabolic disorders. The following products are the best known ones and have been documented to help as part of a comprehensive natural antifungal program.

Beet root powder is particularly high in carotenes, iron, calcium, potassium, niacin, copper, vitamin C, folic acid, zinc, manganese, magnesium, and phosphorus. It is effective as an all-purpose antifungal nutritional supplement. Beet powder enriches the blood and is a good general tonic. Aside from eating the real thing, the most optimal way of deriving the benefits of beet root is to swallow capsules of beet root live food concentrate capsules.

Betaine and pepsin hydrochloride, as well as other stomach acidifiers like glutamic acid and stomach bitters, dissolve Candida and fungi in the stomach. One reason antacids and acid-suppressing drugs like cimetidine and ranitidine lead to fungal infections is because they eliminate the fungal-protective effect of hydrochloric acid. Excess acid, however, can cause severe heartburn and lead to gastritis or peptic ulcer disease. The need for acid supplementation should be determined by tests ordered by a natural health-care practitioner. One good test is the CSDA (comprehensive stool and digestive analysis).

Bile salts are made by the liver and secreted into the intestinal tract to help correctly digest and assimilate fats. They are crucial in preventing essential fatty acid deficiency and the resulting fungal infections. Supplements may be required by certain biochemically unique individuals and those with liver and gallbladder abnormalities.

Biotin is one of the B-complex vitamins. It is important particularly for the health of the hair, skin, and nails. It inhibits the conversion of the benign yeast form of Candida to the invasive mycelial form. The usual effective therapeutic dose in adults is 1 milligram or more daily.

Essiac (also known as Flor-Essence, Native Legend Tea, Can-Aid) is a popular herbal combination made up of slippery elm, burdock, Turkish rhubarb, and sheep sorrel. Sheep sorrel (*Rumex acetosella*) appears to be the most powerful antifungal and anticancer component of the four-herb tonic. Researchers report that sheep sorrel is effective in breaking down tumors, soothing ulcers, and helping a long list of skin diseases. It contains carotenoids; chlorophyll; B complex vitamins; vitamins C, E, and K; calcium; iron; magnesium; silicon; copper; iodine; manganese; and zinc. Its mode of action may well be through chlorophyll to provide more oxygen to tissue cells. Oxygen in higher amounts counteracts cancer cells, viruses, fungi, and other infections and may be the sheep sorrel mechanism of immune system optimization.

Burdock root (*Arctium lappa*) has long been recognized by herbalists as a blood purifier. It, too, contains carotenoids, B-complex vitamins, vitamins C and E, chromium, magnesium, potassium, silicon, zinc, calcium, copper, manganese, selenium, and iron. Up to 45 percent of burdock may be made up of a substance called inulin. Inulin is thought to be responsible for this herb's curative powers by combining with white blood cells. Japanese scientists have also discovered a chemical in burdock root that can reduce cell mutations and have named this antitumor chemical "Burdock Factor."

Slippery elm (*Ulmus fulva*) is one of the better known herbal remedies. It has traditionally been used as a treatment for ulcers, burns, cuts, hemorrhages, and other wounds. Its active component is a mucilage (soluble fiber) similar to the mucilage in flaxseed. Other components of slippery elm are gallic acid, phenols, tannins, starches, carotenoids, B-complex vitamins, vitamin C, vitamin K, calcium, magnesium, chromium, selenium, silicon, and zinc. Slippery elm is a natural antacid, an antibiotic, and a regulator of intestinal flora. It contains chemical components known to have antifungal and antitumor effects.

Turkish rhubarb (*Rheum palmatum*) has strong bowel detoxification effects. In all forms of cancer and fungal infections, the elimination of toxins from the body is crucial to recovery. Its primary use is to help cleanse the blood of various toxins. Turkish rhubarb has a gentle laxative action, cleanses the liver, and supports the secretion of bile into the intestine. It contains carotenoids, B vitamins, vitamin C, calcium, magnesium, copper, iodine, manganese, potassium, silicon, sulfur, and zinc. Some of its active components include gallic, malic, oxalic, and tannic acids; bioflavonoids; pectin; resin; starch; and volatile oils. Turkish rhubarb also contains rhein, a chemical member of the anthraquinone family. Rhein has the ability to inhibit the growth of several pathogenic bacteria, parasites, and Candida in the intestinal tract. This may help explain its ability to fight a wide range of infections. It has also been shown to have antitumor properties.

For a full explanation of how this herbal combination works, testimonials, history of its development, and all the other controversies surrounding its use, see the book *The Essiac Report* by Richard Thomas.

Flaxseed oil is a good source of omega-3- and omega-6-EPA fatty acids. Evening primrose oil, borage oil, and black currant seed oil are excellent sources of omega-6-EPA fatty acids. All are antifungal. Flaxseed oil has many important roles in the creation of health. Its major properties are:

- natural anticoagulant: helps prevent blood clots
- reduces risk of heart attack and stroke
- protects arteries from damage
- reduces blood triglycerides
- lowers LDL blood cholesterol

- lowers blood pressure
- improves symptoms of rheumatoid arthritis and other autoimmune diseases like lupus, multiple sclerosis, and scleroderma
- helps migraine headaches, asthma, gastritis, and colitis
- anti-inflammatory agent
- prevents cancer

Glutamic acid hydrochloride is a stomach-acidifying digestive aid that works better in some individuals than betaine hydrochloride. It is usually effective for improving the absorption of trace minerals and killing off unfriendly microorganisms in the gastrointestinal tract.

Glutamine (L-Glutamine) may be very important for those Candida cases where leaky gut syndrome has been identified, such as in severe cases of chronic fatigue syndrome or fibromyalgia. Glutamine is produced primarily in skeletal muscle. Its mechanism of action is to work as an inter-organ nitrogen and carbon transporter. Glutamine is traditionally classified as a nonessential amino acid because it can be made in the body from other amino acids. Regardless of this classification, glutamine is essential for maintaining intestinal function, immune response, and amino acid homeostasis during times of severe stress or greater physical activity. Glutamine is an important metabolic fuel for all the white blood cells, fibroblasts (cells involved in tissue repair and healing), and enterocytes (cells lining the gastrointestinal tract). Glutamine also functions as a precursor of other amino acids, glucose (blood sugar), purines and pyrimidines (DNA and RNA), and glutathione, the body's most important self-generated antioxidant.

Glutamine can also be an effective treatment for sugar cravings, hypoglycemia, peptic ulcers, depression, moodiness, poor memory, irritability, anxiety, insomnia, short bowel syndrome, and Crohn's disease. It also has been shown to enhance stamina and exercise performance. The usual aches and pains after heavy exercise are significantly reduced by regular use of this supplement.

Glutamine is used for HIV wasting, abnormal intestinal permeability in people with HIV, chemotherapy-induced mucositis, protection of the immune system and gut barrier function in people with esophageal cancer undergoing radiochemotherapy, cystinuria, ulcerative colitis, and sickle cell anemia; for improving recovery after bone marrow transplant; and for alcohol withdrawal support. Glutamine is also used for preventing morbidity in trauma patients and preventing infectious complications in critically ill patients.

Glutamine helps sustain mental ability, regulates brain metabolism, and, along with glutamic acid, is used as a brain fuel. Glutamine is used in the treatment of alcoholism and can protect against alcohol poisoning. It has been documented to benefit both schizophrenia and senility.

Studies show that glutamine is well tolerated and without side effects in doses up to 40 grams per day.

Lemon juice is a good stomach acidifier. In cases where other stomach digestive aids such as apple cider vinegar, glutamic acid hydrochloride, or betaine hydrochloride are poorly tolerated, the citric acid derived from lemon juice is a good alternative. It can be diluted as needed for better tolerance.

Pancreatic digestive enzymes are a line of protection normally found in the body. These enzymes (amylase, lipase, protease, and others) can be supplemented to increase the control of fungal growth in the gastrointestinal tract. Both plant- and animal-source (beef, pork, lamb) digestive enzymes are available without prescription from any health food store or pharmacy. Some brands are combined with bile salts (to help emulsify fats) and lactobacillus acidophilus (to help crowd out fungi). No significant side effects occur with any of these; a trial therapy is certainly worth a try, especially with symptoms such as gas, bloating, diarrhea, or constipation. The need for pancreatic enzyme supplementation can be determined by the CSDA (comprehensive stool and digestive analysis).

Many natural health-care practitioners have found plant-source digestive enzymes to work somewhat better than the animal-source variety. The reason is that animal-based enzymes can only work well at a high pH (alkaline) level. The pH in the intestine is alkaline, while that of the stomach is much more acidic. Animal-based enzymes do not work in the low pH, highly acid stomach. Plant-based enzymes work well in both an acidic and alkaline environment.

Papaya (papain) and pineapple (bromelain) are two special plant enzymes with an especially beneficial effect as anti-inflammatory agents in conditions such as tendinitis and bursitis. They are generally well tolerated, except in cases of allergy to papaya and pineapple.

Senna (*Cassia acutifolia* or *angustifolia*) is best known for its purgative effects. Since one of the symptoms of Candida or fungal infections is constipation and resultant toxemia, senna may be a safe and effective therapeutic measure.

Senna is not without side effects and may cause dizziness, abdominal pain, nausea, vomiting, and diarrhea in sensitive individuals. Most tolerate it very well, for even months of daily use. Prolonged use may lead to colon problems in susceptible individuals. Most believe its use is best kept episodic or infrequent.

Swedish bitters is an excellent remedy for improving digestive function. It contains a combination of aloe vera, myrrh, saffron, senna leaves, camphor, rhubarb roots, manna, theriac venetian, carline thistle roots, and angelica roots. It is available in a liquid form, with or without alcohol. Most people who suffer from fungal infections are best off using the alcohol-free form. It is also available in capsule form. The book *The Family Herbal* by Barbara and Peter Theiss has a chapter devoted to Swedish bitters. Most people know of the beneficial effects of Swedish bitters on digestion; few realize that this combination product has myriad other uses.

Swedish bitters can be safely taken on a long-term basis, provided the user does not suffer from ulcer or hyperacidity problems. This herbal digestive aid increases stomach acidity. If you have diarrhea, bitters may be detrimental because of its laxative effect. As its name suggests, it tastes bitter, but that's just about the only complaint I've heard from patients about the product. For those who despise the taste, it is available in capsules.

Stomach acid is absolutely essential for digesting protein and for the absorption of vitamins and trace minerals. Most people who benefit from bitters have a problem with low stomach acid (hypochlorhydria). Some authorities claim that about half the population of North America is hypochlorhydric.

In my practice I do a test called the CSDA (comprehensive stool and digestive analysis). Low stomach acidity is suggested as a possible problem in over 75 percent of the test results. Stomach acidifiers such as betaine and pepsin HCL, glutamic acid HCL, and Swedish bitters all help to increase stomach acidity. If taken for long periods of time there is no toxicity and no dependence develops. The stomach, in fact, will "learn" to secrete higher amounts of acid on its own, thanks to the supplement.

Low stomach acidity has been associated with a long list of maladies, including anemia; asthma; autoimmune diseases such as vitiligo; spider veins on the face; vitamin B_{12} deficiency; deficiencies in iron, copper, zinc, manganese, and calcium; food allergies; Candida syndrome; parasites; and other gastrointestinal conditions—the list goes on. This is the reason for the many testimonials on the benefits of bitters on a wide range of conditions seemingly remote from the digestive system. By increasing stomach acidity you get at the physical root cause of many diseases.

ABOUT DIGESTIVE AIDS

BY JEANNE MARIE MARTIN

Some people avoid digestive aids because they do not think they are natural or beneficial. When possible they can be avoided, but natural digestive aids are not harmful in any way for the body if used correctly. It is better to use them to digest and assimilate foods than to be unable to handle the foods you need to eat in order to heal. Ask your doctor to help you determine which digestive aids are best for you.

Using too many digestive aids can overprocess foods so that they are too quickly absorbed and the body cannot extract and utilize the needed nutrients. One can become hungry a few hours after a full meal or wake up hungry in the middle of the night. Some individuals lose weight from too many; since excessive weight loss is common with some people during Candida treatment, this added weight loss is not beneficial.

Taking too many or taking the wrong kinds of digestive aids for you may cause an increase in excess stomach acid, irritation, or a burning sensation in the stomach or digestive tract. Some individuals must eat a very large meal or a hard-to-digest food such as popcorn before they require a digestive aid. Others require several digestive aids to help process even a small amount of food. Even if digestion is usually normal, some individuals require digestive aids because of the added stress on the body during Candida treatment.

Digestion is always assisted by chewing food thoroughly, almost to water, before swallowing, especially for those who have trouble digesting.

Sometimes you have to experiment to see what works for you. Start with one small dose and monitor the results, especially if the digestive aid has not been doctor recommended. Even doctor-recommended digestive aids may require adjusting and should only be altered after consulting with your doctor.

Outside of stomach upset or temporary runny stools, there are generally no major side effects from digestive aids. In the case of stomach upset or a burning sensation, eat a little plain yogurt (acidophilus yogurt) or cooked tofu. A starchy food, like a bit of warm whole grains, tender cooked yam, or winter squash, may be eaten instead; eat 4 ounces, or about ½ cup or more. In the rare event that major side effects do occur, consult your doctor.

Digestive aids are particularly helpful for heavy or large meals, meats, dairy products, legumes, popcorn, and fatty foods. See individual digestive aids listed here and recipes as a partial guide for how to use them. It is best to consult your doctor before purchasing or using any digestive aids.

WHERE TO GET CANDIDA TREATMENTS

Natural Candida treatments and food remedies can be purchased at most health food stores. Garlic and food treatments are more beneficial if they are organic. Most natural herbal treatments and special nonprescription remedies are available from a holistic pharmacy or naturopathic physician. However, some physicians will only sell treatments to their own patients. Prescription drugs must, of course, be prescribed by a medical doctor and can be purchased at any local pharmacy or drug store.

CANDIDA TREATMENTS FOR INFANTS AND CHILDREN
BY DR. ZOLTAN P. RONA

Candida or fungal infections in infants and children usually manifest in the vaginal (vaginitis) or rectal area (diaper rash, pruritis ani, or hemorrhoids). They can usually be treated successfully by changing to a high-fiber diet and using natural remedies, especially lactobacillus acidophilus and bifidus. Spirulina, chlorella, barley green, and other green foods are easy to take for infants and children and are good immune system boosters. Topically, creams containing calendula, zinc oxide, and aloe vera are often effective.

The usual cause of the problem is the high sugar intake found in commercial infant formulas or "unsweetened" fruit juices. Even if juices are freshly squeezed and consumed immediately, the average glass of apple or orange juice has the equivalent of five or more teaspoons of sugar. Cow's milk, soy milk, rice milk, and even goat's milk can increase the total daily sugar intake to fungal growth–stimulating levels in susceptible individuals. Switch to water until the infection clears, then use these beverages sparingly, if at all for older children. For infants, switch to yeast-free, sugar-free formula and rotate types of milk. See Beverages for Babies in Chapter 12).

In the case of vaginal infections, make sure that underpants are loose and allow the passage of oxygen. Fungi are difficult to eradicate from underwear even if they are machine-washed with detergents. In persistent, recurrent vaginal yeast infections, placing the moistened underwear in a microwave oven and turning the setting to high for five minutes destroys all traces of Candida. Placing underwear on a clothesline in the sun for one hour will also kill Candida. Sitz baths with Epsom salts or magnesium sulfate are soothing for the inflammation, often the cause of severe itching in Candida vaginitis.

Echinacea, goldenseal, calendula, ginger, pau d'arco, and aloe vera can be consumed in liquid form as herbal juices or tinctures. Lactobacillus products can be taken in a powdered form, as can buffered vitamin C. Children often seem to respond better to homeopathic remedies like cantheris (123 or 6C) and sulfur (303 or 9C) taken three or more times daily.

Recurrent or resistant Candida/fungal infections in children should alert one to the possibility of an underlying diabetes or immune system problem. A medical doctor can order appropriate tests that confirm or rule out underlying diseases requiring medical treatment. (See Children and Candida at the end of Chapter 8.)

Chapter 4

HERBS AND FOODS FOR THERAPY

THERAPEUTIC FOODS

BY DR. ZOLTAN P. RONA

Many different whole foods and herbs are effective treatments against Candida and other fungal infections. Whenever possible, use whole-food concentrates rather than single-nutrient tablets or capsules. When one isolates a single component from a food, many benefits of the complete food are lost. Supplemental vitamins and minerals cannot duplicate the mixture of nutrients and many still-to-be-identified substances found in natural foods. Whole foods contain phytochemicals, linked to the prevention and treatment of major degenerative diseases such as heart disease, stroke, high blood pressure, and cancer. The only way to get these phytochemicals is from eating whole foods or live whole food concentrates.

Some of the best-known phytochemicals are:

Indoles and isothiocyanates are found in cruciferous vegetables like broccoli, brussels sprouts, cabbage, cauliflower, kale, bok choy, rutabaga, and turnips. They help protect against colon cancer. Evidence is mounting that these phytochemicals also help in the prevention and treatment of other cancers, most notably breast cancer. All are antifungal.

Isoflavones, such as genistein, are found in soybean products like tofu and soy milk. Isoflavones offset the negative effects of excessive estrogen in breast and ovarian cancer. They are antifungal.

Limonene is found in citrus fruits, which produce enzymes that eliminate cancer-causing substances from the body. Citrus fruits are known for their high content of vitamin C and bioflavonoids, vital for optimal immune system function.

Phytosterols are found in soybeans, which can lower the absorption of cholesterol from the diet and prevent colon cancer.

LIVE WHOLE-FOOD CONCENTRATES

Under survival conditions when people do not have access to live whole foods, live whole-food concentrates may be the only option. Live whole foods can be converted to live whole-food concentrates at temperatures below 100°F, thereby maintaining the "life" of the food. The temperature during the process is the crucial deciding factor that distinguishes a "live" from a "dead" food. Shelf life can be at least 10 years.

Major advantages of live whole food concentrates:

- naturally occurring high vitamin and mineral content with highly bioavailable antioxidants
- naturally occurring, highly concentrated phytochemicals
- naturally low calories, fats, salts, and sugar
- naturally occurring live active enzymes and soluble fiber
- rapid and convenient source for the vital 5 plus daily servings of fruits and vegetables
- pesticide- and herbicide-free

Green food supplements are effective against Candida and fungi, primarily because of their immune system–boosting properties. Their high chlorophyll content prevents the spread of fungal or bacterial infection and promotes the growth of friendly colonic bacteria. Some of the best known and documented beneficial green foods are barley green, chlorella, spirulina, blue green algae, and green kamut. High-quality popular brands that contain a mixture of green food products are Greens Plus (Supplements Plus) and Green Life (Bioquest).

Some sensitive people are better off using singular green food products, one at a time, and rotating.

Blue green algae, spirulina, chlorella, barley green, green kamut, and other concentrated green foods are excellent sources of high-quality vegetable protein, complex carbohydrates, essential fatty acids, essential amino acids, phytochemicals, chlorophyll, vitamins, minerals, and fiber. These whole foods plus water provide enough nutrition to help sustain life for years. All green foods have the quality of being natural appetite suppressants, are rich in beta-carotene and other carotenoids, have a high bioavailability (easily digested and absorbed compared to synthetic vitamins and minerals), and have strong antioxidant properties. Some of the many beneficial effects of green foods include higher energy, greater physical stamina, improved digestion and elimination, allergy relief, and immune system boosting. All these green foods are compatible with each other and with all the other supplements on this list.

Kelp, dulse, bladderwrack, and other seaweeds are exceptionally good anti-fungal whole foods. They are rich in iodine and selenium, minerals known for their ability to inactivate fungi.

Seaweeds are high in sodium alginate, calcium, phosphorus, magnesium, iron, sodium, potassium, sulfur, and vitamins C and B_{12}. It is an alkaline-forming food that replenishes glands and nerves, particularly the thyroid. It is a good source of trace minerals and has traditionally been used in the complementary medical treatment of obesity, goiter, hypothyroidism, anemia, emaciation, impotence, nervousness, a weakened immune system, and hair loss.

Saw palmetto, also known as *Serenoa serrulata, Serenoa repens,* or *Sagal serrulata,* may be an important remedy for men with prostatitis associated with Candidal infection. It works as a diuretic, nerve sedative, expectorant, general nutritive tonic, urinary antiseptic, gastrointestinal stimulant, muscle builder, and circulatory stimulant. Saw palmetto has traditionally been used in the complementary medical treatment of prostate conditions (benign prostatic hypertrophy, prostatitis), enuresis (bed wetting), stress incontinence, infections of the genitourinary tract, and muscle wasting diseases of any kind.

Other whole food concentrates may include aloe vera, beet root powder, cloves, onions, garlic, golden seal, and pau d'arco.

CONTROVERSIAL FOODS FOR CANDIDA TREATMENT

BY JEANNE MARIE MARTIN (WITH DR. RONA)

There are a number of herbs and foods whose value in treating Candida is debated among health professions. When it comes to herbal remedies, let your holistic doctor help you decide which herbs to take and how to take them, if any. When it comes to foods, experience may be the best determining factor as there is sometimes evidence for and against the same foods. Certain individuals with certain body types respond better or worse to particular foods. This may be determined through allergy testing and other diagnostic tests or by practical day-to-day experience.

Some common Candida food controversies are discussed here. Decide with the help of your health-care specialist(s) which foods are right for you to enjoy or avoid.

Apple cider vinegar: This is controversial as an antifungal remedy. Many authors, including Dr. William Crook (see *The Yeast Connection*), advise against it in the diet but recommend it as a vaginal douche for yeast infections. Marjorie Hurt Jones (*The Yeast Connection Cookbook*) recommends apple cider vinegar as a vegetable wash, for removing bacteria from raw vegetables before making salads (2 tablespoons per sinkful).

On the other hand, authors such as D. C. Jarvis, M. Hanssen, and C. Scott have written a great deal about the therapeutic effects of ingesting apple cider vinegar. Apple cider vinegar is made by fermenting the juice of whole, fresh apples. It is high in calcium, potassium, sodium, phosphorus, and other trace minerals. It has an average acetic acid content of 5 percent and has been used as a food and a medicine.

Published research indicates that apple cider vinegar inhibits diarrhea due to its astringent property; it helps oxygenate the blood, increases metabolic rate, improves digestion, fights tooth decay and intestinal parasites, and improves blood-clotting ability. It also seems to help bad breath. Many people over age sixty suffer from a lack of stomach acid. Supplementation of 1 to 2 tablespoons of apple cider vinegar with each meal aids in protein digestion and prevents many vitamin and mineral deficiencies. Apple cider vinegar can be used as a mouthwash and throat gargle for antiseptic purposes. It has no significant side effects, is safe for diabetics, and, despite its sodium content, is suitable for those on low-sodium diets.

A long list of conditions can benefit from apple cider vinegar supplementation, including obesity, infections, allergies, arthritis, fatigue, circulatory disorders, and thinning hair. It is true that apple cider vinegar can increase the body's acidity, but in many individuals this produces a beneficial effect, especially for those with Candida who often do not have enough stomach acid. In others, the excess acidity makes their symptoms worse. Some people are allergic to it, and in some cases apple cider vinegar has no effect whatsoever. It's a matter of biochemical individuality. Its low toxicity and potentially spectacular health effects make it worth trying for those suffering from a wide range of suboptional health conditions, including Candidiasis and other fungal infections.

The consensus, however, is to avoid apple cider vinegar for Candida, and because some people are not affected positively by it, apple cider vinegar has been omitted from all recipes in this book. You may decide, with your doctor's approval, on a treatment that includes apple cider vinegar if it suits your body's needs.

Honey, maple syrup, fruit concentrate, fruit juice, sweet fruits, and sugar: No sweeteners are recommended for any Candida treatment diet, and sugar and artificial sweeteners are the worst offenders. A large percentage of people are allergic to sugar, and for the yeast it is their "sweetener of choice." There is growing evidence of brain tumors, thinking difficulties, and multiple side effects from artificial sweeteners, especially aspartame. Still, one of the best Candida books to date is by Dr. Dennis Remington, *Back to Health,* where he states groundbreaking ideas. One in particular relates to sweeteners: "A very small amount of sweetener is acceptable when mixed with a whole grain (complex carbohydrate). . . ." This backs my experience that minute amounts of sweetener cooked into large batches of food are spread very thin when mixed with other carbohydrates and if they are well cooked, they are not capable of feeding the yeast.

I recommend using no more than 1 teaspoon of sweetener for one large recipe that yields no less than 4 to 6 cups; that recipe must be cooked 20 minutes or more to prevent yeast growth. This small amount of sweetener is used as a flavor balancer rather than a sweetening agent and helps to balance and enhance a recipe's taste. Try it for yourself. I believe this is better for individuals with Candida than the sweet bananas, mangoes, and tropical fruits that most Candida books say are "okay occasionally." This is erroneous, in my experience with thousands of students and clients. Sweet fruits greatly hinder healing, and yeast thrive on them. (See chapter 20.)

Lactic acid–fermented vegetables including sauerkraut: These are also very controversial healing foods. Like vinegar and miso, they contain wonderful live enzymes that assist digestion, they are mildly detoxifying, and they can be helpful for Candida provided yeast, sugar, or vinegar are not used in making them. Check with your holistic doctor to see if these are beneficial for your digestion and body type or if they may not be helpful for your particular health problems. (See page 71 under Diet for more on sauerkraut.)

Mushrooms: Mushrooms are not recommended in any of the Candida treatments in any books, so it was surprising to find them used in almost all the Candida cookbooks. It seems that they "sneaked" into a few recipes. But a little bit of a bad thing is not okay on a Candida diet.

A few specialists say shiitake mushrooms are okay (because they are high in germanium, which is high in oxygen), but I hold to the popular premise that no mushrooms are acceptable in any of the Diet Phases until Phase IV (see chapter 10), which is after treatment; even then, cooked mushrooms are okay but not raw mushrooms. No recipes in this book contain mushrooms, nor are they a recommended food. Many tasty substitutes for mushrooms exist, such as sautéed onions, which turn naturally sweet after being cooked for a long time, and sautéed water chestnuts, which also take on a pleasant mushroomy flavor when cooked with toasted sesame oil and tamari or Mock Tamari Soy Sauce. See the substitution chart for more ideas. Kombucha mushroom liquid is said to be beneficial for Candida by a few health specialists but not the majority. Dr. Rona and I do not recommend it for Candida.

Milk: About half the Candida books say milk drinking is okay in moderation; the other half say none at all. The milk sugar, or lactose, makes it an impossible food for Candida; however, small amounts may be cooked into foods on occasion. Like sweetener, cooking and dispersing milk in larger amounts of other foods effectively counteracts possible Candida growth. Of course, those who are allergic to milk should avoid it. This book has some recipes with milk options, so the choice is yours. Note: If all dairy products are eliminated from the diet for six months to two years, a person may lose the ability to digest them, so keep a little dairy, preferably yogurt, in the diet once weekly (or twice monthly) to retain the enzymes needed for future dairy consumption. Since some dairy allergies can be healed, retaining even a little dairy in the diet allows a choice to be had in the future.

Yogurt: Some books say yes, some say no. Natural, plain yogurt may be cooked into other foods or eaten with acidophilus powder or lemon (or lime) juice to counteract bacteria that may be present. (See "Healing Foods" later in this chapter for more information.) I say yes to yogurt, the best dairy product that can be had as long as precautions are taken. Use or omit it, based on your body's requirements and your personal desire to eat or avoid dairy. (See Milk note on previous page.)

Soft cheeses: All Candida books say no to hard cheeses, with or without rennet enzymes. I agree. Some books allow soft cheeses, including cream cheese and cottage cheese. These often have aggravating additives, as well as being high in bacteria, and can be hard to digest, so I say no. However, higher quality soft cheeses, including goats' milk feta, farmer's cheese, ricotta cheese, and quark may be used sparingly (about one to two times weekly) if well cooked into recipes for all Phases, if your doctor permits.

Eggs: These are included in just about every Candida cookbook, although they are not recommended. Eggs must be very well cooked to be safe for Candida treatment. No soft-boiled, sunny-side up, or quick-cooked eggs, and certainly no raw eggs should be eaten. One to two servings per week are okay for most individuals unless allergic. (See chapter 14 for egg options.)

Tamari soy sauce and miso: These two fermented soy products are generally banned during Candida treatment. My experience, and that of most of my clients, shows that tamari may be enjoyed if precautions are taken, with no advancement of yeast growth. East Asian cultures have thrived on these products and used them for healing (as in macrobiotic cooking, for instance). Macrobiotic healing, discussed by Annemarie Colbin in *Food and Healing,* suggests that excessive amounts of ingested sugar can be neutralized with miso and/or tamari.

Real tamari soy sauce is a great deal different than the quickly processed soy sauces found in supermarkets and many Asian markets and restaurants these days. Commercial versions are made from caramel coloring and flavoring, preservatives, and sometimes MSG and other harmful additives. Real tamari soy sauce is naturally fermented from six months to two years, usually in wood, and made with natural ingredients that complement good health. All tamaris are soy sauces, but not all soy sauces are real tamaris. Always use real tamari soy sauce and accept no inferior soy sauces on a Candida diet. Tamari soy sauce is used in a number of recipes. My experience shows that if real tamari soy sauce is used, kept refrigerated after opening, and simmered 4 to 6 minutes or cooked into foods for 20 minutes or more, it has no ill effect on the body and does not feed the Candida yeast.

Miso is a fermented bean paste (usually made from soybeans, sometimes chickpeas) and is not used in this book. It is more beneficial if not boiled; if used raw, it may feed Candida. However, some health specialists feel that the high enzymes in miso make it a perfect healing food for some body types during Candida treatment. Natural miso assists digestion and is high in many amino acids (7 percent to 18 percent protein, depending on the type of miso) and also very high in minerals, including: calcium, magnesium, manganese, phosphorus, potassium, iron, zinc, and sodium. Keep it refrigerated and always use it in cooked recipes. It is more beneficial heated and if kept just under a boil. Use it occasionally (about 2 to 8 times monthly) if your doctor/ Candida specialist permits. Use it in soups and sauces by first mixing it in a little hot water or broth with a fork, adding to the recipe and simmering in recipes for 5 to 10 minutes.

For those allergic to soy or squeamish about using it, a Mock Tamari Soy Sauce recipe was created for this book, which tastes similar to real tamari and is made from black beans. (See recipes.) Bernard Jensen's Quick Sip and Bragg's Liquid Aminos may be substituted for tamari if they are refrigerated, simmered 4 to 6 minutes, or cooked into foods for 20 minutes or more. If adding to raw recipes, simmer right before use. For recipes that are cooked more than 20 minutes, tamari, Quick Sip, or the Liquid Aminos do not require pre-simmering. You decide, with your doctor, and alter the recipes accordingly.

Tofu and soy products (and popcorn and corn): Most books reject soy products because they are hard to digest; then they often turn around and say eat lots of popcorn, which is much harder on the digestive tract, in my opinion. Popcorn for breakfast? Only if you have nothing important to do that day. Because of the starch content and how difficult it is to digest, corn is not used in this book. Fresh, non-microwaved popcorn, eaten alone, is suggested one to four times a month as a "treat." Digestive aids can be taken with it, if needed.

Soybeans and soy flour can be used if not allergic, if they are cooked properly, and if they are eaten only occasionally. Tofu is generally much easier to digest than whole beans. The problem is possible bacteria from processing.

Avoid raw tofu entirely. Tofu recipes in this book are well cooked. Sometimes the tofu is pre-steamed five minutes or more if it is stir-fried or cooked lightly in a recipe to ensure that any yeast-feeding bacteria will be killed. Fermented soy tempeh is not recommended for Candida diets.

Safflower oil: A beneficial food, claimed to be reactive for many with allergies. Dr. Rona and I feel that it is quite healing for Candida albicans, if it is naturally pressed without solvents and you are not allergic to it.

Stevia, or honeyleaf Stevia: Stevia is 200 to 300 times sweeter than sugar. A mere liquid drop or a pinch of the powder is sweeter than spoons of sugar or natural sweeteners. It has varying sweetness and a slight licorice-like flavor that takes getting used to for some people, while others dislike the taste. It is virtually calorie-free and is said to prevent cavities and not trigger a rise in blood sugar. Although research claims it does not feed yeast or other microorganisms, Dr. Terry Willard, herbalist and founder of Wild Rose College in Canada, has said that he could culture and grow lots of Candida by feeding it stevia. He advised against using it. Its importation to the United States for use in foods is banned, and there are problems getting it into Canada as well. Stevia has not been used in this book, as its sweet taste and use in desserts using flours and other Candida-prohibited foods may ignite cravings and receptivity for other sweets. In the same way that other yeasts may not affect Candida but are avoided because it makes one predisposed to Candida yeast, stevia is avoided here. Also Dr. Rona and I are inclined to agree with Dr. Willard. Consult your doctor as to whether stevia would be a wise choice for your Candida diet. If using it, avoid liquid varieties that contain alcohol.

Vegetable bouillon cubes and vegetable broth powder: These contain many items people may be allergic to: corn, peanut oil, lactose, and sometimes MSG or hydrolyzed vegetable protein. In the same way that a bit of sweetener may be used in some recipes if cooked, these items may be used if cooked 20 minutes or more (unless you are allergic to any ingredients). For those who prefer not to use store-bought cubes and powder, natural recipes are in chapter 19.

Certainly, there are other controversial foods, and as time goes by more foods good or bad for Candida yeast growth will be recognized and require exploration. Other controversial foods are mentioned in chapter 10 and other parts of this book. If unsure about whether a certain food is right for you, consult your doctor or health specialist.

HEALING FOODS

BY JEANNE MARIE MARTIN

Your doctor may recommend certain foods for therapy, or you may ask him or her about these special treatments. The average medical doctor may not know about or appreciate the use of food remedies, so it is best to consult a holistic M.D., naturopathic doctor, qualified herbalist, or holistic nutrition consultant for advice on healing foods.

The following is not a complete list of ways to use healing foods. A complete list would require a full-length book! These treatments are among the most popular, easy, and beneficial remedies for Candida treatment.

These foods present few problems or side effects for most people and can easily be incorporated into a routine for a short period of time. The great thing about using foods as therapy is that it is difficult to overdose on wholesome foods, and no lasting damage can be done unless misused for long periods of time or you are allergic.

Note three extremely important points:

1. Do not use these food remedies if you are sensitive or allergic to these foods.
2. Get your holistic physician's approval before adding these during, or even before or after, your doctor's recommended treatment program.
3. It is imperative not to take too many healing herbs, foods, and treatments at once. Some people make themselves quite ill by "overtreating" Candida. See Regulation of Treatment in chapter 5. Avoid excessive remedies that may weaken the immune system further and actually delay or prevent healing.

FOODS FOR FIGHTING CANDIDA

Having a reaction to an herbal or food remedy does not always denote an allergy or sensitivity. Sometimes one has a reaction to treatment because it is doing good, by killing or agitating parasites that then react within the body. The yeast may get upset when certain herbs, foods, and remedies are frequently ingested. Dying yeast respond by making the body host agitated, nervous, nauseous, angry, hyperactive, and/or irritable, among other symptoms. While good foods are being ingested, harmful body toxins are being expelled, and this may create symptoms known as "healing reactions."

Discuss unpleasant reactions or side effects with your holistic doctor. If severe reactions occur, treatment with special herbs, foods, and remedies must be lessened, rotated, or discontinued with medical advice to minimize repercussions. Some treatments need to be gradually reduced before stopping them. Problems like these can be avoided if you get a doctor's advice before taking special treatments. (See chapter 5 for tips on how to lessen or eliminate some unpleasant side effects.) Remember not to take too many different treatments at one time.

Garlic

One of the most powerful everyday foods is garlic. It is easily available and usually well tolerated. When used in cooking, the beneficial effect is minimal. Eaten raw, it provides positive healing reactions. During colds, flus, or Candida problems, raw garlic, chewed, kills bacteria and fungi in the mouth and throat. This can be easily accomplished by adding raw garlic to a salad or salad dressing. Raw garlic can be added to recipes like Lowfat Falafel Spread, Black Bean Dip, and other appetizers, soups, and main dishes. (See recipes.) Or garlic can be chewed all by itself and the pulp spit out. Unfortunately, one does have to deal with garlic breath after chewing raw garlic. Chewing raw parsley shortly after a meal that includes raw garlic can help reduce the smell (and taste).

Another way to ingest garlic is with supplements. However, even the most potent capsules are limited in their capacities because the garlic must be processed, which destroys certain qualities of the garlic yet to be medically determined. Certain other qualities may be enhanced by processing.

One potent method of taking garlic is to eat it raw without chewing it! Special precaution must be taken to avoid stomach upset with this method. Take one medium clove of garlic and chop or mince it very finely. Do not press or crush it! This releases the precious juice, which contains healing allicin. Allicin is the essential element in garlic oil, responsible for the healing properties of garlic that give it antibacterial and anti-inflammatory qualities. Garlic also helps to normalize blood sugar.

Never take raw garlic this way on an empty stomach! Halfway through a regular meal, take chopped garlic on a spoon and put it on the back of your tongue. Wash it down with water, without chewing, so the precious juice remains in the garlic until it reaches the small intestines, where it can do the most good killing Candida and other parasites. (Carbohydrate-digested foods like garlic break down mainly in the small intestines.) Avoid putting garlic on the front part of the tongue if you want to reduce the strong flavor and avoid garlic breath. Many of my clients and I, personally, have taken one to three cloves daily for weeks or months at a time with no garlic breath. After ingesting the garlic, continue with your meal.

This special garlic treatment can be effective in reducing Candida yeast and other intestinal parasites as well. It works best when taken daily for periods of one to three months (usually 30 to 60 days is enough). Do not exceed this time period, however; overextended use of garlic (as with other natural remedies) can contribute to garlic sensitivities or allergies and anemia.

One may experience healing reactions or seeming side effects while taking garlic this way. These reactions usually denote that the garlic is doing its work and the parasites are reacting to it. As a test for parasites I sometimes suggest that clients who appear likely to have Candida or other parasites take a medium clove of garlic daily for at least 10 (to 14) days. If they have no reaction, they usually do not have a yeast or parasite problem.

Often, within 3 days of garlic eating, sometimes as many as 7 or 10, an individual with Candida problems (or parasites) becomes nervous, irritable, hyperactive, easily angered, emotional, and/or queasy in the stomach. This may denote a yeast problem and almost always these suspicions are confirmed by their doctors.

Use only the regular type of garlic (not elephant garlic) and be sure it is organic. Organic garlic often has a purplish color in the outer skin, though this is not always so. Nonorganic garlic may have been treated with formaldehyde and other unnatural additives and pesticides.

Lemon Juice

Lemon juice is a potent antibacterial, cleansing, and healing food. It can kill bacteria and fungi, especially in the mouth, throat, and a little bit in the stomach. Unfortunately, it loses full potency by the time it reaches the intestines. Many people mix lemon juice in hot water, which reduces its value even more. To be effective, lemon juice (or lime juice, which is equally effective) must be ingested full strength.

Hand-squeeze one small lemon or one-half of a large lemon and drink the juice straight down. Do this on an empty stomach. It can be drunk first thing in the morning after water only, or midmorning or mid-afternoon; never at night! Do not leave juice in the mouth any longer than necessary (about ½ hour), as it can strip enamel off teeth if left on them for long periods of time on a regular basis. The juice may be drunk with a straw, if desired, but is best if gulped quickly by itself.

After drinking the juice, take two to three sips of water and notice how sweet the water tastes in your mouth. This treatment is often effective for avoiding minor throat irritations that can lead to coughs and colds. It is most effective if the treatment is taken for 7 to 21 days in a row. One may notice a metallic taste on the tongue after several days of this treatment, as lemon juice is a potent expeller of heavy metals from the body. If a metallic taste occurs, gargle with sea salt water, aerobic oxygen in water, or antibacterial mouthwash or other cleansing gargle to remove traces of metals being brought up in the mouth for the body to eliminate.

After drinking the lemon juice, followed by a few sips of water, do not eat for at least 15 minutes! Only tart or subacid fruits may be eaten, alone, after the lemon juice, or wait 30 minutes or more to eat breakfast or any other foods.

If slight dizziness occasionally occurs after taking the lemon juice, it is a natural sign that the lemon juice is doing its work. The wave of dizziness is generally quick and temporary. If dizziness persists, eat subacid fruits promptly. When possible, purchase organic lemons if they are good quality, fully ripe, and fresh.

Aloe Vera Gel, Wheat Grass Juice, Barley Green Juice
(And other green foods like: green kamut, spirulina, chlorella, blue green algae, astragalus)

These are listed together as they serve similar purposes in healing; however, it is best to do only one of these treatments at a time. Many people have strong healing reactions to these foods, much more so than to garlic or lemon juice. I personally do not advocate several green food products mixed together except for very hardy individuals. Any of these "green foods" can be beneficial in Candida treatment.

Aloe vera is generally more potent in gel form. Care must be taken to select a product that is full strength, not watered down or processed so heavily that it has lost its medicinal properties. Ask your health-care specialist for rec-ommended brands. Aloe vera is a wonderful stomach soother and is claimed to heal ulcers and internal and external wounds. It works better on minor burns than vitamin E when applied externally. My clients and I have used it to remove warts without scarring and heal blisters almost overnight. (Specific methods are required for this and may not work for all individuals.) Aloe is also good for diaper rash. As with some controversial foods, aloe vera and some other green foods are not right for everyone. Since aloe vera has an astringent effect, it is not always beneficial for those with dry skin, those on fat-reduced diets and for some body types. Get checked and tested by your health-care specialist to see if it is right for your body type and health concern.

Barley green juice and wheat grass juice work similarly; barley is preferred, as wheat is a common allergen. These have been used for cancer treatment, cleansing, and healing diets. They contain high amounts of chlorophyll, protein, and beta-carotene, with some vitamin C, B_{12}, and other trace nutrients. Barley green is particularly high in potassium and calcium, and wheat grass has more iron. Take these healing "green drinks" (the aloe may be clear but comes from a green plant like the others) preferably 30 to 60 minutes after meals to lessen reactions. Start with ½ ounce or 1 tablespoon at a time; increase to 1 ounce or more if tolerated and approved by your doctor or health-care specialist. Take the small (1 tablespoon) dose for two weeks or more before increasing amounts. Stay with the new amount for at least two weeks before increasing. For green powders, start with ¼ teaspoon or less and increase after two weeks only if very comfortable with this amount. Adjust amounts to a comfortable level or leave at a small dose. To stop taking green drinks, slowly reduce treatment by cutting it in half every three to seven days, until amounts are 1 or ½ tablespoon liquid or ⅛ to ¼ teaspoon powder, as preferred.

Using one type of green food at a time is more beneficial than taking some of these green mixtures with a dozen or even 60 different green foods and other additives: natural and sometimes unnatural. Many of these mixed greens also contain a good amount of sweetening—here again, sometimes natural, sometimes not. These products do not agree with many people, especially those with food sensitivities, allergies, and many other health problems. Some people get a "buzz" from taking green products for the first several months or even longer; this often goes away once the body gets enough of the green nutrients that it has usually been deficient in. North Americans do not usually eat enough green vegetables and green herbs in their diet. It is best to use one green product at a time, for 30 to 60 days, then skip a couple weeks and switch to another type of green. Rotate different greens for a variety of benefits unique to each green product. Remember to slowly build up green food dosages and slowly decrease before stopping for a while.

Sea Kelp, Dulse, and Other Seaweeds

These are natural antifungal, heavy metal–expelling treatments, foods used widely in East Asian countries like China and Japan. Unfortunately, in tablet or raw form they may actually contribute to Candida yeast problems: Bacteria can be high in seaweeds in raw form. (Consult your holistic doctor.) It is best to use these cooked into foods during Candida treatment. Sea kelp is used to assist weight loss, help heal the thyroid, and regulate metabolism.

Sea kelp contains iodine and high amounts of magnesium, calcium, phosphorus, and potassium as well as sodium and trace B vitamins. Other seaweeds have the same nutrients, in lesser amounts than kelp, with no recognizable magnesium but higher iron content. Dulse has the least value, with only calcium and iron as special nutrients. Seaweeds have been used as healing foods for centuries. Note: These food products are not recommended with certain types of thyroid medications! Consult your doctor if taking prescription thyroid drugs.

Cayenne Red Pepper

Cayenne is a good stimulant, beneficial to the circulation and heart. It assists in keeping the arteries clear and blood flowing smoothly. It is also good for ulcers. Dr. John Christopher, who was one of the world's most renowned herbalists (whom I studied with), dedicated a book to the wonderful benefits of cayenne entitled: *Capsicum*, which is another name for cayenne.

Cayenne agitates and offends the yeast; they do not like spicy foods. Spices have been used for centuries to preserve foods, long before refrigerators came to be, especially in hot countries. Note the traditional spicy hot foods of the Middle East, India, Thailand, Mexico, and Caribbean countries in particular. Spicy foods like cloves, ginger, garlic, horseradish, and cayenne fight the yeast and some other parasites as well. Consult your holistic doctor before taking regular amounts of ginger or clove supplements or teas.

Cayenne is a food that can be used almost daily in cooking and recipes. Use it frequently in recipes and sprinkle it in herb teas occasionally to break up mucus in the throat. Or take it in capsules, on a full stomach; it may feel like you swallowed a bomb if you take cayenne capsule(s) on an empty stomach. Your eyes may water and it can bring on a downpour of tears as well as temporary stomach pains. As with garlic, have cayenne capsules halfway through a meal or take immediately, right after a meal. Remember not to take extra cayenne supplements if you are already taking enough other Candida treatments.

Yogurt

Cultured milk is one of the most digestible dairy products that can be eaten. Real, plain, natural yogurt contains live enzymes that are "friendly bacteria" for the body and help counteract Candida yeast growth. Unfortunately, not all yogurt is natural and contains real live enzymes. Stick with the brands mentioned in chapter 11 or choose a type of yogurt that can be used to make yogurt from itself. These are the only true yogurts. Once fruit is packaged with yogurt, the live enzymes are no more. In picking real yogurts, note if the fruited variety has yogurt mixed with fruit or fruit on the bottom. If fruit is on the bottom, usually the yogurt will be "real" and contain live enzymes. Some people who are allergic to other dairy products can tolerate real, plain yogurt.

Eaten with certain other foods, yogurt helps to break them down and make them more digestible. Yogurt can be eaten with other protein foods and with beans and legumes. Yogurt may be eaten occasionally with tart/subacid fruits at certain stages of Candida treatment for Phases I, III, and IV. Most yogurt is store-bought, from containers, and/or is stored for long periods in the refrigerator; it may contain bacteria from packaging and storage. This problem can be alleviated by adding a bit of acidophilus powder, about ¼ to ½ teaspoon per cup of yogurt, to ensure that any bacteria in the yogurt is counteracted. See the Acidophilus Yogurt recipe in this book. Add lemon or lime juice to yogurt to counteract bacteria in packaged and stored yogurt if acidophilus is not used.

Other Foods for Candida

Many other foods can help speed healing during Candida treatment: vegetables (especially onions), legumes, and whole grains can be especially helpful. Only specific, powerful yet gentle, antifungal healing foods have been mentioned here. Other special foods and herbs are discussed elsewhere throughout this book.

How foods are prepared and eaten can have everything to do with whether they benefit Candida treatment or not. Many foods have to be cooked or prepared a certain way to be beneficial. See the Foods To Enjoy list in chapter 10, Phase II Diet, for a complete list of healing foods and the proper form in which to consume them.

Chapter 5

YOUR DOCTOR'S ROLE DURING TREATMENT

CHOOSING A DOCTOR

BY DR. ZOLTAN P. RONA

Most victims of Candida/fungal overgrowth or sensitivity can get significant help from a naturopath or nutritionist. Naturopathy is a system of treating disease that avoids drugs and surgery and emphasizes the use of natural agents. Naturopaths believe that disease happens when natural defense mechanisms are overpowered by stress, poor lifestyle, and poor nutrition. They believe that the body works best when allowed to heal itself without drugs or surgery. Most naturopaths will work in cooperation with medical doctors (allopaths), but the reverse is often not the case.

Complicated or more severe cases of Candida may need the help of a medical doctor. Many medical doctors are skeptical, opposed, or antagonistic to treating Candida other than with prescription antifungal creams for vaginitis. Finding a medical doctor who supports trying natural treatments first can be difficult. Holistic physicians treat individuals as partners in health care and acknowledge a body-mind-spirit connection to health. Some holistic medical doctors offer nutritional medicine. Many do not. Some holistic doctors discourage the use of vitamin and mineral supplements, though this is not common. Some offer psychotherapy; others focus on visualization therapy, yoga, meditation, acupuncture, homeopathy, and over 30 other modalities. Look carefully into the philosophy of health care you believe in. Holistic medical doctors will usually work with naturopaths if necessary.

Check the credentials of anyone with the labels holistic practitioner, wellness counselor, iridologist, reflexologist, homeopath, or acupuncturist, and any label without the initials M.D., N.D., D.C., or R.N. Many who claim to do natural therapeutics are neither an M.D., nurse, chiropractor, or naturopath. Such lay practitioners may only have taken a weekend seminar in nutrition, iridology, or homeopathy. Their intentions may be good, but their training is not at a professional level. Some practitioners are wise beyond such training, but this is not the rule. If you are looking for an alternative practitioner, consult a professional.

Beware of an ever-growing army of lay practitioners dispensing advice on natural therapeutics. What took a naturopath or medical doctor five years or more to learn cannot be obtained from a seminar or paperback health book. If you use a lay practitioner, verify it with your medical doctor, chiropractor, or naturopath. It is within your rights to question practitioners about their training and licensing background.

Several resource groups in the United States and Canada can give you information on the availability of various therapies or practitioners. Some can help you find a practitioner in your area.

American Holistic Medical Association and American Holistic Nurses Association
4101 Lake Boone Trail, Suite 201, Raleigh, NC 27607
800-878-3373 or 919-787-5146

American Association of Naturopathic Physicians
P.O. Box 20386, Seattle, WA 98102
800-235-5800

Canadian Naturopathic Association
Box 4520, Station C, Calgary, Alberta, Canada T2T 5N3
403-244-4487

CFIDS Association (for information on chronic fatigue syndrome)
P.O. Box 220398, Charlotte, NC 28222-0398
800-442-3437 or 900-988-2343 (information line)
This is the largest organization of its kind. It dispenses information on CFS and immune dysfunction syndrome.

International Bio-Oxidative Medicine Foundation
P.O. Box 13205, Oklahoma City, OK 73113-1205
405-478-4266
This organization provides information on chelation therapy, H2O2, ozone, and other oxygen-related therapies.

National Health Federation
P.O. Box 688, Monrovia, CA 91016

World Research Foundation
15300 Ventura Blvd., Suite 405, Sherman Oaks, CA 91403
818-907-5483; fax 818-907-6044
This organization provides information on therapies inside and outside mainstream medicine for any health condition.

Consumer Health Organization of Canada
280 Sheppard Ave. E., #207, P.O. Box 248, Willowdale, Ontario, Canada M2N 5S9
416-222-6517

REGULATION OF TREATMENT

BY JEANNE MARIE MARTIN

For many people with Candida, treatment is simply a matter of taking the remedy prescribed by their doctor and sticking (as much as they are able) to the basic diet outline that has been suggested. A few finish treatment, achieve a desired cure, and go on their way, often returning to their old living and eating habits. The majority have recurrent problems within six months to three years.

Some need stronger treatment, some need it for longer periods of time. Sometimes a different treatment is required. Sometimes after one type of treatment, a different follow-up treatment is a good idea. Rotation of treatments is required for some: a different remedy each day for four days or so, then repeated. Sometimes multiple treatments of two or more remedies are most effective. Your doctor can help you determine what works best for you. Also see: Rotating Treatments by Dr. Rona near the end of chapter 3 in this book.

Some individuals respond well to prescription drugs, while others require natural treatment. Some patients deal with the treatment process easily; the majority have side effects that make treatment uncomfortable and even agonizing for a few. It is hard to predict and monitor the type and amount of treatment an individual can tolerate. Many find they cannot handle the prescribed amount given by their doctor or recommended by the product's directions.

In my nutrition counseling sessions I have heard from clients that some doctors are unsympathetic, unaware, and/or uninterested in the fact that they have been given higher doses of Candida treatment than they can handle. Certain treatments "blow their circuits," make them nonfunctional, or make them "wish they were dead." Some patients "put up with" the treatment for "as long as I can stand it," then decide to give up completely rather than suffer anymore. Many do not return to their doctors or even tell them they are having problems. Some do and are told, "Live with it and it will get easier."

Reduction of a treatment or trying a different treatment will often work, rather than discontinuation. In Dr. Dennis Remington's *Back to Health* Candida book, he says: "Some people can tolerate only as much powder (nystatin) as they can fit on the end of a flat toothpick!" He suggests finding the amount of treatment that produces only mild side effects. Once that is found, stick with it.

People are not always told by their doctors that Candida symptoms will usually get worse during treatment before they get better. As the yeast die off, the body is filled with their poisons. This weakens the entire body, making all symptoms worse for a while. This is one reason for side effects. Another is that your "treatment" may not be right for you. I have found that many sensitive people, those with allergies or food sensitivities, chronic fatigue syndrome, low blood sugar, or other health concerns besides Candida, cannot tolerate nystatin, ketoconazole (or Nizoral), and other prescription drugs. These people may respond more favorably to natural, nondrug treatments.

If you are seeing an M.D. who only uses drugs, you may have to make an appointment with a holistic M.D. or naturopathic doctor to acquire natural treatment recommendations. Health food stores sell some treatments suggested by Dr. Rona. **People with severe health problems must consult with a qualified doctor before taking any treatment on their own.** Ask your doctor if a natural remedy is safe to try. If the doctor feels one or more of the natural treatments presents no harm to you, proceed with them. Consult your doctor if problems occur.

Most natural treatment products are harmless in small doses. You may begin with minute amounts and slowly build up until slight side effects are noticeable. (When the yeast die, expect discomfort in the first week or so of treatment. A slight increase of side effects is a sign of progress.) Gradually, symptoms should decrease and natural treatments can be increased slightly as tolerated.

Side effects during treatment may also occur due to withdrawal symptoms from coffee, alcohol, chocolate, dairy products, sugar, wheat, or the yeast—to name a few. The Phase I Diet for reducing these foods is important. Follow and finish it before the Phase II Diet is employed, with treatment, to avoid side effects from food withdrawal. The Phase I Diet also provides time to adapt to new foods and see if you have allergic reactions or digestive problems before treatment actually begins.

A few individuals think healing is quicker if you suffer worse side effects during Candida treatment. Suffering does not speed healing! It may hinder it because it weakens the immune system and other body systems so much that they cannot function properly and the body may become more susceptible to bacteria, viruses, disease, and injury. This leads to emotional problems, physical setbacks, digestive troubles, and slower elimination by the body of poisons accumulated as a result of Candida overgrowth. For treatment to be successful, you are not supposed to suffer horribly!

While doing Candida treatment, it is not a good time to take up new, strenuous forms of exercise, like skydiving, scuba diving, long distance running, or any more strenuous exercise than you have previously been doing. Present forms of exercise and work levels are better if decreased, at least slightly, during treatment. Candida treatment is like a cleanse and puts extra stress on the body, which can contribute to lower disease resistance and more of a predisposition to possible physical injury.

Treatment for Candida is a healing phase for the body and requires quite a bit of extra energy. Expect to feel tired and require additional rest or sleep. If you overextend yourself too much, you may become hyperactive, depending on your body type and its response to the extra stress. Treat yourself gently. If you are a woman, treat yourself as if you were pregnant or at least suffering from PMS. If you are a man, treat yourself as if you were in training for an athletic event and rest and eat as though you were running 10 or more miles or kilometers every day.

Some discomfort is inevitable (except with very mild cases). Properly regulated treatment allows you to function as you did before treatment, except possibly during the first 4 to 8 days. Expect an adjustment period that may be temporarily more uncomfortable. If this goes beyond 8 days (or 10 days) or if symptoms are severe, consult your doctor immediately! Symptoms should lessen with proper treatment, after 8 to 10 days.

Side Effects

Most individuals will experience a few side effects or symptoms during Candida treatment. There are ways to minimize these discomforts. Following is a short list of common problems and possible solutions or methods of partial relief. Be aware of your body, and when tensions and pressures build, they can be alleviated before they grow to proportions that cause major stress, mental or emotional eruptions, extreme physical problems, pain, or dysfunction.

Rest and relaxation are essential to healing and reducing symptoms. When you feel tension and stress building, stop what you are doing and take time to recharge. See chapter 7 on the immune system and healing. If you have already gone too far and the body is in the midst of side effects, slow down and deal with them before they get worse. Here is a partial list to assist you in dealing with symptoms. **Consult your doctor if major symptoms occur.** Do not take all the supplements suggested at once. Carefully choose one or more of the recommended aids with the help of your holistic health care practitioner(s).

Allergy reactions These often may increase during Candida treatment or if you never had allergies or food sensitivities before, they may temporarily crop up during this time. Avoid reactive foods and follow food combining. Take digestive aids if needed. Extra vitamin C, echinacea, B_{50}-complex, and energizing supplements can be helpful for some people. Avoid toxic air, artificial clothing, dust, and unclean places. If reactions are severe, see your doctor. Get a balance of exercise and rest. Avoid extra stresses. Be sure to prepare and cook foods properly.

Anger and aggression Take extra vitamin C. Enjoy an Epsom salt bath. Take a walk, exercise, or do deep breathing. Use digestive aids if constipated or if digestion is sluggish. Take acidophilus powder (½ teaspoon or so) in water or 2 acidophilus capsules with water on an empty stomach, or some other flushing agent (like oxygen or psyllium capsules) to relieve internal pressure that can stimulate anger. Eat cleansing/flushing foods like yogurt, grated raw beets with lemon juice (or carrot/beet juice), miso soup (if allowed), or tender cooked veggies. Anger and agression can be common during treatment. Tolerance levels seem lower. One reason may be that the yeast are agitated; they in turn agitate you, and you pass it on. During treatment, quick anger is generally a body response—not a real emotion. For extreme anger, take one 300 milligram capsule (containing .9 milligram of hypericin) St. John's wort (if not conflicting with any prescription drugs), with a flushing agent or digestive aid to speed its action. (Take a maximum of 3 to 300 milligrams St. John's wort capsules daily, *only* as needed. It may cause tiredness or grogginess if taken in excess.)

Bloating This is common during Candida treatment and cleansing. There is a battle going on in your digestive tract against the yeast/parasites and that contributes to bloating. Also, the extra stress on the digestive tract may cause food sensitivities or allergic reactions even if you do not usually react to most foods. Sometimes the bloating can be decreased with the help of easier-to-digest foods or with digestive aids or laxatives. However, expect bloating to a greater or lesser degree during probably the entire treatment. Fear not; it usually disappears a week or more after treatment, provided you properly flushed all the Candida from your body and eased slowly into the Phase IV Diet.

Blood sugar problems If you already have low blood sugar or diabetes, these may become more problematic during Candida treatment. If you don't, you may still experience more dramatic blood sugar swings due to the extra stress of treatment. Foods like Jerusalem artichokes, asparagus, garlic, onions, and hearty legumes such as soybeans, chick peas, black beans, and pinto and kidney beans help to stabilize blood sugar levels, as do dandelion and burdock. Blueberry leaf tea reduces high blood sugar. The Phase II and III diets in this book are perfect (with a very few changes) for these diets. B50-complex, biotin, chromium, and L. glutamine (if your doctor approves) are very helpful supplements. (See also chapter 23 for more information on low blood sugar and diabetes.)

Bruise easily Usually only very sensitive people have problems with this. Avoid quick movements and a hurried pace. Use tea tree oil on bruises, applied immediately after or as soon as possible several times a day until bruise disappears, which is usually within 24 hours if used right away and often. (Tea tree oil also helps swelling and is better on burns than vitamin E or aloe vera for first- or second-degree burns only. [Run burns under cold water first, then apply tea tree oil generously several times during the first hour and then often daily until healed. Temporary stinging shows it is working and killing infection.])

Colds When body defenses are lower (as during Candida treatment), you may be more susceptible to colds. Protect yourself by avoiding drafts and damp places. Dress warmly and avoid people with colds and flu. If you feel a cold coming on, drink straight fresh lemon juice (on an empty stomach) or swallow a raw, chopped garlic clove (halfway through a substantial snack or meal); take extra vitamin C and echinacea; avoid dairy products; drink hot herbal tea with fresh lemon, lime, or a dash of cayenne; and get extra rest. Keep warm and dry but make sure there is enough moisture in heated rooms. (See chapter 4 for more information on how to take garlic or lemon juice for colds.)

Cold extremities Hands, feet, and the entire body can easily get cold when body circulation is poor. Exercise every day; eat warming beans in easy-to-digest soups or casseroles at least five times per week. Walk after eating or do self-massage, tensing and relaxing techniques, and breathing techniques. Get a massage or chiropractic adjustment if possible. Use hot and cold packs or showers, and, of course, dress warmly (include gloves and socks). Avoid drinking cold beverages or eating cold foods. Take cayenne in warm herbal tea or 1 to 2 capsules with a meal. If you are over forty, some North American ginseng or gotu kola can be taken in the morning. Ginger and/or horseradish cooked in, added raw, or powdered with a meal can also help stimulate circulation.

Crying This may occur more frequently because of the stress of treatment. It's okay! Realize you will be more sensitive during this time and allow yourself a little harmless release, provided it is not excessive. Many toxins are released in tears, so this may assist cleansing. See also the following section Emotional Experiences. Get sufficient rest and get support from family and friends. Get counseling and/or see your doctor if crying is excessive.

Constipation Eat raw grated beets (about ½ to ¾ cup) with lemon juice or drink a glass of carrot and beet juice (Use a 1 to 1 ratio). Eat four to six servings of vegetables daily, mainly cooked. Eat no raw vegetables except juices after lunchtime. Yogurt may be helpful. Use digestive aids (plant enzymes, HCL, or psyllium, etc. See Digestive Aids in chapter 3), laxative teas, and/or acidophilus as needed. Avoid stir-frys, fatty foods, nuts, and seeds (unless tiny amounts of ground or buttered nuts or seeds are cooked into other foods). Drink club soda and avoid sparkling bottled waters. Add ground flaxseeds to foods and eat yogurt if allowed. (See the following section on Indigestion and chapter 9 on digestion.)

Coughs Use the same treatment as for colds and sore throats. Realize that some coughs can develop from excessive parasites in the body or can occur as you are killing parasites.

Cravings See How to Handle Constant Cravings at the beginning of Chapter 13.

Depression Eat properly. Take extra vitamin C, B50-complex, and calcium/magnesium. Royal jelly, ginseng, ginkgo, melatonin, and/or chromium may help. If depression is severe, get qualified counseling and call your doctor. If minor, talk to friends, rest, relax, or do something special for yourself. Raise body energy levels with meditation, deep breathing, tensing and relaxing techniques, yoga, tai chi, exercise, massage, and/or chiropractic care. Take an Epsom salt bath to relieve pressure. Be careful not to overdo it. Ease up on self-demands and reduce workload or, if not busy enough, get busy with work, arts and crafts, a garden, or better yet—cook! St. John's wort may also be helpful. (See the previous section on Anger and aggression for proper usage.)

Diarrhea Avoid eating beets. Avoid ginger and ginger teas, citrus fruit, and cleansing herbs or teas. Eat lots of well-cooked whole grains, yams, or winter squash. Complex carbohydrates can help ease diarrhea. Eat salads. Eat whole cooked beans. Drink lots of liquids without foods. Chew on a few roasted carob pods. Chew all foods extremely well. Peppermint, raspberry leaf, and/or slippery elm teas are helpful. Take doctor-recommended aids for diarrhea.

Energy lows Eat properly. Take extra vitamin C. Royal jelly, ginseng, gotu kola, echinacea, melatonin, or ginkgo may help in the morning. Raise body energy levels with meditation, deep breathing, tensing and relaxing techniques, yoga, tai chi, exercise, massage, and/or chiropractic care. Get enough exercise daily (early in the day is best), or you may feel sluggish. Do not work too much or too little. Eat properly and get enough strength and endurance foods, like well-cooked legumes and whole grains, daily.

Emotional experiences Eat properly. Take extra vitamin C, B50-complex, and calcium/magnesium. Sometimes royal jelly, ginseng, ginkgo, or chromium can help. It is natural to revive or relive emotional experiences during treatment, especially experiences that reflect the same energy levels that you have during cleansing. Do not be surprised if old loves, old hurts, and old feelings resurface. Spend time releasing, forgiving, and letting go. Do deep breathing and meditation, take reflective walks, chat with friends, and/or get qualified counseling if needed. Do not wallow in the past or get depressed about it. See this cleansing time as a time of renewal and recharging, a "cocoon time" in preparation for your emergence as a "healthy butterfly."

Headaches Take simple pure aspirin, white willow bark, or feverfew herbs (choose one of these per headache). Take lots of vitamin C, (especially hypoallergenic C from sago palm, if available). Put a hot or cold pack (or alternate them) on your forehead or headache spot. Do self-massage, or get a massage or a chiropractic adjustment. A headache is a signal from the body that something is wrong. Did you eat enough today? Did you eat improper food or food with toxic additives? Did you rest enough, rest too much, overwork, or overexercise? Did you inhale smoke or other air pollutants? If one of these rings a bell, the solution is obvious. Eat if you are hungry or rest if you need it. A hot, then cold shower or Epsom salt bath can also help relieve pressure. Take B_{50}-complex if your headache is due to stress, St. John's wort if stress is extreme. (Pasta, seafood, junk foods, and low-nutrient foods often cause headaches in average people not on a Candida diet!)

Hyperactivity During treatment, this may occur when overworking or overplaying is done. Calm yourself by resting, taking a walk, doing slow, deep breathing, or whatever calms you. Slow down! Not enough food or too high a Candida treatment dosage can lead to hyperactivity, too. Make sure your schedule is balanced and do not overdo. Take St. John's wort (see previous section on Anger and agression) if very "hyper" and stressed. Parasites can contribute to this, as they are greatly agitated during treatment. Get sufficient rest and sleep. Take B_{50}-complex daily, or even three times a day, and extra calcium/magnesium supplements.

Indigestion Follow the food combining, meal planning, and menu guidelines in Part II. See chapter 7 for information on self-massage, self-burping, deep breathing, and tensing and relaxing techniques. Use digestive aids, laxative teas, and acidophilus as needed. If digestion is very bad, eliminate raw vegetables except for juices, and eat only tender cooked vegetables and blended soups at meals for a few days. If all else fails, ease up on treatment a little bit. Do a one-day Veggie Fast if discomfort is not alleviated.

Lack of coordination May occur more often during treatment. Take extra vitamin C, echinacea, and B-complex. See sections on Stomach Agitation, Hyperactivity, and Bruising.

Mental confusion, spaciness Eat two to three full meals daily and snacks as desired. Eat one serving of legumes and at least two servings of well-cooked whole grains daily. Get enough sleep and exercise each day. Take vitamin B50-complex and calcium/magnesium daily. Reduce Candida treatment(s) slightly if confusion is extreme. Do not overwork or overplay.

Mucus Spit it out. The body expels mucus as parasites die. Gargle with sea salt water, aerobic oxygen in water, or other antibacterial mouthwash. Brush your tongue when brushing teeth and remove all white film. Take propolis or slippery elm lozenges or tea. Take lemon juice or garlic (see chapter 4) for one to three days as added help, if desired. (See Oral Hygiene in chapter 7.)

Nausea Avoid citrus foods, cleansing teas, and raw salads. Eat well-cooked whole grains, yams, or winter squash to settle stomach. Eat yogurt or take acidophilus. Do slow, gentle deep breathing or take a slow walk. Take one to two vitamin B50-complex and extra B_6 or ginger capsules. Drink mint, ginger, or red raspberry herbal tea or drink club soda alone or with a slice or two of fresh ginger root added to calm the stomach. An Epsom salt bath can help by relieving body pressure. Lie down for a while if needed, with the head elevated and a cool cloth on the forehead. Parasites can cause nausea when they are disturbed and dying from Candida treatment. Also, excessive food, sometimes mixed with fatigue or stress of treatment, may contribute. Take digestive aids daily or with each meal if needed. (See Digestive Aids in chapter 3.) Also, strong smells/odors, smoke, or toxic fumes may contribute to nausea when one is more sensitive, such as during treatment. If fumes have been inhaled, turn on an air purifier if possible, do gentle deep breathing, and take vitamin C. Avoid boating, amusement park rides, and excessive car travel.

Paranoia Temporary mental problems and confusion can be caused by parasite treatment. The poisons being eliminated can flood the body and brain and may contribute to creating delusional thoughts and emotions. Reduce treatment if side effects are too severe. Consult a doctor or a qualified counselor if mental anguish is not improved within 24 or 48 hours of reduced treatment OR contact IMMEDIATELY if anguish is unbearable! Make sure you are NOT constipated. If so, use fast-acting laxatives. Take an Epsom salt bath immediately to help relieve pressure or, if not possible, a steam bath or hot/cold shower. See sections on Constipation, Mental Confusion, and Emotional Experiences for aids.

Skin problems Purging the body of poisons that accompany parasites may contribute to skin irritations or rash. If toxins are not effectively eliminated through the proper channels of the elimination organs, especially the liver and small and large intestines, poisons may back up and exit the body through the skin. Be sure to chew food extremely well, follow food combining, get proper exercise and rest, and use digestive aids and/or laxatives as needed. See also the sections on Indigestion and Constipation. Use aloe vera, calendula, or tea tree oil on some rashes; sometimes goldenseal (mixed with water) in a paste form can be a helpful salve. If symptoms persist, see your doctor. Staph (*staphylococcal*) or other infections may require more aggressive treatments. Also, temporary food intolerances may become evident during Candida treatment. One could become agitated by dairy foods, tomatoes, meats, nuts, or many other foods you are not normally allergic to. Try eating separately any foods you think may be causing reactions and rotate (eat only every other day, or third day, etc.) or eat sparingly any foods that appear to cause problems.

Sleeplessness Do not eat fruit at night or take vitamin C, echinacea, acidophilus, strong digestive aids, royal jelly, ginkgo, ginseng, or dong quai too late at night. Take melatonin (on an empty stomach one hour or more before bedtime or with a digestive aid [or use sublingual brand] for 15-minute action). Do not eat hard-to-digest, upsetting foods like corn chips, legumes, meats, oily foods, raw vegetables, or nuts late at night. Some people need a little food in their stomach to sleep well; others cannot sleep at all when they do. Find out what works best for you. If you have not had at least two full meals during the day, the body may not let you sleep restfully, long, or at all. Do not drink too many liquids late at night. If you are sedentary all day and exercise at night, that may also keep you awake. If you nap too much during the day or do not exercise at all, you will be sleepless at night. Too little fresh air or too much can affect sleep. Take vitamin B50-complex and calcium/magnesium supplements close to bedtime. Skullcap leaf tea may be drunk occasionally to assist sleep. Other sleep aids that can be tried individually (not with drugs) are: valerian root capsules, kava kava (mild aid), Hyland's Calms (homeopathic), and, if upset as well as sleepless, St. John's wort. (See section on Indigestion.)

Sore throat See section on Colds. Also try slippery elm lozenges and propolis in lozenge form, in tablets (crushed in mouth), or opened capsules. Gargle with salt water, aerobic oxygen, or another antibacterial mouthwash a few times daily to kill bacteria that help cause a sore throat. Straight lemon juice taken alone, once or twice early in the day away from food and followed by only a few sips of water, also kills bacteria and speeds healing. Use the juice of ½ large lemon or one whole small lemon. (See Oral Hygiene in chapter 7).

Stomach agitation Parasite movement can cause stomach upset, throbbing, and even insomnia. Also, the extra stress of parasite cleansing overburdens the digestive and elimination tracts, often contributing to upset and possibly even nausea. See sections on Nausea, Indigestion, Insomnia, and Hyperactivity for helpful aids.

Teeth hurting/toothaches When this happens during treatment (but not normally and you have no real dental problems), it is sometimes a sign that you are not eating enough of the right foods or you are not assimilating them well enough. It may denote that your body is very low on energy or needs "endurance proteins." Make a hearty, blended bean soup and eat it for at least three days in a row. Switch from raw to well-cooked vegetables for a few days but still enjoy raw vegetable juices. Chew foods well. Eat two to three full meals daily. Take extra vitamin C and calcium/magnesium. Get sufficient rest and moderate work and exercise. Take digestive aids if not assimilating foods well. For actual toothaches or infection, chew a garlic clove and spit out the pulp (the juice kills the bacteria/infection that causes pain); swish a tincture of goldenseal and myrrh in the mouth 1 to 3 times daily; or, most effectively, use peelu extract swished in the mouth and spit out once a day 1 to 3 times a week. (See Oral Hygiene in chapter 7.)

Throbbing See sections on Stomach Agitation or Headaches.

Weight gain This is not common during Candida treatment. The reverse is more likely. However, in the event this occurs, be careful not to stuff yourself with food each moment you have a craving. Limit your meals to three per day plus one to three reasonable snacks. Avoids lots of high-calorie foods with oil, dairy, nuts, seeds, and meats. Follow food combining. Do not sleep or lie down too soon after eating, as this increases calorie absorption. See How to Handle Constant Cravings in chapter 13. (See previous section on Bloating.)

Weight loss (too much) Be sure to eat three full meals a day and one to three snacks as desired. Eat legumes and at least two servings of whole grains daily. Chew foods slowly and well. Do not take too many laxative teas and digestive aids. Rest right after eating. Do not consume excessive amounts of yogurt, blended foods, club soda, or beets.

Chapter 6

CASE HISTORIES

MEDICAL CASE HISTORIES: DR. RONA'S FILES

These case histories illustrate the fungal/Candida connection in chronic degenerative diseases. By no means is this the only factor in the treatment of the diseases of civilization; still, the fungal connection cannot be ignored. Cancer, heart disease, high blood pressure, arthritis, gout, multiple sclerosis, migraine headaches, and mental illness can improve or disappear when the fungal infection is treated.

CASE 1 MR. K.: PROSTATE CANCER DISAPPEARS

I first saw Mr. K., an otherwise healthy British man in his early sixties, about two years ago. He had been told by his urologist that he had cancer of the prostate; that he required radical surgical excision, radiation, and chemotherapy; and that he would "suffer a miserable death" if he did not follow this advice. He was given a few months to live. Despite these dire predictions, he refused to have anything further to do with the conventional medical system.

Mr. K. instead did a great deal of reading and visited holistic doctors, naturopaths, and alternative medical specialists. He followed a completely plant-based (vegan) diet, received colonic irrigation, had intravenous chelation therapy, and took a long list of herbs, vitamins, and food supplements. Even after all this, his PSA (prostate-specific antigen) remained at 34, which indicated that his prostate cancer was still quite active. He came to see if I could offer him any other treatment that might help his problem.

I advised Mr. K. to continue with most of the natural treatments he had been taking. He discontinued chelation therapy and I added a more aggressive antifungal program (see chapter 3), including the prescription drug ketoconazole in high doses. He had no side effects to any of the treatments. Within six months his PSA was down to 10, with no detectable traces of cancer. He has remained on low-dose ketoconazole, a vegan diet, and nutritional supplements. Both his family doctor and his specialist know of his amazing recovery, and both remain skeptical about natural treatments.

CASE 2 MR. P.: THE VEGAN WITH HIGH BLOOD PRESSURE

Mr. P. is a fifty-year-old black man with a long history of high blood pressure (200/100 or higher at times). He had tried many different drugs over a period of five years, prescribed by his family doctor and two cardiologists. All the prescribed drugs had intolerable side effects, including impotence. His major complaints were dizziness and headaches. After extensive medical investigations, he was given the diagnosis of "essential hypertension," a fancy label meaning high blood pressure without any known cause.

Prior to seeing me, he put himself on a strict vegan diet for several months. His blood pressure remained sky-high. He did not use any salt in his diet. When I first started seeing him, I recommended garlic, parsley, green food concentrates, and high doses of antioxidants, including beta-carotene, vitamin C, and Coenzyme Q_{10}. His blood pressure continued to be high, in a range of 160/100, but his symptoms disappeared. One winter, vacationing in the Caribbean, he came upon a holistic clinic that offered intravenous ozone therapy. He took a four-week course of daily ozone injections, which dramatically lowered his blood pressure to 120/80. Unfortunately, shortly after his return to Canada, the pressure jumped up again to the 160/100 range.

Mr. P. had developed what appeared to be a fungal rash in the region of his belly button. I decided to give him a trial therapy with an oral ozone-liberating product called Bioxy Cleanse and the prescription antifungal drug ketoconazole. Within two weeks the rash disappeared and his blood pressure was suddenly down to 120/74. He is no longer dizzy and continues to follow a natural antifungal regime of diet and herbal remedies.

Case 3 Mr. R. G.: Kidney Stones and the Fungal Connection

Mr. R. G. is an aspiring thirty-two-year-old Caucasian actor with a history of recurrent kidney stones and kidney infections. He had been on a long list of antibiotic drugs and analgesics, but his back pain attacks continued relentlessly. He had not been given any dietary advice except to stay away from dairy products and drink lots of water. When I first saw him, he had just come off antibiotics. I ordered a kidney ultrasound, which showed the presence of several kidney stones. His uric acid and cholesterol levels were both elevated. High cholesterol and uric acid are often signs of an underlying fungal infection.

He was placed on a vegan diet and prescribed the following natural supplements in high doses: Greens Plus, folic acid, vitamin C, magnesium citrate, vitamin B_6, echinacea, and lactobacillus acidophilus. Folic acid and vitamin C are antifungals and indirectly lower uric acid and cholesterol levels. Magnesium and vitamin B_6 have been documented to reverse kidney stones.

After three months, his symptoms completely disappeared and his cholesterol and uric acid levels returned to normal. A recheck ultrasound showed no evidence of kidney stones and he was discharged by his specialist, who announced that the "antibiotics probably cleared everything up." Mr. R. G. had taken no antibiotics for the six months while he was under my care.

Case 4 Ms. D. D.: Rheumatoid Arthritis and Alternative Medicine

Ms. D. D. is a twenty-nine-year-old Caucasian woman who came to see me several years ago for natural treatment of rheumatoid arthritis. She had been told that her arthritis was severe enough to require gold injections and anti-malarial drugs to suppress the disease. She refused this option and referred herself to my office.

At the time the only medication she was taking was aspirin. Blood and stool testing revealed the presence of a heavy growth of Candida, geotrichum (another fungus), and several parasites (*Blastocystis hominis* and *entamoeba coli*). She had numerous food allergies and a long list of vitamin and mineral deficiencies. She was prescribed a strict antifungal diet; avoidance of allergic foods, including the nightshades; antioxidant nutritional supplements; and natural and prescription antifungals, as well as antiparasitic herbs.

With excellent compliance to diet and supplements, Ms. D. D.'s arthritic symptoms disappeared entirely within six weeks. Two years later she is symptom-free. She continues to follow a healthful, high-fiber diet and takes only a green food supplement.

Most cases of rheumatoid arthritis, like all autoimmune diseases, respond very well to a hypoallergenic diet and antifungal treatments. Some require prescription antifungals but the majority will settle nicely with diet changes alone.

Case 5 Mrs. N. S.: The Saved Thyroid Gland

Mrs. N. S. is a fifty-six-year-old Caucasian woman who came to see me about four years ago. Her thyroid specialist told her that she needed to have her thyroid gland excised. She had developed a goiter, bulging eyes, high blood pressure, and generalized rashes. Conventional medications had failed to control the overactive thyroid and she was frightened of radioactive iodine treatments.

Lab testing done through my office showed the presence of numerous food allergies and Candida. An aggressive antifungal therapy was started with a high-fiber, hypoallergenic diet; nutritional supplements (flaxseed oil, evening primrose oil, garlic, antioxidants); and oral ketoconazole. It took four months for the signs and symptoms to be reversed with this approach. For a few months, she was also prescribed low-dose lithium carbonate, a mineral that, in larger than RDA doses, slows down an overactive thyroid gland.

The exact role of antifungal therapy in this case is uncertain, but the patient continues to follow a sugar-free, yeast-free, high-fiber diet. She has been stable with no symptoms for over three years. Her thyroid specialist recently retired, and I continue to monitor her thyroid function tests every six months.

Case 6 Ms. N. R.: Migraine Headaches and Candida

Ms. N. R. is a thirty-seven-year-old teacher who consulted me about two years ago to see if alternative medicine held any answers to her twenty-year history of migraine headaches, fatigue, and an abnormal craving for sugar. She was not a diabetic, nor did she have any other significant medical history; she did have a history of being on the birth control pill, for at least 15 years. There was no history of excessive antibiotic use. She also suffered from recurrent vaginal yeast infections, for which she used prescription antifungal creams of various kinds. Her headaches were "under control" with three different prescription drugs taken on a nearly daily basis.

Testing done at my office showed no abnormalities except for low levels of red blood cell magnesium and multiple food allergies to common foods she ate or drank nearly every day, especially yeast, sugar, caffeine, and dairy products. She was advised to eliminate all her allergic foods and take a high magnesium-containing green foods supplement, antioxidants, D,L-phenylalanine, and the herb feverfew for pain control.

In the first week migraines intensified and she became more fatigued than ever. She had only a limited response from her prescription medications, one of which was a narcotic analgesic. I gave her a series of two magnesium sulfate injections weekly for three weeks and encouraged her to continue her nutrition program. After three weeks her migraines were under better control, but she continued to suffer from severe fatigue and food cravings, especially for sweets and baked goods. After a month I prescribed the antifungal drug itraconazole (Sporanox). Two weeks later her symptoms abated and she was able to get off all her prescription drugs. She remained on itraconazole for a month.

After two years Ms. N. R. has no symptoms except when she occasionally goes off her healthful diet and pays the price with a migraine headache and fatigue. She continues to use natural food supplements but no longer needs prescription medication to control symptoms.

CASE 7 MS. S.: BREAST CANCER AND ANTIFUNGAL PROGRAM

Who Gets the Credit?

Ms. S., age forty-two, one of my breast cancer patients, recently visited her oncologist for a routine follow-up examination. I had placed Ms. S. on a low carbohydrate, low-fat, high-protein diet as well as oil of oregano and other antifungal remedies. The specialist seemed very pleased with her progress, commenting that she was healing from surgery and radiation far better than expected.

Elated at this news from the usually grimly serious oncologist, Ms. S. volunteered that she had been seeing a holistic medical doctor, had changed her diet, and was taking several vitamin, mineral, and herbal remedies. At this news, the specialist turned noticeably red in the face and blurted out: "If you remain cancer-free, then who gets the credit, him or me?"

I believe that neither gets the credit. Doctors, whether conventional (allopathic) or holistic (naturopathic), do not heal anybody. It is only the individual who can heal him- or herself. If Ms. S. remains cancer-free for the next decade or longer, she has only herself to credit. All the doctors did was to guide Ms. S.'s energy to heal herself. The desire to be healed and the release of any resistance to doing so are the true anatomy of a cure.

NUTRITIONAL CONSULTATIONS: JEANNE MARIE MARTIN'S FILES

These nutritional case histories show the importance that diet plays in healing Candida albicans and other diseases and health concerns. The stories support the fact that proper diet is one of the major components of good health. All of the people here were also under a doctor's supervision and made no major diet changes not accepted by their doctors.

Case 1 Judy: Recurrent Candida Yeast Problems

Judy is a twenty-two-year-old student. Besides Candida yeast problems, she had suspected allergies and mineral imbalances. Her diet looked like this:

Day 1 Breakfast: bagel, jam, yogurt. Snack: fig bars. Lunch: pita pockets with cheese, spinach, and cauliflower. Supper: pasta with onions, spinach, mushrooms, and butter.

Day 2 Breakfast: oatmeal and banana. Lunch: two granola bars, two rye crackers with butter, two carrots, one banana. Snack: granola bar. Supper: apple.

Day 3 Breakfast: oatmeal and orange juice. Snack: nectarine. Lunch: Greek salad (tomatoes, cucumber, green peppers) with oil and cheese dressing. Snack: apple. Supper: two power bars. Snack: plain cooked brown rice.

I took her off wheat and oranges and limited dairy (including butter) to every other day. Cheese was allowed in small amounts, if well cooked. Oatmeal was changed to hearty millet or quinoa cereals. As protein deficiency was evident, salmon and white fish were added to her diet two to three times weekly. Legumes and other whole grains were added, along with three servings a day of vegetables. Fruit was temporarily eliminated; the bananas especially were not helping the Candida. Her health improved within the first week of diet changes and most symptoms disappeared even before new Candida treatment was begun.

CASE 2 ANDREW: CHRONIC CANDIDA FOR TEN YEARS

Andrew is an average man, age thirty-six, who suffered from asthma, gas, bloating, sleep difficulties, food allergies, and digestive problems. He had had no success with multiple Candida treatments over a 10-year period. He lived in a damp basement apartment. His diet looked like this:

Day 1 Breakfast: lemon juice, apple, three slices spelt toast, and two scrambled eggs. Lunch: water, dahl (red lentils and rice), papadam (lentil and spice flat-bread), and chapati (wheat) bread with butter. Snack: two oat bran muffins. Supper: soup with beef, vegetables, and noodles with corn chips.

Day 2 Breakfast: lemon juice, apple, four slices spelt toast. Lunch: suji (semolina with butter, cream, and sugar), papadam, and chapati. Supper: two banana oat bran muffins. Snack (11:00 P.M.): grapes.

Day 3 Breakfast: lemon juice, apple, four slices spelt toast. Lunch: carrot, lemon, apple juice. Supper: steamed beans, raw carrots, green peppers, two scrambled eggs with margarine. Snack: grapes, corn chips.

Andrew was making classic mistakes made by many Candida sufferers. He thought this diet was pretty good. Like many people with food allergies, he assumed that if he avoided the foods he was allergic to (wheat and dairy), he could eat almost anything else. He thought the Candida would go away if he just stopped eating desserts during Candida treatment.

The early-morning lemon juice was an attempt at a healing remedy—but did little good when followed by toast. Andrew had trouble digesting raw vegetables so these were changed to steamed vegetables and more tender, cooked vegetables, four to six servings daily. Morning apples were also eliminated.

East Indian foods, which Andrew said were not typical of his Western Canadian diet, were eliminated. He had a wheat allergy, so chapatis and suji were not acceptable foods. More well-cooked whole grains and legumes were added to his diet. The red meats he had trouble with were eliminated temporarily. Fish and free-range chicken were added, two to three times per week. Eggs were limited to four per week.

Andrew's late-night grapes and corn chips were keeping him up at night. Grapes are loaded with fruit sugar. (Eat no raw fruits at night!) Corn chips are hard to digest; they agitate the digestive tract and interfere with restful sleep. Although he was not eating sweets, the fruit and muffins were not helping the Candida. All these foods were eliminated from his diet. An apartment change was also suggested, as dampness breeds perfect conditions for continued yeast growth.

With these dietary changes the Candida finally showed substantial improvement and most of the allergy symptoms disappeared.

CASE 3 EILEEN: EXCESSIVE HAIR LOSS AND LOW BLOOD SUGAR

Eileen is an office worker, an attractive woman in her thirties who appears to be in excellent health. Her recent Candida treatment was prolonged and ineffective; she had problems with hypoglycemia, toxic liver, and poor digestion. Her main concern was hair loss; she claimed about one-third had been lost. She had made rounds with several doctors and after expensive allergy and diagnostic testing and numerous supplements, still found her hair to be falling out at an alarming rate.

A hair analysis test was suggested. I suspected high copper and low calcium amounts in her system and the test confirmed this. Calcium and zinc supplementation along with a major change in diet plan stopped the hair loss. She had been a vegetarian for three years, with a diet centered on pasta, cereal, rice, fruits, and vegetables. The addition of legumes to her diet, as well as the removal of coffee and too many fruits, helped her condition. Hypoglycemia is no longer a problem and Candida treatment was swift and successful. Eileen says her energy levels are higher than ever and she feels terrific mentally and physically.

CASE 4 LARRY: MILD CANDIDA PROBLEMS AFTER ILLNESS AND ANTIBIOTICS

Larry was a handsome, successful businessman in his forties. His doctor put him on a rigid Candida diet and gave him nystatin to help him overcome fatigue and headaches brought on by Candida, which had developed after a recent illness. He had been bedridden for a couple of weeks and taking large doses of antibiotics.

By all appearances he was healthy, with no digestive problems and only slight side effects from Candida. The acidophilus recommended for him upset his stomach. I suggested he take acidophilus capsules 15 to 30 minutes after meals (rather than the usual 1 to 2 hours after). He had high stomach acid, unlike many Candida sufferers, and needed food in his stomach to counteract the acidity created by the acidophilus. I put him on a diet similar to the Phase III Diet, only a little more relaxed, and allowed him cooked cheeses and nonyeasted breads and crackers. After about two weeks of treatment the Candida problems were easily overcome.

CASE 5 ANDREA: DIABETIC, UNABLE TO HOLD A JOB, SEVERE EMOTIONAL DISTRESS

Andrea appeared for her consultation looking tired, upset, and ready to cry. It took a short while before she was in tears, bemoaning her sad condition. She was in her late forties, slightly overweight, and could not work, think straight, or function well. It was all she could do, for the day, to show up for her hour and a half consultation with me. Andrea was diabetic and did not ask for much, just to be able to do a little work and not be depressed and crying all the time. She stuck to the main rules for a diabetic diet and limited her amounts of fats, white bread, fruit, and sweet intake. She kept craving milk, shrimp, and junk foods and munched all day without eating one really good meal. She had no idea how she could stay with a Candida diet when her diet was already so restricted.

I placed her on two to three full meals a day: 50 percent vegetables, 20 to 25 percent complex carbohydrates (in the form of cooked whole grains only: no breads, pasta, crackers, or potatoes), 15 to 20 percent legumes, and occasional lamb, eggs, and three servings a week of salmon and/or white fish.

After one week of sticking with the diet, she stopped crying. In the second week, with her doctor's approval, she was able to reduce her insulin amounts by one half. *The Wellness Encyclopedia* from UC Berkeley states: "Diabetics who eat a substantial amount of beans require less insulin to control their blood sugar." Shortly afterward, she was able to begin Candida treatment, which was highly successful. Within the next three months she was organizing her own business and successfully launched it one month later. Andrea went from barely functioning to managing her own business and employees within four months!

CASE 6 MARY: FIFTEEN YEARS OF CANDIDA, CHRONIC FATIGUE SYNDROME, CAR ACCIDENT

Mary is a slim forty-six-year-old who says her diet looked like this for five years: Breakfast: tea. Lunch: stir-fry with green onions, red peppers, carrots, and imitation crab or Chinese soup with seafood, pork, or beef along with rice bread and tofu cheese. Snack: chocolate bar or potato chips. Supper: tea and rice bread, corn chips, or potato chips, apple or orange and nuts. Late snack: orange or lemon juice or clear soda pop (like ginger ale).

Mary had mononucleosis twenty years ago and a severe car accident ten years ago, after which she began to exhibit signs of chronic fatigue syndrome and allergies. She spent time on work disability and welfare, had no energy, had stomach pains, suffered from chronic digestive problems, and craved meat and chocolate. Mary's medical doctor suggested a vegetarian diet and sent her to see me. She was put on a diet similar to Andrea's, along with small amounts of Flor-Essence or Essiac liquid for increased energy. (Only small, regular doses—2 tablespoons daily—increase energy. Too much causes major cleansing reactions.) Oranges, pop, meat, corn chips, potato chips, and nuts were eliminated completely, ending the stomach pains. Nuts especially are like "bombs to the digestive tract." Only those with excellent digestion should eat whole nuts.

Mary now works a job she enjoys, has fewer thinking difficulties, and has more energy and stamina.

CASE 7 ROB: SEVERE DIGESTIVE PROBLEMS AND FOOD ALLERGIES

Rob was a man in his middle sixties with chronic allergies and severe digestive problems. His diet was perfect—for an average healthy person—but he was making no improvement with it. His health, energy levels, and sleep patterns were erratic. Rob's desserts included normally wholesome items like oatmeal cookies and rice milk ice cream, and he enjoyed sweet fruits daily, like cantaloupes and mangoes, and a glass of wine or beer three or four times per week. He drank water frequently between and during meals. He ate lots of raw and cooked vegetables, legumes, whole grains, and occasional corn chips and avoided most meats.

From his stories and symptoms, a wheat allergy was likely, besides the dairy and environmental allergies already known, so I took him off wheat products. He was put on a strict rotation diet with 50 percent vegetables, all cooked or raw-juiced, as he had severe stomach upset when eating raw vegetables. The whole grains and legumes required longer cooking times than he was accustomed to and were blended into soups or mashed into burgers and casseroles instead of plainly prepared with bland seasonings, undercooked, and chewy as he had previously prepared them. Flavorful foods are easier to digest. Mealtime water and all alcohol were eliminated from his diet. Candida was suspected; all desserts, fruits, and corn chips were eliminated, and he was placed on a natural, mild Candida treatment. Some digestive aids were recommended.

Within a week of the changed diet, digestive problems and Candida side effects were reduced more than 75 percent. Reduction of allergy symptoms has been consistent and the Candida is now under control.

CASE 8 SEAN: FOOD ALLERGIES, SENSITIVITIES, AND SEVERE CANDIDA

Three-year-old Sean had a difficult birth, was constantly crying, insisted on being carried and held all the time, was sensitive to light and sound, and slept poorly. He had no interest in potty training. His typical daily diet included banana, pear or plums or berries, dry cereal, apple juice two times, orange juice, popsicle, cheese, cow's milk, cake or chocolate cookies, corn chips or popcorn, wheat crackers, mushroom soup, occasional chicken (one to two times per week) with cut green pepper, a small carrot, a potato, and some green beans spread throughout the day with no real mealtimes.

There was not much worth saving in that diet. He was taken off all fruit juices. Fruit was limited to one nonsweet fruit serving daily. Dairy was rotated so he only had cow's milk and cooked cheese every other day. Soy and almond milk were rotated on dairy-free days. (Goat's milk was later used as an alternative to cow's milk. Approximately 50 percent of those allergic to cow's milk can tolerate goats' milk, as it is closer to human milk in composition than cow's milk and more digestible.) Wholesome cooked and blended soups using vegetables, whole grains, and legumes were added daily, and occasional casseroles with the same ingredients well mixed and mashed. Tasty steamed vegetables were added daily, and raw vegetables were limited to one serving every other day. On off-days he had vegetable juices instead of raw vegetables. Lunch and supper times were established.

Candida looked evident, so yogurt was added and bifidus powder was mixed in a little water and given once or twice daily between meals and snacks. Improvement was immediate after dietary changes. There was less crying and irritability and a longer attention span. Digestion got better and sleep was less often interrupted by noises and sensitivity. Doctor's follow-up tests confirmed wheat and dairy allergies and Candida albicans.

Chapter 7

THE IMMUNE SYSTEM AND HEALING

THE IMMUNE SYSTEM

BY DR. ZOLTAN P. RONA

The immune system is composed of many different cells and tissues that facilitate the reaction of the body to substances that are foreign or are interpreted as being foreign. It is one of the most important body defenses against disease (infections, cancer) or the actions of certain poisons. The mechanisms by which all this takes place are complex. In brief, they involve the thymus gland; the bone marrow; the lymphatic tissues; the different types of white cells such as macrophages, killer T cells, helper T cells, B cells, and others; and the antibodies produced by the white cells. These cells all have different functions in protecting the body from invasion by viruses, bacteria, fungi, cancer, and other foreign matter. They work in concert and communicate with each other in a very organized fashion.

Natural immunity is an inborn protection. Acquired immunity occurs as a result of antibodies produced by the white cells. This latter form of immunity comes in two types: active and passive. Active immunity results when a person produces his or her own antibodies in response to the presence of an antigen (foreign substance), such as while recovering from an actual infectious disease. Artificial active immunity can be produced by vaccines containing antigens that, when introduced into the body, cause the production of antibodies.

Passive immunity results when antibodies are introduced into the body from an outside source (for example, breast milk antibodies). Since no antigen is introduced, there is no stimulus for the production of new antibodies.

Passive immunity is of short duration, lasting only as long as the introduced antibodies remain active in the body.

Immune System Supporters

Emotional/Spiritual: positive attitude, self-love, laughter, affirmations

Visualization/Relaxation: yoga, breathing, meditation, aerobic exercise

Healthful Diet: hypoallergenic (rotation, if possible), low fat, low sugar, chemical-free, filtered or purified water, adequate digestive function, adequate stomach acid and pancreatic enzyme function, dietary enzymes like plant-source amylase, protease, lipase, bromelain, papain, trypsin, and others

Herbs and Other Nutrients: garlic, licorice, echinacea, goldenseal, ginseng, DMG, CoQ10, germanium, thymus glandular, zinc, selenium, copper, vitamin C, bioflavonoids, vitamin A, beta-carotene, vitamin E, B-complex vitamins, essential fatty acids, protein, and special amino acids (arginine, ornithine, carnitine, cysteine, glutathione, lysine, taurine)

Over the few past years there has been a great emphasis in many health journals and books on dealing with conditions caused by an unhealthy immune system. I am referring here to the broad categories of infection and allergy.

It may be important to treat these conditions directly with medical or nutritional intervention, but focusing on the disease alone is never enough. The infection or allergy either recurs or becomes chronic. Classic examples are the Candida/fungal-related complex, 20th-century disease, and chronic fatigue syndrome. These diagnostic labels are useful, but none would have come about if the immune system were functioning at an optimal level in the first place.

Optimizing immunity is possible by maintaining a positive balance between the effects of immune system supporters and suppressors. To begin the task, take stock of several key areas. The most obvious are your diet and lifestyle habits. Nutritional excesses as well as deficiencies can have a remarkable impact on the likelihood of infections. It is well known that starvation (particularly protein deprivation) causes a lower production of antibodies and a greater risk of developing infections. For the immune system to function optimally, the body requires adequate (at least RDA levels) amounts of zinc, vitamin C, vitamin E, vitamin A, iron, copper, folic acid, vitamin B_{12}, and all essential amino acids.

Studies have shown that refined carbohydrates (glucose, fructose, and sucrose) have a depressant effect on the immune system, as early as an hour after eating them. A diet high in saturated animal fats impairs immune function, while a higher intake of the omega-3-EPA oils (found in halibut and cod liver oil) and gamma linolenic acid (flaxseed oil, evening primrose oil, black currant oil, and others) enhances it. A higher protein intake is helpful simply because it enhances antibody production.

Alcohol and other drugs (such as birth control pills, antibiotics, steroids, and analgesics) deplete the body of B vitamins and zinc and indirectly suppress immunity. An alteration of the normal bowel flora (the balance between friendly and unfriendly bacteria and yeast in the large bowel) may result from taking these drugs, predisposing the individual to infections. Cigarette smoke is a well-known suppressor of the immune system, and the large number of chemicals in our food, drinking water, and air (70,000 at last count), depletion of the ozone, and destruction of the rainforests negatively effect immunity. Even the chlorine in ordinary drinking water can have a negative effect because of its ability to destroy friendly bacteria in the large bowel.

It would be ideal to avoid these toxins altogether, but living in a city can make this impossible. A number of antioxidant nutrients can be supplemented to offset environmental assaults, including beta-carotene, B-complex vitamins, vitamin C, vitamin E, selenium, zinc, bioflavonoids, and amino acids such as cysteine, alanine, arginine, and ornithine in proper balance. Studies show, for example, that smokers who supplement their diets with large doses of beta-carotene have a lower incidence of lung cancer than those who do not. Live yogurt, which contains the friendly lactobacillus acidophilus, helps balance the large bowel flora in favor of protection against harmful bacteria, yeast, and fungi. Garlic and onions have natural antibiotic and antifungal activity and contain many natural antioxidants such as vitamin C and bioflavonoids. Fresh air (if you can find it) and regular exercise have a positive effect on immunity.

Immune System Suppressors
alcohol
aging
allergies

chemicals (phenol, formaldehyde, hydrocarbons)

air and water pollution

surgery, radiation, chemotherapy

prescription drugs: cortisone, steroids, including the birth control pill, NSAIDS (nonsteroidal anti-inflammatory drugs)

recreational drugs: marijuana, nicotine, cocaine, amphetamines

lack of sleep

airplane travel

stress (social, work, financial)

depression

overeating

high-fat diet

excess iron

malnutrition (deficiencies in protein; vitamins A, B-complex [especially B_5], folic acid, B_6, B_{12}, C, and E; selenium; zinc; essential fatty acids)

IMMUNE-ENHANCING SUPPLEMENTS: IMPORTANT

The supplements discussed in this section are recommended for use by children, nursing mothers, and adults of any age. While generally regarded as safe and effective, these nondrug alternatives to vaccines should be used as directed on the labels or as recommended by a natural health-care provider. Dosages will vary according to age and other factors, including past medical history, current nutritional status, and weight.

VITAMIN A

Supplementation with vitamin A has been shown to reduce the severity of measles infections. Vitamin A deficiency increases susceptibility to any infection. For most children, the best source is cod liver oil (one tablespoon or three capsules daily). Adults can take twice this amount, especially if they are prone to infections or exposed often to individuals with flu, colds, or other infections. Cod liver oil has the added benefit of the essential fatty acid omega-3, known for its anti-inflammatory benefits.

Vitamin A can only be reliably obtained from animal sources. Fruits, vegetables, and other plant sources contain no vitamin A but are high in beta-carotene (pro-vitamin A). The body can usually convert plant-source carotene into vitamin

A. In some people who are hypothyroid or deficient in zinc, copper, iodine, selenium, or the amino acid tyrosine, this conversion does not take place and carotene accumulates, leaving the skin with a yellow-orange pigmentation. The use of beta-carotene may act to prevent the development of various cancers. Beta-carotene is not toxic to the liver even in high doses. Large doses of beta-carotene increase the body's demands for vitamin E. If you take 50,000 to 100,000 units of beta-carotene per day, increase vitamin E to 1,000 to 2,000 units per day.

Bovine Colostrum

See Colostrum/bovine colostrum under Natural Antifungal Treatments in chapter 3.

Probiotics

Supplementation with probiotic products provides another unique type of protection against most common infections, allergies, and cancers. Probiotics is the name given to the "friendly" bacteria that maintain a healthy intestinal flora, an essential aspect of overall health.

Probiotics prevent the overgrowth of undesirable intestinal bacteria and microorganisms that produce putrefactive and carcinogenic toxins. If harmful bacteria dominate the intestines, essential vitamins and enzymes are not produced, and the level of harmful substances rises, leading to cancer, liver and kidney disease, hypertension, and arteriosclerosis.

Well-known probiotics include *lactobacillus acidophilus* and *bifidobacterium bifidum*. Another probiotic that has recently generated a great deal of interest is the friendly yeast known as *saccharomyces boulardii*, an organism that belongs to the brewer's yeast family. *S. boulardii* is not a permanent resident of the intestine, but taken orally, it produces lactic acid and some B vitamins and has an overall immune-enhancing effect.

Probiotics are considered to be very safe and well tolerated in the usual dosages prescribed. Highly sensitive individuals have reported the occasional occurrence of indigestion (nausea, heartburn), which disappeared when the supplement was discontinued or the brand of probiotic was changed.

Sugar, caffeine, alcohol, chlorine, tobacco, prescription antibiotics, steroids, vaccinations, and x rays inhibit probiotics. Some evidence exists that casein, a milk protein found in most commercial dairy products, inhibits probiotic growth. The antibiotics found in dairy products are also a factor in suppressing probiotics. A diet high in complex carbohydrates (vegetables, fruits, whole grains, legumes) encourages the proliferation of most probiotics.

Nondigestible food factors that selectively stimulate the growth and activity of probiotics in the gut are referred to as "prebiotics." The best example of a prebiotic is FOS (fructo-oligosaccharides). This substance is found naturally in many vegetables, grains, and fruits, including Jerusalem artichokes, chicory, burdock, garlic, and onions. In Japan, FOS is widely used as a sweetener.

Cultured dairy products like yogurt, acidophilus milk, buttermilk, sour cream, cottage cheese, and kefir are the best-known sources of friendly bacteria. Equally effective probiotic sources include cultured/fermented soy products like soymilk, tofu, tempeh, and miso. Other, lesser-known food sources of probiotics are sauerkraut and sourdough breads. If dietary sources are not easily available, supplemental probiotic powders and capsules are good alternatives.

Larch Arabinogalactan

See Larch Arabinogalactan under Natural Antifungal Treatments in chapter 3.

Interferon Boosters

Using a combination of vitamins, minerals, herbs, and other food factors that increase interferon production can further bolster immunity. Interferon is produced naturally by the body's white cells to fight and prevent viral and other infections, as well as cancer, allergies, and toxic poisoning of the body. A fever stimulates the body to make more interferon, one of the reasons why naturopaths recommend against the use of drugs to suppress fevers. Interferon can stimulate the immune system to produce more of the disease-fighting T cells.

Many natural substances have been shown to stimulate the body's natural production of interferon. Some of the best known and documented ones are listed here (in alphabetical order). See chapter 3 for more information on the following interferon boosters:

Astragalus	Pau d'arco
Boneset	Vitamin A
Echinacea	Beta-carotene
Germanium	Vitamin C
Licorice	Bioflavonoids
Medicinal mushrooms	Wheat grass

OTHER NATURAL IMMUNIZING AGENTS

See chapter 3 for information on the following:

Oil of oregano
Colloidal silver

NATURAL WAYS TO SPEED HEALING

BY JEANNE MARIE MARTIN

Healing Candida albicans can be assisted by a variety of different methods. Ask your health-care specialist or an expert in these areas to help you decide which of the following healing aids might benefit you most. There are many powerful ways to speed healing. Note the items on this list that interest you. Read about these healing aids and utilize some of them in your treatment program. It is not necessary to do "everything." Simply employ whatever healing aids listed here are appealing and/or helpful to you.

Affection	Hot and cold packs	Shower filter
Air purifiers	Laughter and play	Skin cleansing
Cleanliness, household	Massage	Stability and
Cleanliness, personal	Meditation	support
Chiropractic care	Oral hygiene	Steam bath
Deep breathing	Positive thinking	Strengthening
Dehumidifier	Rest	techniques
Diet and Nutrition	Sauna, dry	Sunshine
Ear candling	Sauna, wet	Tai chi, Qi
Exercise	Self-burping	gong or yoga
Fresh air	Self-massage	

Affection As warm-blooded mammals and humans, we require love and affection for optimum well being and good health. Candida symptoms may increase when we lose a loving relationship with a mate or even a family member, or if a major personal relationship in our lives alters significantly. During Candida treatment, it is helpful to have the love and support of a mate, family, and/or other intimate friends.

Air purifiers Unless you live in an unpolluted country area with abundant fresh air, an air purifier is a wise investment. For less than $80, you can buy one large enough to clean the air in a one-bedroom apartment. Replacement filters are only $10 to $20 per year. These compact appliances fit almost anywhere and measure about 1¼ feet in length and less in height. They remove some dust, pollen, smoke, and other air pollutants. This improves your air quality and can assist speedy healing. If you get one with an air ionizer, this adds energizing negative ions to your air supply, perfect for daytime. At night, while sleeping, turn the air ionizer off. You do not want to feel energized while sleeping; it may wake you. The average air-purifying unit can be kept on through the night (without the ionizer). It helps to prolong the life of the machine if you can find a few hours a day to turn it off and let it rest. You may notice you feel better, day and night, when using an air purifier. Find a high-quality model that suits the area you want to have cleaned for proper air purifying with full effectiveness.

Cleanliness, household It is essential to live in a clean living space with as little dirt, dust, and clutter as possible. Buy antibacterial dish soaps and other cleaning products to reduce germs that may contribute to yeast growth. Clean all areas that have mold, mildew, and grime with rubber gloves and effective cleaning products. Scrub sinks, bowls, and tubs twice weekly with antibacterial cleaners. Keep your home well vacuumed and ventilated. Air the entire place out at least once per day. Do not use strong-smelling cleaning agents that agitate allergies or Candida. (See list of equipment and household products in chapter 11.)

Cleanliness, personal For personal cleanliness, bathe or shower daily. Change to fresh towels regularly (at least two to three times per week). Do not take long hot baths, as they can weaken you and your body can absorb pollutants from the water such as chlorine, copper, and bacteria that collect in water pipes, bathtubs, and around bathing areas. Try a 15- to 20-minute maximum Epsom salt bath or hot-cold shower. (For baths, make sure the tub is thoroughly clean and properly rinsed before filling the tub.)

Epsom salt bath Put about two cups of Epsom salts into a bathtub under hot water as it fills. Swish it around before getting in and then soak away. Skin toxins are purged; this bath can relieve all-over body pressure and bring soothing relief to sore body parts. After the bath, rinse off with cool water. (See Shower filter, for important information on filtering bath water to avoid pollutants.)

Dr. Roger Rogers, M.D., a Vancouver disease expert, suggests that women not urinate before bathing or swimming; a little urine in the bladder helps prevent bacteria and pollutants in the water from entering the bladder and contributing to infections.

A hot-cold shower A shower is stimulating and invigorating for daytime bathing. (Stick with a moderately hot or warm shower before bedtime.) Take a warm shower, not too hot. When ready to step out, gradually turn the water cooler and cooler until it is as cold as you can stand it. Imagine a waterfall! If done gradually, it will not shock the body and you will feel energized and tingly all over. This can stimulate the immune system. Hot and cold treatments—packs, baths, or showers—can help send blood to needed areas of the body and help circulation. Do not just have a hot shower and expect to feel active and invigorated! Hot treatments invite sleep and slow the body down. (See Shower filters.)

Chiropractic This is a drugless healing art that can assist body healing and boost energy levels by adjustment of the spinal column. Chiropractic or spinal manipulation is based on the principle that the major cause of disease is disturbance in the balance between activating and inhibiting nerve impulses transmitted to affected body areas. The spine and other body parts can be adjusted or manipulated to remove interference of nerve impulses that weaken the body by inhibiting the flow of natural energy currents or "life force" in the body. Regular chiropractic adjustments during Candida treatment can increase energy levels and minimize unpleasant symptoms. I highly recommend it for most individuals. Choose a chiropractor carefully. Find one who meets your personal needs and whose style of adjusting works well for you. As with all professions, quality of care varies widely as do the benefits. Besides my own researched definition of chiropractic, I am including a quote from an expert chiropractor, Dr. Aaron Hoy of Vancouver: "Chiropractic health care is a branch of the natural healing arts. Its premise is based on academics, philosophy, art form and technique. Once a diagnosis is made, the treatment given can be a combination of the following: chiropractic manipulation; soft and deep tissue techniques, exercise, ergonomic and nutritional counseling. Chiropractic stimulates the nervous system and helps direct the body's natural response to heal and maintain itself."

Deep breathing Breathing is essential for human life. Many people breathe too shallowly and this can lead to lower energy levels and increased health concerns. Do your own treatments of "ozone therapy" by practicing deep breathing techniques. (I am still alive today due to deep breathing. A certain type and length of deep breathing can replace sleep and reduce pain; I used these to heal when doctors said my case was hopeless. These methods must be taught individually by professionals. See the next sections.)

Everyone can practice simple breathing techniques that work wonderfully to increase energy and reduce Candida treatment side effects. Some beneficial techniques are explained here.

Pranic breathing Lie down or sit in a chair or sit cross-legged with the spine straight. Put one hand on your stomach and one on your chest so you can feel them rising and falling, until you learn how to do it correctly; then your hands can be at your sides or in your lap. Take in a deep, s-l-o-w breath through the nose; let the stomach push out a bit. Continue breathing in until you feel the chest rising, too. Take in as much air as you possibly can without straining or forcing. Breathe in very slowly and deeply, never quickly! Now reverse the process by slowly exhaling, feeling the chest drop first and then the stomach area retract a little. Do a second breath the same way and continue. Do at least eight slow deep breaths; build up until you can do 5 to 10 minutes maximum. Practice at least once a day or anytime you are overstressed, upset, spacy, over-tired, anxious, have low energy, or you just need to relax and let go.

This technique helps you digest food by gently massaging your insides and helps to move digestive organs in a way that stimulates digestion. It will not cure indigestion, but it can help if done 30 or 60 minutes after eating. Do not do deep breathing right after eating or before sleeping!

Sleep-enhancing breathing Do this technique lying in bed, just before sleeping. Do the pranic breathing (above) with one difference: Exhale through the mouth. This can relax you and help bring on restful sleep. Only do 5 to 10 deep breaths, no more. Too much will keep you awake. Start with 5 until accustomed to this and increase to 10 if that works well for you. Remember to breathe slowly and deeply.

Many other types of deep breathing can be beneficial to healing Candida, but these methods should be taught by a professional. Attend a beginners' hatha yoga class, a low-key Iyengar yoga class, or a yoga class that stresses gentle, easy breathing rather than fast, pushed, or forced techniques. Make sure your teacher is qualified.

Dehumidifier Damp, cold weather or damp rooms, sleeping quarters, or basement apartments can contribute greatly to Candida problems. If you live in a damp climate (such as parts of Kentucky or Tennessee, Oregon, Washington, British Columbia, or certain parts of South America), buying a dehumidifier can be a wise investment in your health as it will remove excess water from the air. Candida breed in damp places. They die in hot, dry air (like that of Arizona, New Mexico, and similar climates). This does not mean to turn the heat on high and leave it there; that would create opposite problems and could be damaging. If you are sleeping in the basement of a house, move your bedroom upstairs. Make sure towels and clothing are thoroughly dry before using or wearing. Keep yourself warm and dry, both during and after Candida treatment.

Diet and nutrition A healthful diet and supplements are essential in boosting the immune system and promoting healing. The main message of this book is how to eat correctly and take proper supplements. See the book lists for books on vitamins and herbs.

Ear candling (coning) Candida can collect in the ear canals. You would be amazed at the amounts of white, cottage cheese–like material that can clog the ears, besides just wax. If you want to try ear candling, find someone with experience and references to give you a treatment. Some people advocate weekly treatments forever, but I disagree. In taking proper care of your health, one to four sessions a year (or less) should be adequate for the average person (unless your health problems are severe). Some healthy individuals may never require ear candling. I am, however, no expert on this particular subject; you may want to do your own exploring. Some doctors discount this treatment; others think it is beneficial. (I have used it successfully.)

Exercise Some people avoid exercise when they do not feel well: this slows down the healing process! The body needs stimulation to heal effectively. Even bedridden individuals can exercise by moving different body parts slightly and tensing and relaxing them. (This method is explained under Strengthening techniques.) Exercise must be done daily for optimum healing. It does not have to be strenuous. At least take one 15-minute walk daily or ride a bike at a casual pace. Indoor stationary bicycles, walking machines, rowing machines (for the stronger), or other exercise equipment are options. It is best to exercise for at least 30 minutes; this may be broken into two 15-minute segments. If you are accustomed to more exercise, do it. Only minimums are stated here. An absolute minimum of 15 minutes per day is required for optimum healing. Yoga, tai chi, and swimming are other forms of easy but extremely beneficial exercise if done moderately. Do not remain sedentary all day and exercise at night; it may energize you so much as to keep you awake much of the night. During Candida treatment, as during all cleanses, it is best to exercise just a little less than usual *if* you are an avid exerciser/sports participant. (Some less energetic people will require an increase in exercise!) A 10 to 25 percent decrease in vigorous exercise is recommended, as the body is stressed during treatment and requires more rest. Also, it is easier to strain yourself or pull a muscle while cleansing. This is not the time to take up a *new*, strenuous, or over-exerting sport or hobby like sky diving, scuba diving, hang gliding, boxing, or long-distance running. Take it easier during treatment and for several weeks following treatment as well, so your extra energy can go to optimum healing.

Fresh air Get country-fresh, mountain, seaside, or ocean air whenever possible. Avoid polluted areas, smoky rooms, strong-smelling cleaning products, dusty or musty rooms, strong or offensive perfumes or colognes, and anything that smells offensive to you or aggravates your healing. (See Air purifiers.)

Hot and cold packs A hot water bottle (or well-padded heating pad) can be used on body parts that are especially sore or agitated during Candida treatment, to relax and stimulate them. The hot treatments are even more effective if rotated with cold packs. A bag of frozen peas wrapped in a thin dish towel is the perfect ice pack. It is flexible enough to mold to different body parts and not as freezing as a solid block of ice. The cold forces blood to an area and improves circulation. Apply hot first for 5 to 15 minutes; rotate with cold for about the same length of time, or a little shorter. Try two to four rotations.

Laughter and play They say: "Laughter is the best medicine." This is definitely true. Read Norman Cousins's *Anatomy of an Illness*. He used funny movies and comedy shows to laugh his way to health. A good belly laugh stimulates all your major organs like a wonderful massage. Laughter helps to raise your energy levels. "Laugh and the world laughs with you," said poet Ella Wheeler Wilcox. Play is essential. Go to the park or beach with your children, or borrow someone else's children. They know how to play. Roll down a grassy hill, tickle someone—just a little—or let them tickle you, play a game, fly a kite, cuddle a teddy bear, gently and lovingly tease someone or be teased. Forget to be serious for a while. I decree at least 15 minutes daily of pure fun and play. Choose your favorite toy and let the games begin!

Massage This can help to relax you, strengthen and tone the body, help circulation, stimulate organ functions, and help to move poisons out of the body. Thirty to 60 minutes or more one to two times per week is ideal; however, even twice a month is better than nothing. Be sure that overly aggressive techniques are not used, or your body may be stimulated to release more poisons than it can handle removing at a time. Too many massages or massages that are too long can do the same thing. Massage is a wonderful aid in reducing body pressures and side effects while healing. Used wisely, it will help speed healing and make the treatment process more pleasant. Avoid massages during viral infections or avoid massaging infected areas, as this may stimulate or agitate the infection.

Meditation This is a great way to relax and reduce stress if practiced moderately. Daily or frequent meditation three to six times per week for 5 to 15 minutes a time is ideal. There is no need to overdo it. Extended meditation times have proved distressing to inexperienced meditators, but small periods of meditation can benefit almost anyone. There are thousands of ways to meditate. Anything that brings you a relaxed, peaceful feeling of serenity qualifies as a meditation technique, according to the foremost teachers of the art. A contented walk at sunset or a relaxing, quiet bath can be called meditating if done serenely.

One can sit quietly in a chair or cross-legged with the spine straight and employ one of many concentration techniques: the main purpose is to lead you to that "ah" place of serenity. The "ah" place or state of mind is what meditation is about. The moment may last a few seconds or longer. Just let go. Allow nothing to affect you (momentarily) and feel content, serene. This is true meditation.

Try reading positive, inspiring books about good people, angels, or inspirational stories, then reflect on them. Repeating positive statements like, "I am healthy, happy, and wonderful" is another technique. See one of the many books on the subject, especially *How to Meditate* by Lawrence LeShan, for a practical approach to meditation that almost anyone will enjoy. The main reason for meditating: It makes you feel good! Feeling good speeds healing.

Oral hygiene Candida breeds and multiplies readily in the mouth, especially around dental work and on the tongue. Brush the teeth thoroughly, at least twice daily with a gentle/medium brush and a peppermint, peelu, tea tree oil, or baking soda toothpaste, preferably one recommended by your Candida specialist. Do not use the citricidal toothpastes, as they may strip tooth enamel and cause the teeth to become super-sensitive. Also, brush the tongue at least once daily, preferably in the morning, as toxins and Candida coat the tongue more heavily during Candida treatment. Brush vigorously the middle to front of tongue, removing all white coating, if any. No need to brush the edges of the tongue. Use a natural, antibacterial mouthwash at least once daily as well—one with aloe vera, tea tree oil, or aromatherapy oil. Aerobic oxygen (see bottle directions) may be used; or a drop or two of tea tree oil in water; or sea salt in water; or a clove of garlic could be chewed and the pulp spit out to kill bacteria occasionally. Sometimes diluted colloidal silver can be used, though not daily. It is best not to use just one mouthwash. Check with your health food store and/or doctor for other alternatives. Variety is best for better antibacterial potency. For bad breath (halitosis), use bee propolis to kill infection and purify the breath. Take powder with water, chew a tablet, or open a capsule in the mouth daily and continue until breath improves.

Positive thinking You are what you think. You have to want to be healthy and see yourself that way to escalate healing. Depression lowers healing capabilities. Keep positive and support yourself. Surround yourself with supportive ideas and people.

Rest Most people need seven to nine hours of sleep each night while healing. Too much sleep makes you groggy and keeps your energy low and may interfere with the quality of sleep you get. Too little can make you hyperactive, punchy, agitated, and argumentative. If you nap in the daytime, you need less sleep at night. Some people who nap in the daytime have trouble sleeping at night.

Every hour you sleep before midnight can be more beneficial to you and is often better quality sleep. Each body is different; you must find your own healthful rhythm. If you are the overactive type, take several times a day to slow down and relax and do nothing, or read a book or watch TV. If you are the inactive type, make yourself take walks, do household chores, arts and crafts, garden, or cook. If you do not sleep well, you cannot digest your food. If you do not digest your food well, you cannot sleep. This can be a vicious cycle for some individuals, especially those with allergies, chronic fatigue syndrome, low blood sugar, and other ailments besides Candida. The cycle must be broken in order to heal.

Sauna, dry This helps eliminate poisons/toxins like pesticides, preservatives, and heavy metals through the skin and can help reduce the pressures of Candida cleansing. A good sweat flushes/cleanses the body, speeds up the metabolism, and kills harmful bacteria and some viruses. It helps speed healing and increases immune response. Dry sauna, wet sauna, or steam baths are extremely beneficial, especially four to six times monthly or about every 5 to 7 days for 30 minutes or more for dry sauna and 15 minutes or so for wet sauna or steam. See the following.

Sauna, wet Same as dry sauna except water is usually poured on hot rocks to create steam at self-regulated intervals. The use of hot steam helps cleanse the body in half the time, or less, than dry sauna with most of the same benefits. After (or halfway through, in-between) either dry or wet sauna, it is beneficial to soap off toxins exiting on the skin and end with a cold shower, or, if possible, a roll in the snow, as is traditional in Finland where saunas were first developed. No, you won't freeze! A 15-minute or longer hot sauna usually keeps your body hot even in snow for up to 30 minutes afterward. A steam bath is like a wet sauna, only the steam is continuous. Temperatures vary. See previous entry.

Self-burping Babies require burping as they are new to digesting foods. While Candida is healing, digestion may become sluggish or hindered. You may need a kick-start with digestive aids, self-massage (see following section), or self-burping. How do you burp an adult? You do not want someone else to do it for you, once you reach a certain age. You can burp yourself from the front quite easily with this special technique. With the flat palm of your hand, strike yourself quite briskly and solidly in the middle of the sternum or chest plate (as my chiropractor taught me to describe it), about one to two inches below the collarbone on the chest plate, just above the breast. Give yourself about seven good whacks. Repeat the seven whacks one to four times, pausing between each set. If done correctly, no hurt whatsoever will be caused, and you will likely find yourself giving up a few healthy burps that will ease digestion and stimulate energy to the digestive tract. This technique can be done as many times daily as desired, within reason. Usually, one to three times per day is enough.

Self-massage When no one else is around to do it for you, self-massage is an effective release of body pressure, especially on the head or neck to help reduce headache symptoms and around the digestive tract, liver, gallbladder, spleen, and colon. No special techniques are required. Just use your hand to knead the skin around these areas, gently at first, then more deeply as you proceed. It is a good idea to wait at least 30 minutes after a meal before doing this on the digestive tract and do not do it too hard if you have eaten within the last 2 hours. Knead, rub, press, stroke, and jiggle with the fingertips for 2 to 3 minutes, up to 10, or until you feel some benefit and release. This is a simple, yet powerful and effective, technique for self-healing. Do it one to three times daily or as needed. As always, do not overdo it.

Shower filter These wonderful gadgets can remove chlorine, lead, copper, asbestos, and other contaminants from your shower water and can also be used to fill the bath. Pollutants can more easily enter all over the skin, especially during a long, hot shower. (Also, if you have soft water, it often eats away at pipes, usually made of copper and soldered with lead, adding these toxic metals to the water.) Sensitive people may experience slight faintness or dizziness from the chlorine. Even healthy individuals are affected by chlorine and other heavy metals; although it may only be slightly, there is a build-up over time. For about $15 to $40 a small shower filter cylinder can be purchased and easily installed for 6 months to 1 year of pure showers, depending on how much you use it. Shower water decreases when the filter is old, so it's easy to know when to replace it. If you prefer to filter the entire household's water, almost all major water filter companies have small to large household units at varying prices.

Skin cleansing During any kind of cleansing, including Candida treatment, it is imperative that poisons exit the body speedily to avoid constipation or blockages that slow or impede the healing process. There are many ways to remove toxins from the skin's pores. They include: saunas, steam baths, Epsom salt baths, hot/cold showers, dry brushing, wet brushing, using a loofah, and the "scrape" method. One of the last four methods should be employed even if one or more of the other methods are also used. Special natural bristle brushes can be purchased at health stores and some pharmacies to help brush off dead skin that may clog pores. It is best to do this all over the body (get instructions, usually with the brush or from a health specialist). However, I feel that this method should be done in a bathtub before showering in the morning so the body does not get overstimulated at night. Some people use a dry brush while walking around the house, which allows dry skin to fall all over and feed dust mites, and other microscopic bugs and bacteria. The same type of brush can also be used for wet brushing in the shower; however, use one brush for dry use only and a separate brush for wet use if you want to do both. The third way of skin brushing is by using a loofah sponge, softened by hot water in the shower or bath to scrub off dead skin and toxins. Get these at any health food store, corner drug store, and most bath shops. The fourth method requires only that your fingernails are not too jagged. Use the nails to scratch or "scrape" off dead skin and toxins wherever you feel a buildup (all over the body, including the face) while showering or bathing. Using one of these four skin "rubbing" methods regularly gives the skin a healthy, youthful glow and appearance.

Stability and support It helps to have regular patterns of daily activities to keep yourself grounded and secure while healing. Surround yourself with stable conditions, friends, and family, especially those who want to assist your healing process and offer support (such as helping you prepare food, exercising with you, talking about what you are experiencing). Ask those close to you for help, so that your task is shared and easier. (See Affection.)

Steam bath See Sauna, wet.

Strengthening techniques The tensing and releasing method of strengthening and relaxing muscles is a powerful yet gentle way of exercising if you are too tired for traditional exercise or are bedridden. It can be used as a way to relax and release tension. It is often taught in yoga classes. Lie down on a comfortable bed, sofa, or mat and place the feet a foot or two apart; arms at your sides, palms slightly turned up; head centered. Start with the toes and feet. Squeeze them up tightly for 5 to 10 seconds, then release and wiggle them around; let them come to rest. Repeat the tensing-relaxing process with both legs. Then the buttocks. Take in a deep breath and push your stomach out like a balloon. Hold the air in 10 to 15 seconds, then release with a big gush through your mouth. Take another deep breath; this time push out the chest, hold 10 to 15 seconds, and release in one gush through the mouth again. Next, tense the shoulders for 5 to 10 seconds, shrug them a few times, and relax. Then both hands and then both arms: tense, wiggle, relax. Last, squeeze the whole face and head as if you were going to squeeze them into one tight knot on your nose, release; roll the head, wiggle the face, relax.

Sometimes this helps to induce sleep. If you cannot or will not do any other kind of exercise, do this two times a day. This can be done in addition to regular exercise. It helps to stimulate body organs, helps circulation, and tones the body internally and externally. It is a fantastic healing aid or beneficial technique—even for healthy individuals.

Sunshine Even in winter, a little sunshine is a good thing. Candida yeast do not like the sun. They "act up" more often and multiply faster in damp conditions and weather; this is why some people move to dry Arizona for their health. Do not overdo the sun, but get at least 15 minutes' exposure daily when possible in the summer (beneficial, provided you are protected so you do not burn); get 30 minutes or more in the winter. Even in winter you can take a walk on sunny days or sit on a sunny porch when weather allows. The sun is a natural healer when used correctly. Sun tanning may be beneficial to some and not to others. Get only as much sun as is beneficial for your body type. Consult your doctor if necessary. Avoid the sun if it harms you. Shark oil is a natural skin protector from sun overexposure (and is also a great anti-wrinkle agent). Apply it generously. It helps with redness, blotchiness, roughness, and dryness, as well as with wrinkling from the sun or aging. One hundred percent tea tree oil is one of the best burn healers, better and quicker than aloe vera, in my opinion; however, it does sting temporarily while it does its healing work, so kids may need encouragement and need to be told that the stinging speeds the healing. Use tea tree oil only when needed, as excessive use has a cleaning effect on the body.

Tai chi, Qi gong, or yoga It is extremely beneficial to practice one of these disciplines throughout your life. The benefits of each are similar. They each provide a gentle stretch of all major body parts and muscles, and they strengthen muscles in ways that vigorous exercise cannot. All give the body and other senses endurance, stamina, vitality, and strength. Practiced regularly, they can help to slow the aging process and keep you flexible and well toned. Any of these can help increase physical energy and improve mental clarity. I have practiced yoga for over 25 years, and my doctors tell me I have the muscle and skin tone of a woman in her twenties! Find a class in hatha or Iyengar yoga, tai chi, Qi gong, or a variation of these taught by a qualified teacher. Practicing three to six times per week for even 10 to 30 minutes brings favorable results.

Chapter 8

SOCIAL GUIDELINES

BY JEANNE MARIE MARTIN

EATING OUT IS NOT ALWAYS EASY. FOR SOME PEOPLE it can be a nightmare, and some say it is not worth the trouble. Life must go on, and there are ways to make eating out not only possible, but comfortable and enjoyable during Candida treatment.

RESTAURANT GUIDE

Unfortunately, the quality of foods in restaurants is inconsistent and questionable. Raw vegetables in a salad bar may have sulfur or other preservatives placed on them for longer-lasting "freshness." Even if they do not, all kinds of bacteria and parasites may get into raw vegetables in commercial, public kitchens. They do not use antibacterial products to soak vegetables (unless they are an extremely rare restaurant catering to those with allergies), so raw foods must be avoided when eating out!

See the lists of Foods to Enjoy and Foods to Avoid in the Phase II and III Diet plans for a complete list of acceptable foods for Candida diets. Remember these when dining out.

The safest bets are cooked foods. If you eat meat, quality cuts of well-done lamb, veal, and beef are possibilities. Have these roasted or broiled for the most wholesome and safe cooking methods. (Grilling is another less wholesome option.) Only eat at quality restaurants where you know they have high cleanliness standards. If you eat salmon, trout, sole, or other fish, choose ocean fish first, if available. Have these steamed, broiled, baked, or grilled.

If you do not eat meat, choices are more limited. Few restaurants serve whole grains and legumes (except for health food restaurants). Do not eat dairy products in restaurants. Eggs are possibilities. Try hard-boiled eggs (served in the shell) and omelets if they are not cooked in meat greases. (Ask the restaurant to use olive oil or butter for omelets.) Avoid soft-boiled eggs, sunny-side up or over-easy eggs, scrambled eggs, or premade frittatas. All can have high amounts of bacteria.

Without meat, fish, or eggs, the main option is vegetables. These can be eaten steamed, baked, broiled, or stir-fried if the chef uses butter or olive oil only. Stick with the vegetables allowed on the diet. It is okay to have a meal of vegetables if that is all the restaurant has that you can eat. Include onions and/or garlic with vegetables whenever possible.

For beverage ideas, see chapter 12. In general, choose club soda or hot peppermint tea. Do not drink plain water unless you are absolutely desperate; then be sure to squeeze 1 to 3 teaspoons fresh lemon or lime juice in it to counteract bacteria. Every restaurant I have ever been to is happy to provide lemon or lime wedges for you. If you think you cannot get these, carry a little bottle of Citricidal (grapefruit concentrate) with you and add a few drops to your water.

If having tea with friends on an afternoon, bring your own snacks to have with peppermint herb tea. If anyone questions you bringing your own snacks, tell them you have allergies and cannot eat anything else.

Most restaurants are supportive and understanding when serving customers with food allergies. Where I live, within the last several years, two individuals have dropped dead in restaurants because they were given a food they were allergic to. It is easier to tell your food servers that you have an allergy than to waste their time and yours trying to explain what Candida albicans is. Restaurants have learned to respect and honor allergy customers.

Be extra kind, courteous, and polite when asking for special foods so they do not resent you and future allergy customers! A generous tip is a wonderful way to say thank you. Your special order does take extra time and effort, especially when the restaurant is crowded. For the most attentive help, visit restaurants during slower times; in some cases it is a good idea to call ahead, make a reservation, and state your special needs over the phone. The chef may be able to prepare something extra special for you when there is more time. This only works in above-average restaurants.

Bring digestive aids to a restaurant if required. It helps to take extra vitamin C before eating out as well. Afterward, take extra acidophilus during the day, or a dose of Citricidal or garlic at night.

WHERE TO EAT

Natural or health food restaurants These can be good bets, but some have low cleanliness standards. Check into this before eating there. Enjoy well-cooked whole grain, vegetable, and legume dishes. Avoid raw vegetables when eating out. If they have fresh vegetable juices prepared on the premises, these can be enjoyed if you squeeze 1 to 2 teaspoons of fresh lemon or lime juice from wedges into a glass before drinking to counteract bacteria on raw vegetables. (If you really want a salad, eat it with 3 to 4 teaspoons of lemon juice squeezed over it and include tomatoes, garlic, and/or real yogurt with it, if possible, to aid digestion and assist in killing any bacteria or parasites.)

Above-average and fancy restaurants These may take the best care of you. Order meats, fish, and vegetables, or sometimes omelets, cooked in butter or olive oil.

Fish houses These are often a good choice for quality fresh fish and good vegetables. Be cautious of sauce ingredients. Use lemon on fish if possible.

Chinese restaurants Unfortunately, their meats of all kinds are often low quality, unless it is one of the fancier restaurants. Enjoy vegetable stir-frys (with added tofu or almonds if desired), and ask them to leave out the MSG! Avoid their soups and all other premade extras.

Mexican restaurants These are some of the few places where you can get beans, usually pinto, kidney, or black. Ask them to "bake" some for you and bake guacamole on top. Stir-frys with green pepper (sometimes red), onions, and other vegetables are good choices. Usually, they only serve white rice; however, inquire if they have brown, just in case. Some will cater to local health food advocates and serve brown rice. Only order rice if they have brown! Avoid all chips and salsa, too, unless they cook/bake the salsa over a dish for you!

East Indian restaurants These are often a good choice. They can serve red lentils, sometimes brown lentils, chickpeas, and/or mung bean dishes.

Sometimes they serve brown rice or basmati brown rice. Avoid chutneys and strong curries. Check out the ingredients in their many mixed dishes. Occasional mild curry dishes are okay. Ask about special vegetable dishes. Avoid deep fried and refined foods.

Greek and Middle Eastern restaurants Greek restaurants are famous for good lamb and they sometimes have fish, too. (No calamari!) Side-dish vegetables must be carefully ordered to avoid potatoes, eggplant, and cheeses. Hummus can be ordered if they will bake it in the oven for you. (Bring your own homemade breads or crackers that are allowed to eat with this.) Falafel must be avoided, as it sometimes contains flours and other additives and is deep-fried. Whole chickpea dishes are possible with vegetables. Sometimes bean fasolada soup is okay if you check the ingredients first. Feta cheese can be had if BAKED over a dish.

Italian restaurants Unless they have good fish, veal, or steaks, these are not the best restaurants to choose. Often, vegetables are limited. However, some restaurants are exceptions and offer good selections for Candida diets.

RESTAURANTS TO AVOID

Fast-food chain restaurants (burgers, fish, chicken, or subs)
Hamburger houses
Chicken "palaces"
Cafeteria-style restaurants
Family-style restaurants
Greasy spoon restaurants
Sandwich and soup shops
Submarine sandwich shops
Pizza places
Pancake houses
Breakfast restaurants
Diners
Delis
Bar and grills
Coffee shops
Japanese restaurants
Thai restaurants
Vietnamese restaurants (with few exceptions)

HELP FROM YOUR FRIENDS

It is immensely important to have support from friends, family, and co-workers (if you are working) during Candida treatment. It is up to you to set the pace and gently inform them of your special diet and lifestyle needs. If your attitude is relaxed, yet you are firm about your needs, they will most likely respect them and offer you whatever assistance they can. It helps during your Candida diet not to have friends pressuring you to cheat on your diet! The people who really care about you and your health will want to help you.

For close friends and family not living in the same household, make a copy of Foods to Enjoy, Occasional Foods, and Foods to Avoid lists in the Phase II and III Diets and add special requirements from your doctor or health-care specialist. Copy favorite, easy-to-follow cooked recipes and give these to friends. Better yet, get them a copy of the book if they are interested or will be responsible for cooking for you often. It is easier not to have them prepare raw foods for you unless they follow all the guidelines.

Make others aware of your cleanliness and lifestyle needs, such as avoiding cigarette smoke, not using microwave ovens, and special dishwashing requirements. Do not be too fussy about cookware used by them for you, if they are only cooking a meal or two for you on rare occasions.

PARTIES, LUNCHES, AND TRAVEL FOODS

Below are special guidelines for parties given and attended, lunch away from home, and travel foods for day trips, holidays, or vacations.

APPETIZERS AND PARTY FOODS

Giving a Party

If you give a party, prepare a variety of foods that you and your friends can enjoy. You do not have to tell them you are serving Candida diet foods. Use the dip and spread recipes given here and put out corn chips, potato chips, and crackers to go with them for your friends.

For yourself, make breads and chapatis from the recipes given here so you will not feel deprived. Make extras—your friends just might like them enough to eat all of yours! Confidently serve these recipes and know that most people will love them (unless they are finicky eaters).

Prepare a few favorite recipes that your friends like and you cannot have. Choose recipes that you do not have to taste-test! Reconcile yourself to all the great foods you *can* have—chances are, your friends will like most of your tasty new recipes! Choose your own beverages from this book and make punches from tried-and-true recipes or buy premade punches, juice, soda, and alcoholic beverages that you know your friends enjoy. Then have a party! Do not emphasize your Candida diet, and no one will resent it or think it is weird. Focus on the positive aspects and your party will be a success!

Attending a Party

If you go to a party, bring your own party platter and drinks. Not everyone has sparkling bottled water or club soda on hand. Ask your hostess (or host) in advance if it is okay for you to bring a dish or two for everyone. If they say no, they prefer to serve only their own creations, you may give a short explanation why you require certain food and drink. If they do not understand, say that Candida is like an allergy. Almost everyone understands allergic reactions.

If your hostess or host prefers that you do not bring food for other guests, tell them you will keep your food to yourself and be discreet while enjoying it. This is a necessity! Do not be tempted to cheat! Do not throw your diet aside for one little party! One party day can set you back weeks or months. It is not worth it.

Avoid excuses like, "A little bit of this won't matter," or "I can make up for it tomorrow." You cannot make up for it tomorrow; you may physically suffer for it tomorrow, and you may set yourself back enough so you have to start all over again! You cannot starve the yeast if you feed them "just a little" every once in a while. There are no new excuses or solutions. My clients have shown me that these comments are necessary to a complete Candida diet book. Once your Candida problem is healed, there will be other parties to attend, when you can eat less restricted foods. Be patient now, so that you can be healthy enough to enjoy future parties.

TAKE-OUT LUNCH IDEAS

Bag Lunches

Pack a salad or cut veggies with an ice pack to keep them crisp and fresh and prevent bacteria growth. A thermos is essential; however, a brown bag is not strong enough to carry it in. A cloth, canvas, leather, or metal lunch box or carryall is best for thermos lunches. Hot soups, stews, and even casseroles can be placed in the bottle or in short canister models. Warm a thermos by swishing boiling water in it before placing food inside. Wash the tall ones with a bottle brush and antibacterial dish soap to clean them properly and eliminate bacteria. Rinse thermos bottles right after using to prevent deep-set, dried-on foods that are very hard to clean, even with a bottle brush, later on.

Most cold foods are a no-no for a Candida diet; choices for bag lunches are limited without a thermos or two. A few types and sizes are a wise investment in your health, especially if you are going somewhere that does not have an acceptable restaurant. (See Restaurant Guide earlier in this chapter.)

Take-to-Work or Friend's-House Lunches

If you eat lunch in a lunchroom or friend's house that is equipped with a hot plate and/or stove, many more lunch options are possible. A main-dish pie can be heated in an oven. A soup or stew can be simmered on a hot plate or stove. A thermos is not required. If your lunchroom has a microwave but no hot plate or stove, do not use the microwave. A microwave does not kill all bacteria and Candida. You can purchase your own hot plate for $20 or even less and leave it at work for regular use. Your friends should understand and will be glad if you take the burden off them by bringing your own lunch over. If they choose to cook for you, see Help from Your Friends earlier in this chapter.

TRAVEL FOODS

Take food with you whenever you go out. Bring your own food stash for purse or pocket. Even if you leave home for an hour, especially if food shopping, bring a snack along. This way, if you see foods you cannot have, you have something to munch on while you tell yourself, "This Candida diet will help me to feel fantastic and healthy. I don't need or want junk anymore. When this is over, I won't even like the taste of some of these junk foods." Or tell yourself, "I can eat goodies when this Candida diet is over."

An over-the-shoulder, insulated, six-pack carrying case is ideal for day-trip snacks and lunches. For longer trips from home, take a larger cooler chest packed with ice and special foods. If staying in hotel or motel rooms, bring a hot plate, covered saucepan, and a few utensils along with brown rice, quinoa, condiments, or other special foods. (I took a hot plate to Hawaii with me once. I saved money by eating one meal a day in my room, as island food prices are high.)

On road trips, carry bottled water in your trunk. It keeps cool and fresh there. Distilled or demineralized/ozonated water is not always easy to find in small towns and foreign countries. Sometimes you may have to make do with bottled spring water. In tropical climates do not drink the local water! Drink club soda or even sparkling mineral water if necessary. For all kinds of climates, travel with lemons, limes, Citricidal, or aerobic oxygen to add to your water (if you cannot find bottled water), in case these items aren't available in travel restaurants and shops. (Bring vitamin C and garlic capsules [and fresh garlic bulbs] for extra antibacterial protection on trips. Also Eucarbon and Vogel's Tormentavina, available at health food stores, can help with diarrhea and parasites while traveling. Take these only if parasite side effects occur.) If possible, boil any questionable water at a furious boil for 20 minutes or more, then cool and strain through a clean travel filter. This kills most parasites.

Always carry emergency food and water; you may get stuck somewhere and the diet may go out the window. Rationalizations such as, "I'm hungry and must eat something. It's only one," or, "I'll make up for it later," do not work on a Candida diet. If you cheat now, you may have to start all over again!

Some foods can be premade and frozen for food safety—for example, legume or tofu dishes. Foods that travel well include stews, soups, and casseroles and sauces. Be prepared at all times. "Bring food, will travel."

If possible, plan your longer trips for a time period after Candida treatment diets. If this is not possible, make the best of it with these guidelines.

FANATICISM

"My way or the highway?" There are many ways to heal every health problem. There are right and wrong ways and there are gray areas in between. Your doctor and/or a specific blend of other diseases besides Candida may require that you take a different approach that is totally your own. Be ready to adapt to a method that suits you. Sometimes a blend of treatments or diets is required. You must be open to doing whatever it takes to regain or attain good health. Sometimes you will need more or less sleep or more or less stringent lifestyle requirements. It is up to you to adjust this book's guidelines for yourself. People with Candida vary so much in their symptoms and severity of disease; you must stick with a program that satisfies your own health goals.

When you deal with other people during Candida treatment diets, it is important not to get fanatical, controlling, demanding, or dictatorial with health-care specialists who are working with you and with friends, family, and co-workers who may not understand what you are trying to do but who have your best interests at heart.

Relax and remember that rigidness is stressful and does more harm than good during Candida treatments or when healing any kind of disease. You will heal faster if you have an easygoing way of dealing with others and are firm yet gentle, consistent yet flexible, when sticking with your course of treatment.

HEALTH HAZARDS

Certain environmental substances and man-made substances can agitate people who are dealing with moderate to severe Candida problems. Here is a partial list of things to avoid. Not everyone will have problems with all these items; however, it helps anyone to avoid these when possible. Follow the tips that are important for you.

AVOID:

Smoke-filled: rooms, elevators, cars, or closed-in spaces.

Car, truck, bus, or plane exhaust.

Areas high in air pollution, factories.

Dusty or dirty rooms.

Pet contact, hairs, litter boxes. (If you have a pet, bathe it frequently or preferably have others do it and have them change litter boxes. Control pet fleas and worms. Have pet-free rooms and areas. Extra cleanliness is a must for pet owners! Some people with persistent or chronic Candida will have to put their pets on a parasite treatment before their own symptoms improve. Sometimes one to two parasite treatments per year are required for pets.)

Dirty toilets, sinks, or bathtubs. (In public washrooms, wipe toilet seats with toilet paper and cover with a double layer before sitting. Always wash hands with soap after using a bathroom.)

Air sprays and fresheners, hair sprays, unnatural or spray deodorants (buy natural ones from health stores or buy hypoallergenic ones).

Moldy leaves or weeds in yards or gardens (use gloves).

Pesticide sprays, garden and soil chemicals, fertilizers, compost, manure.

High-pollen areas or certain flowers or plants in the house.

Paint fumes or fumes from building materials, formaldehyde, creosote.

Unnatural clothing or body-care products (avoid synthetics).

Strong perfumes, colognes, aftershaves, essential oils.

Synthetic fiber: rugs, blankets, bed linens, pillows, furniture, or other items.

Plastic household fixtures, appliances, and containers (when possible, use metal or ceramic fixtures and use glass jars for storage). Plastic can be used for freezing *if* foods are cooled before filling containers.

Fumes and skin irritations from household cleaners, ammonia, laundry soaps, aerosol sprays, office products like white-out formula for paper mistakes, glues, marking pens, and even chalk.

Smell and smoke of fires, incense, and some candles.

Enclosed malls or long periods in large office buildings.

Anything synthetic, strong-smelling, or agitating to the senses.

SEX PRECAUTIONS

Safe sex is an important issue for a Candida book, one that is often overlooked. As far as precautions for AIDS and other diseases, that is not what this book is about. Many of the precautions are the same as for Candida albicans. Many people do not realize that Candida albicans can be transmitted through sexual contact. Candida yeast can be found in many other places besides the digestive tract. Female vaginal yeast infections mean that the yeast are present in the vaginal area and can be transmitted during sex. Males can also carry Candida yeast around and inside their penises, although it is not so commonly recognized or as troublesome. In males, Candida can appear externally as jock itch.

During sex, Candida can be passed back and forth between lovers of both sexes. Wearing a condom can eliminate many transmissions, provided other precautions are taken. Even open-mouth kissing can pass Candida yeast back and forth. Oral sex is another way.

This information is not an attempt to limit sexual freedom; however, these factors must be considered. It is best that you have only one sexual partner during Candida treatment. Even if your partner does not display signs of problems, it helps if he or she takes a small, mild round of treatment for at least part of the time while you are undergoing Candida treatment. He or she should do it preferably at the middle or near the end of the time when you are finishing treatment. One to two weeks should be sufficient. This way Candida will not just be passed back and forth between both of you.

Other things that can help are gargling with sea salt water, aerobic oxygen and water, or another antibacterial mouthwash after sex. Having raw garlic (with other foods or chewed alone and the pulp spit out) or straight lemon or lime juice afterward can also help, if not at bedtime. (Do not leave citrus on the teeth at bedtime, as it may strip enamel off the teeth during extended exposure in the mouth.)

Both partners can wash or bathe right after sex when possible. Women can douche with one part pure apple cider vinegar (some doctors recommend white vinegar) to six to eight parts fresh warm (not hot) water, but not more than once per day (maximum a few times weekly) and preferably not immediately after sex. Wait for an hour or preferably more afterward. Women can also use boric acid vaginal capsules for 1 to 2 weeks to kill the yeast. Your doctor or pharmacist can dispense these without a prescription. Insert one or two capsules into the vagina as directed, preferably before bedtime. Wait at least 12 hours and douche after each use before engaging in sexual activities. (Do not douche too often! This *may* be harmful! Consult your doctor if you are uncertain how often is right for you or if you have problems from douching.)

Do not douche or use vaginal suppositories during the menstrual cycle. When beginning Candida treatment, it is best for women to begin *after* the menstrual cycle ends; never begin during ovulation, PMS, or the week before blood flow begins. The cycle can change considerably during Candida treatment. Blood flow may increase or decrease. Cycle length may increase or shorten. PMS may temporarily worsen as extra toxins are eliminated before blood flow. PMS may continue to be "more intense" until a month or two after treatment ends. The good news is that after 1 or 2 months PMS *may* disappear or the symptoms *may* lessen considerably, due to the cleansing effect of Candida treatment.

When engaging in sex during Candida treatment, change bed sheets more often, at least a few times per week or the next day after each sex act, if sex is less frequent.

Sex is more enjoyable when Candida is not an issue. It is best to deal with the yeast and get it over with. Ask your doctor for suggestions or to answer other questions.

CHILDREN AND CANDIDA

Dr. Rona has provided a wonderful section on treatments for children with Candida in chapter 3. Use the Phase III Diet mainly, with a few alterations. Some children cannot handle or will not put up with a special diet, so it has to have more leeway.

Phase III Diet for Children
Include these changes with the regular Phase III diet:

Include tart or subacid fruits and use food combining.
Occasional yogurt with tart or subacid fruits is okay (if not dairy-allergic).
Use whole grain flours and yeast-free breads, toasted when possible.
Eat yeast-free whole rye crackers and rice cakes.
Avoid wheat (whole grain spelt or whole grain kamut may be used occasionally; no pasta, use spaghetti squash).
Serve whole grain corn chips (unseasoned except for salt), whole grain corn tortillas, popcorn (very occasionally, one to two times weekly).
Use cooked, unprocessed cheeses of all types (except mozzarella, Swiss cheese, processed cheeses; one to two times weekly, if tolerated).
Serve cooked tofu cheese (if tolerated).
Drink acidophilus milk or simmered and quick-chilled goat's or cow's milk, yogurt (unless dairy-allergic).
Make whole grain (not wheat) pancake sandwiches (for lunches, prefrozen and taken out of the freezer in the morning to defrost by lunchtime: use falafel, cooked tuna, or egg salad).
Cook well-blended thin soups with lots of flavor (some kids prefer not to see too many strange things floating in their soup).
Veggie burgers, mock meatballs, and mock meat loaves are special.
Casseroles mashed in a food processor before baking are tastier and easier to look at for many children.

Get thermos bottles for school lunches for soups and lentil stews if
your children like them.

Include unsweetened fruit sauces: Homemade Applesauce and Berry
Berry Sauce on special occasions, or one to two times weekly, if
doctor allows.

Include frozen fresh fruit purees and ices for treats from subacid or
tart fruits.

Include watermelon and sometimes kiwifruits if they agree with
children's treatment.

Part II

DIET PLANS, MENUS, AND RECIPES

BY JEANNE MARIE MARTIN

"There is nothing to eat!" is a common complaint from those with Candida. Other Candida cookbooks offer limited menus with bland-tasting foods, and many contain recipes you can eat after treatment but not during. People want to know what they can eat now.

Here is abundant relief from boring, unappetizing dishes and limited menus. The following chapters are full of a variety of taste-tempting dishes that you can enjoy now, and most likely for the rest of your life, just because they are so delicious. Read on for a brand-new experience in wholesome and delectable Candida cooking.

Chapter 9

DIGESTION, FOOD COMBINING, MEAL PLANNING

H OW YOU EAT YOUR FOOD IS JUST AS IMPORTANT AS what you eat! Have you ever wondered why a friend or acquaintance of yours can get away with eating anything and you cannot? Part of the reason may be how they eat it. Other reasons may include hereditary factors, environment, stress, health history, exercise, attitude, and overall diet.

DIGESTION AND GOOD EATING HABITS

You have to work with your body to find, develop, and instigate eating habits that suit your personal needs and level of health and that will benefit you and complement your lifestyle. Once you understand the principles of wholesome eating, you can devise your own diet plans and experience optimum health and enjoyment from eating. The following sections will teach you important, basic principles of good diets, not just for Candida, but for most healthful diets. Ask your health specialist, if necessary, to assist you in determining your needs.

DIGESTION ENERGY AND HOW IT WORKS

Foods are broken down by the body in two basic ways. Some foods are broken down like carbohydrates (even if they are not completely made up of carbohydrate nutrients), such as vegetables, fruits, legumes, and whole grains, which require a good amount of saliva from the mouth to be mixed with them so that they break down properly when they get to the small intestines, where they are mainly assimilated by the body. These foods pass through the stomach but are not digested there.

Some foods are broken down like proteins: meat, seafood, eggs, and dairy products. These only need to be in the mouth long enough for you to chew them into small bits so that they digest properly when they reach the stomach, where they mainly break down and are absorbed. Steak is one of these foods and takes the longest to digest, up to six hours in the stomach. Acidic fruits like grapefruit, lemons, limes, tomatoes, cranberries, pineapples, and others assist in the breaking down of meats and dairy products.

Food-combining principles work with the body's natural processes. To assist digestion, foods broken down like carbohydrates and those digested like proteins are eaten at separate meals. There are some exceptions. For instance, most vegetables are complementary when eaten with either carbohydrate-digested or protein-digested foods. These guidelines are discussed later in this chapter.

Without proper digestion, healing is slow or impossible. During Candida treatment, the body is under extra stress; it becomes full of poisons while Candida yeast organisms are killed. As they die, their microscopic bodies can pile up and flood the body with poisons unless they are eliminated quickly and efficiently. While they live, they eat your food and defecate inside your system, which creates toxins that can clog the digestive tract or pollute other parts of the body that they inhabit. The more poisons in your system, the more difficult digestion is. The more energy is taken up by digestion, the less goes to healing the body.

Digestion requires a great deal of body energy. In the average healthy individual, it can take up to 40 to 60 percent of the body's physical energy each day. An unhealthy individual, with impaired or extremely poor digestion, may use up to 60 to 80 percent or more of the body's physical energy to digest food in one day.

Once you regain health and are utilizing the principles of good nutrition and digestion, digestion time and energy can be reduced. Excellent digestion requires only 20 percent or a bit more of physical body energy. A very healthy individual does not need to follow food combining to be healthy; however, those with health problems are greatly influenced by using food combining.

Food combining can reduce energy spent on digestion. Be aware that many doctors, even some holistic ones, do not "believe in" food combining. The proof of its value is in its utilization: It works! It does assist those with digestive problems and impaired health! Many different schools of thought exist as to what *is* proper food combining. The methods in this book are tested and have been found quite effective when properly utilized and adapted to the individual.

When I am writing a book, I eat specific foods to assist digestion and provide abundant mental and physical energy so I can work 12 to 16 hours a day (sometimes for weeks in a row) and still feel good. I continue the special diet until weeks after the writing is done, as my energy levels balance out and workdays return to normal. (The Phase II Diet is close to what I follow, only my diet is simpler and the foods are very specific.)

GOOD-TASTING FOODS HELP DIGESTION

Digestion begins in the mouth. If you like the flavor of a food, you salivate more, releasing larger amounts of digestive enzymes into your saliva. I do not believe that a Candida diet should be composed of bland and unappealing foods! You are supposed to enjoy your food, even (and especially) while healing. It is an erroneous belief that you have to suffer and sacrifice to get well! You can eat like a king or queen on your Candida diet. Savor and linger over your food and eat your way to health.

In my experience with nutrition counseling, the individuals who heal from Candida the fastest and enjoy the greatest improvement in health are those who take the time to prepare tasty, enjoyable foods. The individuals who fully explore, experiment, and "get into" the diet and cooking enjoy the speediest and most lasting recovery. They also tend to avoid frequent and devastating reoccurrences of Candida. Remember: Prepare delicious, exciting meals and snacks on the Candida diet (and always!). Chew food well, and mix lots of saliva and digestive enzymes with it for better digestion, less constipation, and less gas.

GOOD DIGESTION TIPS

1. Preparing and eating meals in a positive manner is good for digestion. Foods are harder to digest when one is under stress. Do not eat when upset, angry, or tense. Or, if you must eat, eat lightly and chew foods carefully.

2. Eat in a calm, peaceful atmosphere. Pleasant, low music can be a plus. Avoid watching TV or reading while eating; it takes concentration away from digesting food. Casual, low conversation is fine during eating. Looking at outdoor natural views or scenery is relaxing.

3. Eat only when you are hungry and eat only enough to feel good. Never stuff yourself. It is better to let food spoil in the garbage than let it spoil in your stomach. Spoiled food is perfect food for Candida yeast. Excessive food clogs the system, robs the body of energy, and, of course, adds inches to your waistline.

4. Chew food well. Digestion begins in the mouth. If you eat slower, you generally eat less and absorb more nutrients. This is a proven fact!

5. Do not eat when overtired, restless, bored, or have nothing else to do. Try cooking when you feel like nibbling; the process of cooking satisfies in a way that actually helps decrease food cravings.

6. Do not eat a big meal before sleeping or lying down. Digestion can take twice as long while the body rests. Let your stomach and intestines rest with you. If your body type, health, or low blood sugar require that you eat before bedtime, try cooked yams, winter squash, or a little whole grain cereal, with or without a sauce.

7. After eating, get some mild exercise to help stimulate digestion: walking, casual bike riding, or washing the dishes. If digestion is sluggish, try digestive aids or teas, self-burping, self-massage, or deep breathing for a few minutes, 30 minutes or more after eating. If before bedtime, try the sleep-inducing deep breathing. See chapter 7 for techniques.

SEVERE DIGESTIVE PROBLEMS

Some of my nutrition counseling clients are so ill and have such low energy they require twice or even three times as long as the average person to digest a meal, and even then foods are not completely broken down and utilized. These people may have stools containing chunks of whole foods not able to be broken down. What they had for a meal is sometimes quite recognizable.

Some people have so much trouble digesting, they cannot adjust food temperatures as foods are consumed. Healthy individuals can drink a hot beverage and cool it in their system or eat ice cream and warm it in their system for proper assimilation. Have you ever eaten ice cream and had a momentary response I call "cold throat," when you are eating it too fast and suddenly your whole mouth and throat react? You have to stop what you are doing; it is so cold you cannot stand it. Individuals with severe digestive troubles usually have food allergies and a sensitive reaction to foods that are too hot or too cold. A sip or two of ice water can throw the body temperature off so that these people feel cold for hours. Rotation diets (rotating different foods so that the same ones are not eaten each day) and basic, wholesome foods cooked very simply and eaten not too hot or too cold are required for severe digestive problems.

Quality or organic whole grains, legumes, and vegetables are necessary foods, prepared with seasonings that are not too fancy, complicated, or spicy. Whole grains have to be well cooked with extra water and eaten warm. Blend grains and add them to soup for easiest digestion. Brown, beige, and black (avoid the white) legumes are best, blended into soups or mashed and eaten warm. (These beans are higher in nutrients and less starchy.) It is best to eat singular grains and legumes rather than mix two or more whole grains or two or more legumes together at one meal.

Vegetables must be juiced raw or cooked very tender before eating, by steaming, baking, or broiling. No raw salads, nuts, seeds, wheat, dairy, or meats should be in this diet for severe digestive problems. A few herbs and seasonings are okay; in fact, these are important so that food is tasty and digests better. (Remember, the body digests food better if we like the taste!) As healing takes place in the body, other foods can be re-introduced in the diet.

Exercise, self-massage, deep breathing, and digestive aids are imperative for speedy and complete healing!

CONSTIPATION AND BOWEL DISEASE

A healthy individual who is eating mainly natural, whole foods has three to five bowel movements per day (less if not eating these foods). Healthy, not normal: Many Americans and Canadians think it is normal to have four to seven bowel movements per week, a clear sign of digestive troubles that lead to irritable bowel syndrome, colitis, diverticulitus, chronic fatigue syndrome, other bowel problems, and immune deficiency diseases.

If a sink gets clogged, it backs up and eventually becomes totally closed unless cleaned out. This can happen with the digestive tract. I am amazed at how many people I counsel these days whose doctors recommend partial removal of the colon or a colostomy. According to *Healthy Healing* by Dr. Linda Rector-Page, V. E. Irons (a colon and cleansing expert who lived into his nineties), and countless other health specialists: "Ninety percent of all diseases generate from an unclean colon." Healthy bowel transit time should take about 12 hours rather than the 24 to 48 it takes most people in our society. The longer food takes to process and stays in the body, the more chance there is for putrefaction and disease to grow. (And the more calories are absorbed!) The colon can become a breeding ground for Candida and other yeasts, parasites, bacteria, and viruses.

A serving of white bread (or refined pasta) can make a paste in the intestines that is like glue and clogs the pipes. Not to worry. Many people drink a human variety of liquid Drano, in the form of caffeinated colas and soft drinks. Eating lots of sweets and desserts is the equivalent of feeding a basement full of venomous snakes and then wondering why you cannot use your basement anymore. "Here, yeast, bacteria, and parasites. I have some nice sugar for you, so you can grow up big and strong."

It is no surprise when disease develops. It requires effort to become ill. One has to ignore all natural healing principles, ignore indigestion, gas, stomach upset, headache, discomfort, and pain, the body's warnings that you are on the wrong track and living poorly.

A diet of white bread, pasta, dry breakfast cereal, pastry, potato chips, corn chips, and white crackers has more to do with disease, in particular bowel disease, than occasional meat does. Meat is one of the hardest foods to digest, but it has more nutritional value than refined starches. A healthy individual can digest occasional meat and remain healthy. Eating excessive amounts or poor-quality meat is harmful.

Refined foods are "dead foods" that give the body no vitality. We live in a "cold pasta" generation. Imagine this refined food sitting on a store shelf for months, even years, then sitting in your cupboard for months more; you expect to eat it and feel energized? The body cannot tell the difference between white flour and white sugar. These items are among the biggest offenders when it comes to constipation.

A diet of complex carbohydrates, legumes, and three to six servings of vegetables daily can nearly defeat constipation, unless there is physical damage. If the digestive tract has been severely damaged or is clogged with poisons, these must be flushed out before normal, natural digestion can take place. See a naturopathic doctor or natural health-care specialist about cleansing programs; educate yourself on the pros and cons of enemas, colonics, laxative teas, and other colon-cleansing processes. Some are easy, noninvasive, and highly beneficial if done correctly.

Health experts say, "Death begins in the colon" (as well as "Ninety percent of disease begins in the colon"). Health begins in the colon, too. It is possible to reverse even severe damage, sometimes, if caught before it is too late. I am living proof of this, and many other individuals have experienced miraculous healings—with effort and some natural body wisdom.

Throughout Candida treatment, you must have at least one bowel movement per day, every day. If you do not, poisons accumulate more quickly during the stresses of treatment and if your system gets clogged, especially at this sensitive time, more severe damage can be done to the colon than under normal circumstances! So eat vegetables, raw, juiced, and/or cooked, three to six times daily. If you cannot have a bowel movement, take flaxseed, acidophilus, laxative teas, or digestive aids. Do whatever it takes to bring on a bowel movement as soon as possible; keep them regular. Avoid drugs if possible. If constipation continues for several days and you cannot alleviate the problem, contact your doctor.

FOOD COMBINING

Food combining is a complex issue. Many conflicting points of view exist. The most important food-combining principles are:

1. Eat protein-digested foods separately from carbohydrate-digested foods or starchy foods. This is simple for vegetarians; it is okay to eat legumes and whole grains or starchy vegetables together. Meat-eaters will have to get used to eating meats and proteins without starches on the side. Meats, eggs, and most dairy products are best not eaten at the same meal with starches such as bread, crackers, pasta, cereal, or potatoes. Following this rule helps to speed digestion and healing and keeps one from absorbing as many calories from foods. Meats may be eaten with vegetables (except potatoes), which are less starchy than whole grains.
2. Eat raw fruit alone or first, before a meal, so as not to hinder digestion. The enzymes in raw fruit make them the easiest food to digest. Stomach upset, indigestion, and fermentation of stomach foods may occur if raw fruit is eaten after a meal.

Cooked fruit is like a carbohydrate food and is okay to eat sometimes with and after a meal. It is best, though not essential, to wait 15 to 30 minutes after eating raw fruit before consuming other foods.

SPECIAL FOOD-COMBINING POINTS

1. Eat raw, fresh citrus fruit or juice apart from grains, (preferably 30 minutes or more before, never with or after) as it makes them like lead in the system and increases absorption of calories. (Citrus, except for oranges, are allowed in all phases of the Candida diets.)
2. Raw fruit is limited in all the Candida diets. When allowed in Phases I, III, and IV, do not eat raw fruit at night (or any time after supper). Fruit sugar may keep you awake!
3. A vegetarian diet or a diet of mainly whole grains, legumes, and vegetables greatly reduces the desire or craving for alcohol and cigarette (or other) smoking, according to tests reported by Dr. E. Cheraskin in *Psychodietetics* and other health experts. Remember this if you have to quit smoking during Phase I. A balanced, high complex carbohydrate, low protein/acid diet cuts cravings.
4. Eat the hardest-to-digest food first at most meals. Eat salads and raw vegetables first in a vegetarian meal to help stimulate and assist digestion. Eat meat before salad. Chew foods well to mix in lots of saliva, assisting the digestive process.
5. Avoid drinking liquids with meals. If desired, drink only four to six ounces, in small sips as needed.
6. Plain yogurt can sometimes be eaten with tart or subacid fruits (in Phases I, III, and IV only). Because of its live enzymes, yogurt is the only raw dairy product that is good with legumes; yogurt assists their digestion.
7. A healthy individual generally does not need to follow food-combining principles, if digestion is excellent and weight is satisfactory. During Candida treatment, food combining is very beneficial for the body and can greatly assist healing when the principles are followed daily.

FOOD COMBINING GUIDELINES AND EXCEPTIONS

1. Do not eat carbohydrate-digested foods with protein-digested foods at the same meal or snack. Neutral foods (like most vegetables) may be eaten with protein-digested OR carbohydrate-digested meals.

FOOD COMBINING CHART FOR CANDIDA DIETS

Ⓐ   **Carbohydrate Foods**

Whole Grains (brown rice, brown basmati rice, wild rice, wehani rice, brown pot barley, buckwheat, kasha, quinoa, oats, Scotch oats, rye)

Legumes: Beans, Peas and Lentils (fava beans, soybeans, chickpeas, black or red beans, pinto beans, kidney beans, Romano beans, adzuki beans, mung beans, brown or green or gray or red lentils)

Ⓑ   **Neutral Foods**

Avocados

All Vegetables (yams, green vegetables, carrots, turnips, winter squash, etc.)

Cooked Tomatoes

Cooked Citrus (except oranges) and Tart or Subacid Fruits

Yogurt (fresh only)

Butter (fresh or cooked)

Cooked Nuts, Seeds and Nut or Seed Butters

Cooked Amaranth Seed or Teff Seed Flours

Natural Oils

Cooked Sprouts

Cooked Black Olives

Cooked Water Chestnuts

Cooked Lotus Root

Cooked Bamboo Shoots

Ⓒ   **Protein and Acid Foods**

Yogurt (fresh or cooked)

Cooked Milk (in small amounts mixed with foods)

Cooked Goat's Milk Feta, Farmer's, Ricotta, and Quark Cheeses

Eggs (chicken, duck, goose, or quail)

Fish (especially salmon and ocean white-fish varieties)

Poultry (chicken, turkey, Cornish hens, quail)

Red meats (lamb, veal, beef)

   Complementary Acid Foods:

Raw Tomatoes

Raw Lemons, Limes and White Grapefruit

Left side: DO MIX — YES (between A and B)

Left side: DO MIX — YES (between B and C)

Right side: DO NOT MIX — NO

Key

1. A can be mixed with B but not with C.
2. B can be mixed with either A or with C (either / or, not both).
3. C can be mixed with B but not with A.
4. A, B, and C cannot be mixed all together.

2. Eat raw citrus (except oranges), tart, or subacid fruits alone or with acidophilus yogurt in Phases I, III, and IV only (if allowed), or with avocados
   any time.
3. Raw citrus (lemons, limes, or white grapefruits) or raw tomatoes may be
   eaten with salads any time, even before carbohydrate meals; they assist the
   digestion of raw vegetables.
4. See Meal Planning Guidelines, Glossary, and Candida Treatment Diets for
   more information.

MEAL PLANNING GUIDELINES

1. Approximate overall food ratios for the average Candida diet are: 40 to 50
   percent vegetables, 20 to 25 percent whole grains, 15 to 20 percent legumes
   (and some tofu), 5 to 20 percent other foods (meat, fish, dairy, nuts, seeds,
   fruit, natural oils, and some others).
2. Include the following foods in each meal. Breakfast: whole grains, tofu,
   eggs, or vegetables with optional nut sauce, vegetable sauce, or cooked tart
   or subacid fruit sauce (if allowed). Lunch or Supper: vegetables (40 to 60
   percent of meal) with protein-digested foods (meat, fish, eggs, cooked
   cheese, and/or cooked milk), or carbohydrate-digested foods (legumes or
   whole grains) with optional cooked nut or seed sauces.
3. Enjoy two to three meals per day along with one to four snacks, if desired.
   Some people function better with two meals a day, some with three. If you
   want to avoid breakfast and/or lunch, make sure to have at least one meal
   by noon.
4. Do not overeat any one type of food. No individual food should be eaten
   more than five to six days a week. It is better to have two servings of a food
   every other day than to have one serving every day. Rotate foods for better
   digestion and health and to avoid aggravating or creating allergies.
5. Weekly, include in your diet: 5 to 12 servings of legumes and/or 5 servings
   of meat, 10 to 14 servings of warm whole grains, up to 3 servings of tofu.
   One to three days a week, enjoy up to 6 servings of nuts and seeds in
   cooked foods; different vegetables may be had every day. Avoid foods you
   are allergic or sensitive to.
6. Daily, include: 3 to 8 servings of vegetables (at least two green vegetables,
   one orange and occasionally yellow), 3 to 6 servings of complex carbohy-

drates (warm, cooked whole grains or starchy vegetables like winter squash, yams, turnips, or cauliflower), unless your doctor puts you on a temporary "no" or low-carbohydrate diet (See menus), and 1 to 2 servings of legumes. Optional: 1 serving tofu, nuts/seeds, or meats. (Fruit servings vary with Diet Phases, usually 1 serving every other day.)

7. A serving is: ½ to 1 cup cooked vegetables; 1 cup raw vegetables; ½ to 1 cup legumes or whole grains; 3 to 4 ounces (about 100 grams) tofu; 2 to 4 tablespoons ground nuts or seeds or butters; 4 to 8 ounces meat; ½ to 1 cup fruit.

8. Do not eat too many heavy foods in one meal or you will feel sluggish and your body will be so overloaded it will have trouble healing. About half your lunch and supper, or 40 to 60 percent, should be vegetables. Occasional light sauces and thin soups can help lighten a meal.

9. Create your own menus using these guidelines. For more economical meals, serve the same dish several times in a week or freeze leftovers for later weeks.

SAMPLE MENUS

These menus need not be followed exactly. They are sample guidelines of wholesome meals. Using these suggestions, it is easy to plan meals that include most of the vitamins, minerals, and nutrients that your body requires. Additional menu suggestions are at the end of each main dish and soup recipe. Your health specialist can inform you of any other special food requirements. The Candida Diet Phases contain extra information on which menus are right for you. In the vegetarian (carbohydrate) and meat (protein) menus that follow, recipes found in this book are capitalized. Note that all the vegetarian menus have vegan recipe options included. See Index. Alter the menus to suit your personal needs. Snack ideas are entirely up to you. See Snack recipes.

VEGETARIAN MENUS

Phase I or III / Day 1 / Vegetarian Menu
Pre-Breakfast Fruit (30 minutes before)
Berries, OR nonsweet pear, OR watermelon if allowed

Breakfast
Herb-Scrambled Tofu with Vegetables, OR Avocado Omelet
Optional: Acidophilus Yogurt, and/or Homemade Salsa

Lunch
Great Greens Salad with Italian Herbs and Oil Dressing
Black Bean Vegetable Goulash

Supper
Asian Vegetable Stir-Fry with Tofu
Optional: Broiled Stuffed Tomatoes with Falafel Spread

Phase I or III / Day 2 / Vegetarian Menu
Pre-Breakfast Fruit (30 minutes before)
2 kiwis (high in potassium)

Breakfast
Millet Cereal with Orange Yam Sauce, OR Green Herb and Orange
   Yam Sauce, OR Savory Sweet Onion Sauce

Lunch
Confetti Salad
Fresh Herbs and Oil Dressing
Mock Meat Loaf
Mock Meat Gravy

Supper
Spinach Sunshine Salad
Dilly Cucumber Dressing, OR Fresh Herbs and Oil Dressing
Festival Vegetable Rice Pie

Phase I or III / Day 3 / Sunday or Holiday Vegetarian Menu
Pre-Breakfast Fruit (30 minutes before)
Apple, OR Japanese pear apple

Breakfast
Orange Yam Pie with Crunchy Crust

Lunch
Exotic Greens Salad
Emerald Dressing, OR Tahini Dressing
Broiled Vegetable and Tofu Kebabs
Cooked Brown Rice, OR Basmati Brown Rice

Supper
Zucchini Ribbon and Red Pepper Salad, OR Zucchini Salad
Garlic French Dressing
Mediterranean Vegetable Briam, OR Parsley and Whole Grain
    Casserole
Steamed broccoli

Phase II / Day 1 / Vegetarian Menu
Pre-Breakfast Fruit (30 minutes before)
½ white grapefruit

Breakfast
Scotch Oat Cereal, OR Sweet Brown Rice Cereal
Amorous Avocado Tofu Sauce

Lunch
Sweet Beet Salad, OR Kohlrabi Coleslaw
Italian Herbs and Oil Dressing
Harvest Red Lentil Soup

Supper
Garlic Spinach Soup, OR Great Greens Soup
Quinoa with Zucchini
Steamed cauliflower, OR spaghetti squash
Homemade Tomato Sauce, OR Mock Tomato Sauce

Phase II / Day 2 / Vegetarian Menu
Pre-Breakfast Fruit (30 minutes before)
Lemon juice

Breakfast
Steamed carrots, OR Cinnamon-Baked Squash
Optional: Toasted Sesame Seed Sauce, OR Toasted Almond or Filbert
    Sauce

Lunch
Confetti Salad, OR Sweet Beet Salad
Dilly Cucumber Dressing, OR Yogurt Dill Dressing
Brown Bean and Broccoli Soup, OR Blended Black Turtle Bean Soup

Supper
Wild Rice Celery Soup
Spinach Tofu-Stuffed Zucchini
Homefries, OR Herb Homefries

Phase II / Day 3 / Sunday or Holiday Vegetarian Menu
Pre-Breakfast Fruit (30 minutes before)
½ avocado filled with chopped white grapefruit sections

Breakfast
Amaranth OR Teff Pancakes
Berry Berry Sauce (if allowed), OR Toasted Almond or Filbert Sauce

Lunch
Spinach Sunshine Salad
Velvet Vegetable Dressing, OR Parsley Nut Dressing
Super Sunflower-Bean Burgers, OR Best Bean Burgers
Homemade Ketchup, OR Homemade Salsa

Supper
Orange Yam or Carrot Soup
Asparagus with Parsley-Lemon Butter, OR steamed asparagus with
    lemon wedges
Whole Grain Stuffed Red Bell Peppers

Meat Menus

Phase I or III / Day 1 / Meat Menu
Pre-Breakfast Fruit (30 minutes before)
Strawberries

Breakfast
Zucchini Frittata
Optional: Acidophilus Yogurt, AND/OR Homemade Salsa

Lunch
Great Greens Salad
Italian Herbs and Oil Dressing
Lentil Vegetable Pottage soup
Optional: Whole rye crackers (unyeasted)

Supper
Herb Garlic Chicken
Steamed broccoli and carrots
Optional: Herb and Cheese Stuffed Tomatoes, OR Acidophilus
    Yogurt, OR salad with dressing

Phase I or III / Day 2 / Meat Menu
Pre-Breakfast Fruit (30 minutes before)
2 kiwis (high in potassium)

Breakfast
Millet Cereal with Orange Yam Sauce, OR Green Herb and Orange
    Yam Sauce

Lunch
Warm Chicken Salad

Supper
Zucchini Ribbon and Red Pepper Salad, OR Zucchini Salad
Emerald Dressing, OR Yogurt Garlic Dressing
Mediterranean Vegetable Rice Pie

Phase I or III / Day 3 / Sunday or Holiday Meat Menu
Pre-Breakfast Fruit (30 minutes before)
Lemon juice

Breakfast
Whole Grain Pancakes with Berry Berry Sauce

Lunch
Exotic Greens Salad
Tahini Dressing
Herb and Veggie Burgers, OR Vital Vegetable Nut Burgers

Supper
Layered Vegetable Salad
Tomato and Herb Dressing, OR Tahini Dressing
Stuffed Trout OR Salmon with Sun-Dried Tomatoes
Asparagus with Parsley-Lemon Butter, OR steamed asparagus with
    lemon wedges

Phase II / Day 1 / Meat Menu
Pre-Breakfast Fruit (30 minutes before)
½ white grapefruit

Breakfast
Sweet Brown Rice Cereal, OR Quinoa Cereal
Amorous Avocado Tofu Sauce

Lunch
Kohlrabi Coleslaw
Fresh Herbs and Oil Dressing
Rainbow Barley Soup, OR Marvelous Minestrone Soup

Supper
Herb-Baked Sole OR Cod, OR Baked Salmon Fillets
Steamed cauliflower and zucchini chunks
Homemade Tomato Sauce, OR Mock Tomato Sauce

Phase II / Day 2 / Meat Menu
Pre-Breakfast Fruit
None

Breakfast
Cinnamon-Baked Squash

Lunch
Spinach Sunshine Salad
Dilly Cucumber Dressing
Whole Grain Stuffed Red Bell Peppers

Supper
Mediterranean Chicken OR Turkey Stew
Steamed Savoy OR green cabbage
Carrot-Cauliflower Medley

Phase II / Day 3 / Sunday or Holiday Meat Menu
Pre-Breakfast Fruit (30 minutes before)
½ avocado with chopped white grapefruit sections

Breakfast
Herb-Scrambled Eggs with Vegetables
Homefries, OR Herb Homefries

Lunch
Mexican Layered Salad
Optional: Acidophilus Yogurt, AND/OR Homemade Salsa, OR dressing of your choice

Supper
Roasted Chicken with Berry Berry Sauce, OR Herb-Baked Chicken Kiev
Exotic greens OR spinach
Raw tomato slices AND/OR lemon wedges
Steamed or sautéed snow peas, artichoke hearts, and water chestnuts

All Phases/ Easy-to-Digest Special Menu
Pre-Breakfast Fruit (30 minutes before)
Fresh lemon juice, OR grapefruit juice, OR vegetable juice

Breakfast
Steamed orange yams, OR baked butternut or buttercup squash

Lunch
Digest-Aid-Meal-in-a-Soup

Supper
Steamed carrots, OR cauliflower
Steamed asparagus, OR broccoli OR kohlrabi
Optional: ½ avocado, OR vegetable juice (if not eaten earlier)

Optional Snacks (between meals)
Acidophilus Yogurt
Fresh carrot or beet juice
Steamed orange yams, OR butternut or buttercup squash
Other tender steamed vegetables
Citrus Beet Treat

Low or "No" Carbohydrate Menus*

Breakfast
Broiled Tofu Slices OR Grilled or baked tofu with red bell peppers
OR egg recipe like Avocade Omette

Lunch
Avocado Boat Treat OR a green salad with tomatoes
Oil OR yogurt-based dressing
Baked Salmon Fillets
Optional: Top fish with toasted almonds
Steamed broccoli OR brussels sprouts with butter or olive oil

Supper
Great Greens Soup OR Quick and Easy Artichoke Heart Soup
Warm Chicken Salad OR Herb Garlic Chicken
Steamed asparagus or globe artichoke with butter or olive oil

Optional Snacks (Between Meals)
Acidophilus yogurt
Avocado half stuffed with almonds or warmed almond butter (filbert butter may also be used)
Hard boiled egg OR another type of eggs
Green vegetable sticks with a warmed nut butter (almond or filbert)
Grilled or Broiled Tofu

---

*Only use for 1 to 3 weeks IF recommended by doctor! (Your doctor may alter this menu according to individual needs. Most people with Candida do not require these diet menus, which are for chronic Candida and special cases.)

Chapter 10

CANDIDA TREATMENT DIETS

Candida albicans cannot be cured by diet alone, but treatment without an accompanying yeast-control diet is ineffective and useless. Proper treatment is required to destroy accumulated Candida organisms; a good diet ensures that little or no new growth can occur or become established. Without favorite foods, yeast cannot thrive and multiply. The best way to get rid of an unwelcome guest is to empty your refrigerator. During treatments with yeast killers, Candida yeast will die if you do not feed them.

Stick with the suggested diets and adhere to them completely; at least, do not make major transgressions like eating sugar or mushrooms or drinking alcohol. In my nutrition counseling, many of my clients are already on Candida diets. Probably one-third do not stick with the diet and end up repeating the treatment one or more times, doubling or tripling the treatment time it would have taken if they had stayed with the proper diet in the first place.

Some people think that occasional cheating, having ice cream once or twice a week, for example, is okay. If you wanted to starve someone and fed him or her twice a week, the person might never die. Likewise, yeast will not die if you feed them sweets or refined foods, even occasionally. Many people take large amounts of yeast killers one day, then feed the yeast heartily the next. At this rate, Candida treatment becomes never-ending. If you stay with the diet the entire time of treatment, results are usually swift and effective (unless there is an underlying cause—see chapter 21). Candida treatment time will be shorter and without frequent reoccurrence if diet and treatment are consistently followed. Read about cravings in chapter 13, for advice on dealing with urges to cheat.

CANDIDA TREATMENT DIET PROGRAM

This chapter outlines four phases of diets for Candida treatment: Phase I, Phase II, Phase III, and Phase IV.

> Phase I: Pre-Candida Treatment Diet for Regular or Severe Candida Control
>
> Phase II: During-Candida Treatment Diet for Regular or Severe Candida Control (with yeast control treatment, one to four months)
>
> Phase III: After-Candida Treatment Recovery Diet (immune system boosting diet)
>
> Phase IV: Post-Candida Treatment Diet After Recovery ("The Safe Worldly Diet")
>
> *See Chapter 22 for ways to prevent Candida reoccurrence.*

ALTERNATIVE USES FOR CANDIDA DIETS

Very mild Candida cases: Phase III diet (with yeast control treatment, two to four weeks)

Mild Candida reoccurrence: Phase III diet (with yeast control treatment, two to four weeks)

Moderate to severe Candida reoccurrence: Phase II diet (with yeast control treatment, four to twelve weeks)

Healing diet (during illness or time of excessive stress): Phase I diet initially, then Phase II, or Phase III diet, until healing occurs or body energy rises

Cleansing diets: Phase II or Phase III diet (during body cleansing while taking herbal or other natural cleansing programs)

After cleansing diets: Phase III diet (for one or more weeks after cleanse ends, to build up the immune system), then Phase IV diet (indefinitely)

Healthful-living diet: Phase IV diet (indefinitely) for all health-conscious individuals who are relatively healthy and want to maintain good health

CHOOSING THE PROPER CANDIDA TREATMENT DIET

It is up to you and your doctor to determine which phases of diet are right for you and how much treatment time is required. Generally, pregnant and nursing mothers should avoid Candida treatments unless recommended and monitored by their doctors.

Read my important introduction on Candida and Dr. Rona's vital information on treatments before proceeding with any diet or treatment; they will help you understand the necessity of adhering to each step of the diet plan for maximum results and speedy recovery from Candida yeast symptoms and discomforts.

PHASE I DIET: PRE-CANDIDA TREATMENT DIET FOR REGULAR OR SEVERE CASES OF CANDIDA CONTROL

Two Weeks to Two Months

The Phase I diet introduces food combining. It limits and eliminates certain foods while increasing other foods that you may previously have eaten in smaller amounts or not at all. Most Candida treatment diets are restrictive: sugar, sweets, certain fruits, grain flours, refined foods, coffee, colas, alcohol, smoking, and other foods are not allowed. The Phase I diet helps you ease into changes and allows some cheating with a few treats. A gradual transition is more natural for the body and reduces stress and the anxiety that lifestyle and diet changes can sometimes create. This diet is not for use while taking Candida treatments.

If you are already eating a wholesome natural food diet and the Phase I diet looks too easy for you, skip Phase I and go right to the treatment stage, Phase II, if desired. For wholesome eaters with mild cases of Candida albicans, the Phase III diet may be used instead of Phases I and II diets with Candida treatment, if your doctor permits.

If you are accustomed to eating the average North American diet and generally eat whatever you like at restaurants and at home, it can be a difficult transition to alter your diet and restrict foods all at once. The transition is easier if a less-restrictive diet is followed for one to two months before yeast treatment begins. If you are used to smoking and eating hamburgers, fried chicken, fast foods, potato chips, white bread, candy, desserts, and drinking coffee, colas, and alcohol, you will need more time than others to gradually adjust to the new diet.

Candida treatment puts extra stress on the body while the yeast are being destroyed. Extra body energy is required during treatment to assist healing; therefore, high-nutrient, moderately easy-to-digest foods are required, along with adequate exercise, vitamin supplements, extra sleep, and rest. Read Regulation of Treatment in chapter 5 and Social Guidelines in chapter 8.

PHASE I DIET GUIDELINES
Phase I Diet Fruit:
Reduce fruit intake to a maximum of one serving daily, preferably in the morning. Eat raw fruit according to food combining rules (see chapter 9); eat it by itself, or 15 to 30 minutes before other foods. Cooked fruits may be eaten with other foods. All sweet fruits should be avoided. However, this is a transitional diet; one weekly inappropriate fruit will not be harmful at this stage.

Enjoy:

Apples	Papayas	Strawberries
Avocados	Grapefruit	Blackberries
Nonsweet pears	Fresh lemon juice	Blueberries
Japanese pear apples	Fresh lime juice	Raspberries
Kiwi (tender-firm, not too soft or ripe)	Watermelon	Other berries

Avoid:

Oranges	Peaches	Grapes
Pineapple	Apricots	Cherries
Melons	Plums	Bananas
Mangoes		

Exotic fruits (starfruit, passion fruit, guavas, lychee nuts, persimmons, and others)

Dried fruits (raisins, currants, dates, figs, coconut, and others)

All other fruits not mentioned

Fruit Guidelines:

a. Avoid fruit that tastes too sweet.

b. Avoid fruit with mold on it.

c. Avoid under- and overripe fruits.

d. Raw fruits have live enzymes and are quickly digested when eaten alone. Eaten with other foods, raw fruits take too long to digest and stay too long in the digestive tract, where they become overprocessed and great food for Candida yeast. The live enzymes in cooked fruits have been killed, so they may be eaten with other foods and are digested like other carbohydrate foods. (This is one reason people with Candida have an easier time digesting cooked fruits than they do raw fruits. Raw fruits can upset the stomach when eaten with other foods, and yeast prefer eating raw fruits.)

e. Do not eat raw fruits at night or after supper. The fruit sugar may keep you awake, and fruits are not good for digestion at night. Eliminate chewable vitamin C through all Phases; it is like eating raw, sweet fruit, and it often contains added sweeteners.

PHASE I DIET BREAKFASTS

Two to three full meals a day are required. If breakfast is eaten during Phase I, follow these guidelines:

1. Wean yourself from coffee and black or green caffeinated teas; replace with certain herb teas (see Beverages) and temporarily with dandelion or grain-substitute coffees; these will be eliminated in Phase II.

2. Whole grain muffins, bread, toast, dry cereals, and refined cereals (hot or cold, especially granola), oatmeal and rolled oats, and other rolled or flaked whole grains must be eliminated or reduced to one or two mornings per week. This is preparation for removing these foods completely during Phase II. Pancakes, French toast, and hash browns are included with these and should be eaten without sweetener, served only with cooked fruit or unsweetened applesauce. Avoid jam; use butter or cinnamon instead. Absolutely no refined muffins, breads, pancakes, or white flour pastries of any kind. All grain products or baked goods should be 100 percent whole grain and made with baking powder, preferably without yeast.

3. Eliminate all fruit juices, especially orange juice, which the yeast love. Eat fruits separately, before breakfast or lunch, unless they are cooked. If cooked, eat them unsweetened with foods. Eliminate milk and dairy products except for butter and yogurt. Try yogurt treats (see Snacks and Munchies, chapter 13) or plain, natural yogurt. At this stage, yogurt eaten with cut fruits from the Fruits to Enjoy list are okay without added sweetener of any kind. (Milk can be used occasionally in cooking if tolerated. Feta, ricotta, or tofu cheese can be cooked into foods one to four times per month if desired.) Avoid any of these if allergic.

4. Do not eat bacon, sausage, ham, and all other breakfast meats. Choose eggs instead. Avoid soft-boiled and sunny-side up (higher bacteria count), but enjoy all others. Make sure eggs are fully cooked.

5. Learn to cook whole grain cereals and prepare nut and vegetable sauces to flavor them instead of sweeteners. Use no added sweeteners at all with breakfast.

6. Learn to get along without your microwave. Use the stove, oven, or toaster oven instead.

About Microwaves

Average microwave use does not kill all bacteria in food or kill some parasites that may be found in meat. Use the stove, oven, or toaster oven. Research found in several sources, including Dr. Joseph Mercola's newsletter for June 17, 2000, (http://www.ric1.com/c.e?A6998), gives overwhelming evidence that, among other hazards, people who consume microwaved foods experience increased cholesterol levels and significant changes in their blood; changes also occur in the nutrients of microwaved foods. There are dangers involved in heating baby foods as well. See Dr. Rona's additional information on microwaves in chapter 11.

Breakfast Guidelines:

0 to 2 mornings per week:	1 to 2 eggs, cooked, or 4 ounces scrambled or sautéed tofu
1 to 2 mornings per week:	100% whole grain pancakes, French toast, muffins, breads, or cereals (unsweetened or ½ teaspoon sweetener cooked in each serving)
3 to 5 mornings per week:	¾ to 1½ cups cooked 100% whole grain cereal: millet, quinoa, brown rice, whole oats, scotch oats, brown pot barley with butter and salt, or sauce topping (nonsweet)
0 to 3 mornings per week:	2 or more cups cooked starchy vegetables: Cinnamon Baked Squash, orange yams, carrots, cauliflower, spaghetti squash, or other starchy vegetable

PHASE I DIET SNACKS

a. Enjoy any of the snacks in chapter 13.
b. It is okay to enjoy one to four snacks each day, based on your individual body needs. If you eat three meals a day, limit snacks to one or two. If you eat two meals a day, two to four snacks are okay.
c. Snacks in chapter 20 may be enjoyed many times a week. (If you cheat with honey or naturally sweetened desserts once or twice a week at this stage, you are still doing well. Rice milk ice cream is a wholesome splurge.)

PHASE I DIET LUNCHES

1. Enjoy any of the soup or main dish recipes in this book, along with a salad and/or cooked vegetables. Each soup and main dish recipe offers meal suggestions at the end of the recipe to help you create complete meals. See chapter 9 for food combining and meal planning guidelines. Follow food combining rules: Serve carbohydrates (whole grains and/or legumes) with vegetables, *or* serve proteins (meat, eggs, and/or dairy) with vegetables at one meal.
2. While adjusting to this diet, you may sidetrack just a little, once or twice a week with whole grain pasta, potatoes, or a burger with a whole grain bun.

Whole grain breads, two to three servings per week, should be yeast-free (a piece or two of yeasted bread at this stage is okay). All white breads and refined products must be eliminated now.

3. If you eat lunch away from home, see ideas in chapter 8.
4. Drink beverages a half hour or more before or after meals. Do not drink liquids until over an hour after a heavy meal. During meals, 4 to 6 ounces of water or other liquid may be had if the meal is dry or experience shows it will not interfere with your digestion. When drinking with meals, sip a little at a time. Try dandelion or grain coffees, if desired, in this phase. If you are weaning off milk, one or two servings of milk a week is okay.

Phase I Diet Suppers

a. Follow the same guidelines as for lunch.
b. Depending on your body requirements, try to eat supper four hours or more before bedtime. Some individuals need food in their stomachs to sleep; if so, do not eat a heavy meal and finish eating one to two hours before bed. If you are hungry, have a filling snack one hour before bedtime.

Four- to Eight-Week Program to Convert to New Foods

Try this program if adapting to a new diet creates problems.

Week 1, or Weeks 1 and 2: Add new good foods to your present diet. Experiment with soups, snacks, and main dishes from this book. Do not eliminate anything from your diet yet unless you want to.

Week 2, or Weeks 3 and 4: Continue with new foods, especially for lunch and supper. Start cutting out coffee, extra desserts, and sweet snacks. Try having junk foods and goodies only every other day or every third day. If smoking, quit now and do the 8-week program.

Week 3, or Weeks 5 and 6: Continue with good foods for lunch and dinner and use this book's recipes for those meals, every other day. Concentrate on wholesome breakfasts from this book three to five mornings per week, if you eat breakfast. Cut out caffeine completely and limit desserts and cheat days to once or twice per week.

Week 4, or Weeks 7 and 8: By now you should be completely following the Phase I diet. If you cheat with one or two small foods per week, it is okay for now. Keep expanding your repertoire of recipes from this book. Follow food combining and meal planning guidelines (chapter 9).

After Week 4 or 8: When you can completely follow the Phase I diet without cheating and feel comfortable with it, you are ready to begin Candida treatment with the Phase II or Phase III diet. If unsure, begin the Phase II diet first; once you can stick with it without cheating for a week or two, begin Candida treatment.

PHASE II DIET: DURING CANDIDA TREATMENT DIET FOR REGULAR OR SEVERE CASES OF CANDIDA

One to Four Months, and Up to Six

The Phase II diet is the most important one in the Candida treatment program. If followed correctly and completely, healing is usually speedy and the treatment successful.

Most of the recipes in this book can be enjoyed on a Phase II diet. Avoid the few recipes labeled for Phase I, III, or IV only. Avoid any recipes your doctor says to omit and any that contain items you are allergic or sensitive to—unless you can find suitable substitutes. (See chapter 11 for substitutions.)

Follow food combining and meal planning rules (see chapter 9). Take digestive aids if necessary, when not digesting foods properly. Good digestion is essential for treatment to be successful. If digestion is extremely poor, simplify the recipes and diet, eliminate meats, and avoid raw vegetables except for juices. See your doctor if severe digestive troubles persist.

Follow the Phase II diet while taking yeast control treatment for one to four months or more as recommended by your doctor. This diet works best with treatment when both are followed for six weeks or more; the diet may be followed for up to six months or more. See chapter 5 for information on choosing a doctor and regulating treatment. (Also read chapters 3 and 4 for information on various treatments.) This or any diet alone will not cure Candida.

PHASE II DIET GUIDELINES

Phase II Diet Fruit:

Eliminate almost all fruits during this Phase. If your doctor feels the Candida is not too bad and you can tolerate a few fruits, stick with the nonsweet fruits in Phase III and follow the guidelines for fruit in that section. Most individuals should eliminate all fruit, except for the following:

Enjoy:	*Amounts:*
Avocados	1 to 2 per week
White grapefruit	1 to 2 fresh whole per week, or 2 to 4 juiced (fresh) per week
Fresh lemon juice	1 to 2 servings per day, 3 to 5 days per week only
Fresh lime juice	1 to 2 servings per day, 3 to 5 days per week only
Cooked Berry Berry Sauce or Frozen Berry Sorbet (pages 462 and 461)	4 to 6 servings per month, if doctor permits

PHASE II DIET BREAKFASTS

Two to three full meals a day are required. If you are eating breakfast during this Phase, follow these guidelines:

1. Drink distilled, specially filtered, or spring water on rising.
2. If having citrus juice, herb tea, vegetable juice, or an acceptable fruit or vegetable beverage from chapter 12, have it 30 minutes or more before breakfast. Beverage is optional.
3. No breads, muffins, French toast, rolled oats or oatmeal, other rolled or flaked grains, and especially no dry cereals, refined bread products, or yeast. No flours, refined or whole grain. Seed-flour pancakes with amaranth or teff, from this book only, may be enjoyed as a treat two to four times per month, served plain, with butter or with Berry Berry Sauce. Cinnamon is optional; limit use to one to three times per week.
4. Enjoy cooked whole grain cereals and options in Breakfasts, chapter 14. Try cooked tofu, eggs, starchy vegetables, soups, or casseroles for breakfast.

Breakfast Guidelines:

3 to 5 mornings per week	¾ to 1½ cups cooked 100% whole grain cereal: millet, quinoa, brown rice, whole oats, Scotch oats, brown pot barley with butter and salt or sauce topping (nonsweet)
2 to 4 mornings per week	2 cups or more starchy vegetables: Cinnamon Baked Squash, orange yams, carrots, cauliflower,

	spaghetti squash, or vegetable soup, or Orange Yam Pie, or other main dish
0 to 2 mornings per week	1 to 2 eggs, cooked, or 4 ounces scrambled or sautéed tofu (see recipes)
0 to 1 morning per week	Amaranth or Teff Pancakes with butter or Berry Berry Sauce, cinnamon optional

PHASE II DIET SNACKS

a. Enjoy any of the snacks in chapter 13.

b. It is okay to enjoy one to four snacks per day, based on your individual body needs. If you eat three meals a day, limit snacks to one or two. If you eat two meals a day, two to four snacks are okay.

c. Treats in chapter 20 may be enjoyed one to four times per week, total for all snacks combined.

PHASE II DIET LUNCHES

1. Enjoy any of the soup or main dish recipes in this book, along with a salad and/or cooked vegetables. Each soup and main dish offers meal suggestions at the end of the recipe; use these to create complete meals. See chapter 9 for meal planning guidelines and food combining rules: Serve carbohydrates (whole grains and/or legumes) with vegetables or serve proteins (meat, eggs, and/or dairy) with vegetables at one meal. (No pork, ground meats, luncheon meats, shellfish, pasta, potatoes, flours. See Phase II Foods to Enjoy and Foods to Eliminate lists after the Supper guidelines.) All whole grains and beans must be eaten warm!

2. If raw foods are hard for you to digest, eat these at lunchtime rather than supper. If you cannot handle them at all, have fresh vegetable juice five to six days a week, one glass only per day, away from meals.

3. If you eat lunch away from home, see the take-out lunch ideas in chapter 8.

4. Learn to get along without your microwave. Most microwaving does not kill all bacteria in food. Use the stove, oven, or toaster oven. (See Phase I diet regarding microwaves.)

5. Drink beverages a half hour or more before or after meals, only those allowed in the Beneficial Beverages chapter. Do not drink beverages until over an hour after a heavy meal. During meals, you may drink 4 to

6 ounces of water or other liquids, if the meal is dry or experience shows it will not interfere with your digestion. Sip liquids a little at a time during meals.

PHASE II DIET SUPPERS

a. Follow the guidelines for lunch.
b. Depending on your body, try to eat supper four hours or more before bed-time. Some individuals need food in their stomachs to sleep; if so, do not eat too heavy a meal and finish one to two hours before bed, or have a fill-ing snack one hour or more before bedtime.

PHASE II FOOD LISTS

All foods on the Foods to Enjoy list may be enjoyed raw or cooked unless oth-erwise specified. Occasional foods and foods to eliminate are in following lists. Do not eat foods to which you are sensitive or allergic or that your doctor says to omit. The good news is that the list of foods to enjoy is the longest.

Phase II Foods to Enjoy:

Adzuki (aduki, azuki) beans, cooked only

Agar powder or flakes, cooked only

Alfalfa leaves (dried), cooked only

Alfalfa sprouts (cut off roots and brown hulls and discard), cooked only

Almonds (buy raw, then use in cooking)

Amaranth flour, cooked only

Arrowroot powder, cooked only, in small amounts

Artichoke hearts (packed in water), drained and cooked

Artichokes (globe), cooked only

Artichokes (Jerusalem)

Arugula, raw only

Asparagus, cooked only

Avocados

Bamboo shoots, cooked only

Barley (brown pot), cooked only

Basil, fresh in raw or cooked foods, dried in cooking only

Basmati rice (brown only), cooked only

Bean sprouts (mung bean sprouts), cooked only

Beans (dried), only those listed here

Beans (green, snap), cooked only

Beets

Beet greens, cooked only

Black beans (turtle beans), cooked only

Black olives, canned only, cooked only

Bouillon cubes (home-made, from this book), cooked only

Broccoli, cooked only

Brussels sprouts, cooked only

Buckwheat (contains no wheat), cooked only

Butter (dairy), raw, clari-fied, or cooked

Butters (almond, filbert, pecan, sesame, sunflower, and pumpkin only), cooked only

Cabbage, cooked or juiced only

Carrots

Cauliflower, cooked only

Cayenne pepper

Celery

Chard, cooked only

Chickpeas (garbanzos), cooked only

Chickpea flour (besan, chana, garbanzo), cooked only

Chives, fresh in raw or cooked foods, dried in cooking only

Cilantro, fresh in raw or cooked foods, dried in cooking only

Club soda, with carbonated water and sodium bicarbonate only, no other additives

Cranberry juice (unsweetened), see chapter 12

Cucumbers, raw only

Cumin (seeds or powder), cooked only

Daikon (white radish)

Dulse, cooked only

Eggs, well-cooked only

Exotic mixed greens (minus endive, escarole, and radicchio), raw only

Fava beans, cooked only

Fennel seeds or vegetable, cooked only

Filberts (hazelnuts), buy raw and cook

Fish (salmon, tuna, cod, sole, haddock, trout, and others, preferably ocean variety), cooked only

Flax oil, raw only

Flaxseeds (whole, cooked only; freshly ground, raw or cooked)

Garlic

Gomashio (sesame salt), homemade only; store in freezer

Grapefruit (white only)

Greens (kale, chard, mustard, bok choy, beet, and others), cooked only

Hazelnuts, buy raw and use in cooking

Herbs, fresh, in raw or cooked foods

Herbs, dried, cooked in foods

Herb teas (see Beverage chapter for those allowed)

Horseradish (dried, fresh, or prepared without sugar), cooked unless fresh grated

Jicama, with fresh lime juice only, raw only

Kale, cooked only

Kasha (toasted buckwheat), cooked only

Kelp (sea kelp), cooked only

Kidney beans, cooked only

Kohlrabi

Kudzu (kuzu), cooked only

Leeks, cooked only

Legumes, only those listed here

Lemon juice, fresh

Lentils (red, green, brown, gray, French), cooked only

Lettuce (leaf, red, bibb, and Boston only), raw only

Lime juice, fresh

Lotus root, cooked only

Millet, cooked only

Mung beans (dry or sprouted), cooked only

Nuts, only those listed here

Oats (groats, whole, steel-cut or Scotch), cooked only

(continues)

(continued)

Oil (sunflower, sesame, canola, flax, or pumpkin) natural, cold-pressed, or expeller-pressed only

Oil (olive), extra virgin

Onions (white, yellow, or red)

Paprika, cooked only

Parsley, fresh in raw or cooked foods, dried in cooking only

Parsnips, cooked only

Pattypan squash (scallop squash), cooked only

Peas (fresh, green peas), cooked or raw if tolerated

Pecans, buy raw and use in cooking

Peppers, bell (green), raw or cooked if tolerated

Peppers, bell (red, orange, yellow, purple)

Peppers (hot or chili), raw or cooked if tolerated

Pine nuts, buy raw and use in cooking

Pinto beans, cooked only

Pumpkin seeds, buy raw and home-cook

Quinoa, cooked only

Radishes (red), raw only

Radishes (white), raw or cooked

Red beans, cooked only

Rice (long or short brown, wild, wehani or sweet brown), cooked only

Romano beans, cooked only

Salsa, Homemade Salsa from this book only

Salmon, cooked only

Scallions (green onions)

Sea kelp, cooked only

Sea salt

Seaweed, cooked only

Sesame salt, see Gomashio

Sesame seeds, buy raw and use in cooking

Sesame tahini, cooked only

Shallots, cooked or raw if tolerated

Snow peas (edible pea pods), cooked only

Sorrel

Soybeans, well cooked if tolerated

Soy flour, cooked only

Soy milk, cooked only

Soy sauce, Mock Tamari Soy Sauce from this book, cooked only

Spaghetti squash, cooked only

Spinach

Sprouts (mung beans, alfalfa sprouts), cooked only

Squash (winter), cooked only

Squash (yellow summer)

Sunflower seeds, buy raw and use in cooking

Tahini (sesame), cooked only

Tamari, see soy sauce

Teff (flour or seeds), cooked only

Tofu, cooked only

Tomatoes

Tomato sauce, homemade or Mock Tomato Sauce, cooked only

Tuna, cooked only

Turnips, cooked only

Vegetable broth powder, homemade from this book only, cooked only

Vegetable juices, pure, fresh pressed or heated, canned or bottled (see chapter 13)

Water, spring, distilled or specially filtered

Water chestnuts, cooked only

Wild rice, cooked only

Yams (orange), cooked only

Yogurt, fresh, plain with acidophilus powder, garlic or lemon or lime juice only; plain can also be cooked without extras

Zucchini

Phase II Occasional Foods:

These foods can only be eaten a few times per week or month, if tolerated and your doctor permits. Use only in the form(s) stated. These foods are optional; do not use unless desired.

Apple juice or cider, 1 to 2 tablespoons, can be cooked into recipes, 20 minutes or more

Barley green powder

Beef (chops, steak, roast, or stewing chunks only), cooked only

Berries (raspberries, blueberries, blackberries, strawberries, currants), cooked only (unless doctor permits fresh)

Black or white pepper, use only if allergic to cayenne

Brazil nuts, buy raw and use in cooking; use only if almonds, filberts, and pecans are not tolerated

Canned foods, cooked only: tomato paste, tomatoes, water chestnuts, artichoke hearts in water, black olives, salmon, tuna, unsweetened beans, lotus root, bamboo shoots

Carob pods, whole, roasted

Chicken (free-range or organic is preferred), cooked only

Chili powder, cooked only

Cinnamon, raw or cooked

Curry powder, cooked only

Egg replacer (powdered), use in cooking only

Farmers' cheese, well cooked only (if doctor permits)

Feta cheese, well cooked only (if doctor permits)

Fruits (nonsweet from Phase I diet), if doctor permits: apples, nonsweet pears, Japanese pear apples, kiwi (tender-firm, not too soft or ripe), papayas, strawberries, blackberries, blueberries, raspberries, other berries, not watermelon

Jarred foods, cooked only: unsweetened pure prepared horseradish

Ginger, cooked only

Guar gum, mixed with other foods only

Honey or other natural sweeteners, minute amounts cooked into some recipes, 1 to 2 teaspoons per large recipe, cooked 20 minutes or more to balance flavors and kill yeast (See Honey in Controversial Foods)

Juice (apple, pear, peach, apricot), see apple juice; veggie juices

Lactic acid–fermented vegetables, if doctor permits

(continues)

(continued)

Lamb (chops, steak, roast, or stewing chunks only), cooked only

Lecithin

Lettuce, romaine only

Milk, small amounts in cooking only

Miso, if doctor permits

Mustard (dry only), cooked only

Popcorn, if digestion permits and not allergic, no microwave popcorn or popcorn with additives

Poultry (chicken, turkey, quail, Cornish hens, pheasant); avoid duck and goose

Quark cheese, well-cooked only (if doctor permits)

Ricotta cheese, well-cooked only (if doctor permits)

Sauerkraut (if doctor permits)

Sparkling bottled waters, do not use if constipated

Spices, cooked only, use sparingly

Spirulina powder

Stevia (honeyleaf), minute amounts in cooking only

Tamari soy sauce, cooked in foods 20 minutes or more

Tapioca flour, cooked only, small amounts

Tofu cheese, cooked only (if doctor permits)

Tomato juice, heated only

Turkey (free-range or organic preferred), cooked only

Veal (chops, steak, roast or stewing chunks only), cooked only

Watercress

Phase II Foods to Eliminate:

These foods either feed the yeast or aggravate digestion, allergies, or sensitivities. Do not eat any of these foods, in any form, unless your doctor permits.

Alcohol

Amazake

Apricots, fresh or cooked

Artichoke hearts, marinated only

Artificial flavors, colors or additives in anything

Aspartame in anything

Bacon or Canadian bacon

Baked beans, sweetened or marinated beans

Baked goods

Basmati white rice

Beans, white (dried or fresh), navy, lima, haricots, northern, pea beans

Beans, wax only

Beer

Breads made with refined or whole grains or yeast

Burgers from ground meat

Caffeine

Canned foods of any type unless permitted and cooked (see Occasional Foods), no canned soups, stews, chili, sauces, or main dishes

Cashews

Celeriac

Cereals, refined, dry, puffed, or ground whole grain (unless ground at home from whole grains and kept refrigerated or frozen until cooked)

Cheese, all cheeses (unless mentioned specifically in other sections and doctor permits), "raw" or cooked

Cherries

Chestnuts, tree

Chewable vitamin C

Chicken, breaded or fried

Chocolate

Cocoa

Coconut

Coffee

Colas

Corn

Corn chips or tortillas

Cornmeal

Cornstarch (use arrowroot instead)

Cottage cheese

Crackers, any kind

Cream

Cream cheese

Currants, dried

Dandelion leaves or coffee

Dates

Dried fruit, any kind

Eggplant

Endive

Escarole

Exotic fruits

Fast food

Fatty foods

Fermented foods

Fish, breaded or fried

Fish sticks

Fried foods

Frogs' legs

Fruit juice (any kind, jarred, bottled or fresh), except fresh lemon, lime, or white grapefruit or those allowed in cooking

Figs

Flour, refined or whole grain

Game meats (bear, deer, rabbit, except fowl/poultry)

Grain coffee substitutes

Granola

Grapefruit, pink only

Grapes

Greasy foods

Ham

Herb teas not in Beverage chapter

Hot dogs

Hydrolized vegetable protein

Jarred foods, any type unless permitted and cooked (see Occasional Foods)

Juices, fruit or vegetable (except vegetable juices in Beverage chapter or other juices allowed), heated

Junk food

Kefir

Lima beans, fresh or dried

Lettuce (iceberg or head only)

Luncheon meats

Macadamia nuts

Mangoes

Marinated foods

Meats, cold, processed, luncheon, ground or any with additives, organ meats, fatty meats, poor-quality meats

Melons (honeydew, cantaloupe, crenshaw, muskmelon, watermelon, and others)

Mixed drinks

MSG

Mushrooms

Mustard, prepared

Navy beans

Nectarines

Oatmeal

Octopus

Oily foods

Oils, solvent extracted, refined, regular olive

(continues)

(continued)

Okra

Olives, green

Oranges

Pastas, all

Peaches, fresh or cooked

Peanuts, peanut oil, or peanut products

Pickled foods (beets, onions, peppers, and others)

Pickles

Pimentos

Pineapple

Pistachio nuts

Pizza

Plums

Pops, soda pops

Pork, in any form

Potatoes

Potatoes, yellow sweet

Pumpkin

Radicchio

Raisins

Refined foods of any kind

Rhubarb

Rice, white, basmati white, Thai black or red

Rice cakes

Rolled grains of any type

Rolled oats

Rutabagas

Salad dressings, bottled or packaged

Salsa, except Homemade Salsa in this book

Sausage

Seasoning blends (may contain sugar and additives, mold chance high)

Shellfish: lobster, crab, shrimp, prawns, clams, scallops, oysters, mussels, squid, octopus

Soy nuts

Split peas, dried green or yellow

Squid

Sugar, including artificial

Sweetener, except minute amounts as directed in this book (see Honey in Controversial Foods)

Tabasco sauce

Tacos

Tangerines

Tempeh

Truffles

TV dinners or any store-bought frozen meal

TVP (texturized vegetable protein)

Ugli fruit

Vinegar, any kind, unless doctor permits

Walnuts

Watermelon

Wheat, in any form

White beans (dried or fresh), navy, lima, haricots, northern, pea beans

Wine

Yeast, baking or nutritional

PHASE III DIET: RECOVERY DIET AFTER PHASE II OR DURING CANDIDA TREATMENT DIET FOR MILD OR MODERATE CASES OF CANDIDA CONTROL OR MILD REOCCURRENCE

Two Weeks to Two Months or More

This diet is used as a recovery diet after treatment, for important reasons. After the stricter diet in Phase II with Candida yeast-killing treatment, the body and immune system are weakened and energy levels are low. Destroying yeast is fighting a battle in the body. After the battle, one has to clean up the battle-field. Until the body regains or builds strength, it must be protected with high-quality foods and reduced stress levels. If the body remains weak and you go back to old eating habits immediately, new yeast can easily gain a new foothold in your body!

When your energy is low, conditions are excellent for breeding a brand new crop of Candida yeast. Some people immediately jump back into an "any-thing goes diet" and return to old, bad eating habits; the results are disastrous. All benefits of treatment are quickly lost and you find yourself dealing with the same symptoms and problems six months or more down the road. Then the question is asked: "I did all that work and 'suffering' on the Candida diet, why didn't it work?" It did work, but you did not follow through and complete the process, nor did you take precautions to prevent Candida reoccurrence. One treatment process is not the total solution to Candida problems. (See Keys to Complete Candida Cure in the Introduction.)

A recovery diet is necessary to boost the body's immune system after Candida treatment. One needs to maintain a wholesome diet that is easy for the body to digest and also "loosen up a bit" and enjoy a few more comfort foods. All the recipes in this book, if desired and tolerated, can be used for the Phase III recovery diet. Special foods can be added as listed in the following section.

Use this Candida treatment diet, or healing diet, which is less strict than Phase II with yeast control treatment, for mild or moderate cases of Candida or for reoccurrence of Candida, if your doctor permits. This diet works best with treatment when followed for four weeks or more, and may be followed for up to six months or more. See chapter 5 for guidance on choosing a doctor and regulating treatment. See chapters 3 and 4 for more on various treatments. This or any diet alone will not cure Candida; proper treatment is also required.

PHASE III DIET GUIDELINES

Phase III Diet Fruit:

It is still a good idea to restrict fruit, but not as much as in Phase II. Most Phase I fruits can be enjoyed, with a few exceptions (see below).

Have a maximum of one serving of fruit daily, preferably in the morning. Eat raw fruit according to food combining rules (see chapter 9). Eat fruit by itself, or 15 to 30 minutes before other foods. Cooked fruits may be eaten with other foods. Avoid sweet fruits completely.

Enjoy:

Apples	Papayas	Blackberries
Avocados	Grapefruit, white	Blueberries
Nonsweet pears	Fresh lemon juice	Raspberries
Japanese pear apples	Fresh lime juice	Other berries
Kiwi (tender-firm, not too soft or ripe)	Strawberries	

Avoid:

Oranges	Peaches	Grapefruit, pink
Pineapple	Apricots	Cherries
Melons	Plums	Bananas
Watermelon	Grapes	Mangoes

Exotic fruits (starfruit, passion fruit, guavas, lychee nuts, persimmons, and others)

Dried fruits (raisins, currants, dates, figs, coconut, and others)

All other fruits not mentioned

Fruit Guidelines:

a. Avoid fruit that tastes too sweet.

b. Avoid fruit with mold on it.

c. Avoid under- and overripe fruits.

d. Raw fruits have live enzymes and are quickly digested when eaten alone. Eaten with other foods, raw fruits take too long to digest and stay too long in the digestive tract, where they become overprocessed and great food for Candida yeast. The live enzymes in cooked fruits have been killed, so they may be eaten with other foods and digested like other carbohydrate foods. (This is one reason people with Candida have an easier time digesting cooked fruits than they do raw fruits. Raw fruits can upset the stomach when eaten with other foods. Also, yeast prefer eating raw fruits.)

e. Do not eat raw fruits at night or after supper. The fruit sugar may keep you awake and fruits are not good for digestion at night. Eliminate chewable vitamin C, which is like eating raw, sweet fruit, throughout all Candida diet Phases.

Phase III Diet Breakfasts

Two to three full meals a day are required. If you eat breakfast during this phase of the Candida diet, follow these guidelines:

1. Dandelion or grain coffees can be enjoyed on the recovery diet and healing diet, but not on the mild or reoccurrence treatment diets, unless your doctor permits. Enjoy all the beverages in the Beneficial Beverages chapter.
2. Continue to enjoy whole grain cereal breakfasts. No dry cereals, refined cereals, sweetened cereals (hot or cold, including especially granola or muesli), oatmeal and rolled oats, any rolled or flaked whole grains, or puffed cereal. One hundred percent whole grain (wheat-free) pancakes, French toast, muffins, or breads may be eaten sparingly, provided they are yeast-free, made with Homemade Baking Powder, and sweetened only with cooked, puréed fruits from those allowed in the fruit list. They may be served with homemade applesauce (heated) or Berry Berry Sauce only. No jams or preserves. Butter or cinnamon (sparingly) may be used instead. No wheat whatsoever.
3. Acidophilus Yogurt can be enjoyed alone or in any of the yogurt recipes in this book (unless allergic), if doctor permits. Tart/subacid fruits in allowed list may be occasionally eaten raw, chopped, and mixed with Acidophilus Yogurt as a light breakfast or snack two to four times per week.
4. Enjoy two to four eggs per week if desired. Exclude soft-boiled and sunny-side up (higher bacteria count), but enjoy all others. Make sure eggs are fully cooked. Scrambled tofu is another option. Milk may be used occasionally in cooking, but not drunk by the glass. Feta, farmer's, ricotta, and quark cheeses may be used, if well cooked, in omelets or other recipes (unless doctor objects), one to four times per month.

Breakfast Guidelines

0 to 2 mornings per week	1 to 2 eggs, cooked, or 4 ounces scrambled or sautéed tofu (see recipes)
0 to 2 mornings per week	100% whole grain: pancakes, French toast, muffins, breads, or cereals (unsweetened or ½ teaspoon sweetener cooked in each serving, yeast- and wheat-free), or seed pancakes
3 to 5 mornings per week	¾ to 1½ cups cooked 100% whole grain cereal: millet, quinoa, brown rice, whole oats,

(continues)

	Scotch oats, brown pot barley with butter and salt or sauce topping (nonsweet)
0 to 3 mornings per week	2 or more cups starchy vegetables: Cinnamon-Baked Squash, orange yams, carrots, cauliflower, spaghetti squash, or vegetable soup, or Orange Yam Pie, or other main dish

Phase III Diet Snacks:

a. Enjoy any of the snacks in chapter 13.

b. It is okay to enjoy one to four snacks per day, based on your individual body needs. If you eat three meals a day, limit snacks to one or two. If you eat two meals a day, two to four snacks are okay.

c. Snacks in chapter 20 may be enjoyed many times a week.

PHASE III DIET LUNCHES

1. Enjoy any of the soup or main dish recipes in this book, along with a salad and/or cooked vegetables. Each soup and main dish recipe offers meal suggestions at the end of each recipe; use these to create complete meals. See meal planning guidelines and food combining rules in chapter 9. Serve carbohydrates (whole grains and/or legumes) with vegetables, or serve proteins (meat, eggs, and/or dairy) with vegetables at one meal.

2. One hundred percent whole grain, wheat-free, yeast-free: breads, rye and rice crackers, and rice cakes may be enjoyed occasionally in Phase III. Whole grain corn tortillas and whole meal corn chips may be had one to four times per month but eaten sparingly, as they are hard to digest. I do not personally recommend them; many doctors allow them on these diets. Some do not.

3. If you eat lunch away from home, see the brown bag and office lunch ideas in chapter 8.

4. Do not use a microwave oven for this phase. Most microwaving does not kill all bacteria in food. Use a stove, oven, or toaster oven. (See Phase I diet regarding microwaves.)

5. Drink beverages a half hour or more before or after meals. See Beverage chapter. Do not drink beverages until over an hour after a heavy meal. During meals, you may drink 4 to 6 ounces of water or other liquids, if the meal is dry or experience shows it will not interfere with digestion. Sip a little liquid at a time during meals. (Dandelion or grain coffees are okay for

recovery diets and some healing diets, but not if allergic, and not for mild and reoccurrence treatment diets.)

PHASE III DIET SUPPERS

a. See Phase III Diet Lunches.
b. Depending on your body requirements, try to eat supper four hours or more before bedtime. Some individuals need food in their stomachs to sleep; if so, do not eat a heavy meal, and finish one to two hours before bed, or have a filling snack one hour before bedtime.

EXTREMELY MILD CASES OF CANDIDA YEAST

Add the following information to Phase III if the Candida problem is very minor, you have no food allergies or food sensitivities, and your digestion is not impaired. Sometimes relatively healthy individuals have mild problems with Candida yeast and require only moderate diet changes while taking Candida treatment. This may be due to a recent illness, overwork, recent pregnancy, or extra stress.

1. Candida drug treatments often can eliminate yeast overgrowth and restore body balance in two to four weeks. (If pregnant or nursing, natural remedies are better than drugs and must be monitored by a physician. It is best not to do any Candida treatment while pregnant or nursing and definitely no other body cleansing whatsoever. Vitamin C, multivitamins, acidophilus, and limited other supplements can be had during these times. A doctor must be consulted.)
2. Individuals with mild cases usually have high stomach acid and respond harshly to acid fruits and acidophilus powders. Take acidophilus about 15 to 30 minutes after a meal, unlike the average person who should take it two hours before a meal or one to two hours after.
3. Those with mild cases can be less strict with diet and enjoy whole grain wheat products (yeast-free) and corn products. Well-cooked hard cheeses are sometimes allowed, once or twice per week. Cooked recipes can include milk, green olives, marinated artichokes, tamari soy sauce, and store-bought bouillon cubes (cooked at least 20 minutes), dandelion and grain substitute coffees, and other less restrictive diet adjustments. Ask your doctor for additional diet information for your special needs.

Phase III Food Lists:

Use all the Foods to Enjoy and Occasional Foods in Phase II food lists and add:

Phase III Occasional Foods

Apples

Berries, all types

Breads (whole grain rye, rice, oat, corn, and other), wheat-free and yeast-free, with natural sweetening 2 tablespoons maximum per loaf

Corn chips (whole grain, unseasoned except for salt), if tolerated and doctor permits

Crackers (whole grain rye, rice, oat, corn, and other), wheat-free and yeast-free

Kiwi (tender-firm, not too soft or ripe)

Muffins (whole grain barley, buckwheat, oat, quinoa, rice, and others), wheat-free and yeast-free with baking powder and natural sweetening ½ teaspoon maximum per small one

Papayas

Pancakes (whole grain barley, buckwheat, oat, quinoa, rice, and other), wheat-free and yeast-free (if cooked with natural sweetening 1 teaspoon maximum per 5 or 6 large), can be topped with Berry Berry Sauce (or Applesauce if doctor permits)

Pears, nonsweet varieties

Pear apples, Japanese

Rice cakes (one to three servings weekly, if doctor permits)

Tortillas, whole grain corn, if tolerated and doctor permits

Enjoy occasional foods from Phase II more frequently

All the "Treats That Are Not Too Sweet" in Chapter 20

For recovery diets and healing diets only add:

Dandelion coffees, unsweetened

Grain substitute coffees, unsweetened

PHASE IV DIET: POST-CANDIDA TREATMENT DIET FOR AFTER-RECOVERY DIET (THE SAFE WORLDLY DIET)

Lifetime Diet

It is imperative to let the body return to "normal" or renewed energy levels before attempting to eat "foods that other people eat." Once a person has had a major problem and healing of Candida, this makes them predisposed to the condition and more likely to have future problems with Candida yeast overgrowth.

Special "desensitization" remedies, available from some naturopathic physicians and holistic M.D.s, can help certain people (this works for some individuals and not for others) avoid reoccurrence of Candida, as many people tend to have reoccurrence problems as soon as six months after treatment; sometimes one, two, or several years later. Candida can be picked up on a day-to-day basis; it is essential not to let it gain the upper hand in your body again, unless you want to suffer the consequences.

Food and vitamin supplements can greatly reduce your chances of recurrent yeast overgrowth (discussed in chapter 22). Special foods and special ways to eat them can greatly reduce the chance of return bouts of Candida and definitely diminish frequency. Follow this Phase IV diet plan as much as possible as a "safe worldly diet" for continual protection from Candida reoccurrence.

PHASE IV DIET GUIDELINES

Phase IV Diet Fruit:

a. It is best to enjoy mainly nonsweet (subacid) fruits as recommended in Phase I and III; sweet tropical and exotic fruits may be enjoyed occasionally.
b. Eat sweet fruits with Acidophilus Yogurt (food combining exception) or cut and toss them in fresh white grapefruit, lemon, or lime juice just before eating.
c. Eat sweet fruits only in summer or during warm weather. It is unnatural for the body to eat sweet tropical fruits in winter! Your body cannot process them as efficiently; yeast can "take advantage" of winter sweets and multiply more rapidly in winter than in warm weather.

d. Avoid fruit salads. It is better to eat one or two subacid or sweet fruits whole; you tend to eat less this way and they are easier to digest; also, bacteria increases on fruits that are cut and not eaten immediately.

e. Use food combining rules with fruits; only eat fruit by itself, before other foods, or as snacks between meals. Do not eat raw fruit at night. Cooked fruits may be eaten with meals or as a dessert, even after dinner.

f. Dried fruits should be eaten like other fresh fruits. Eat "raw" dried fruit like raw fruits and do not eat at night. Eat cooked, dried fruits like other cooked fruits. Do not eat too many dried fruits, especially in winter. Do not eat cooked dried fruits at night unless you brush your teeth afterward.

PHASE IV DIET SWEETS

1. Use natural sweeteners, rather than refined and artificial sweeteners, at least most of the time. After a Candida treatment program, you will enjoy less-sweet desserts more than fancy ones, and desire less as long as you continue to eat a well-balanced, wholesome diet! Avoid aspartame and sugar and use honey, maple syrup, molasses, stevia, and other natural sweeteners instead.

2. Eat desserts one hour or more after a full meal of wholesome foods. Do not eat desserts on an empty stomach! You actually absorb more calories when desserts are eaten first or alone. If you are trying to lose weight and keep yeast growth to a minimum, avoid desserts on an empty stomach.

3. Keep sweets, sweet fruits, and dessert consumption down. If you maintain a good diet, you should not desire lots of sweets unless your body is off-balance, sick, or you are over-tired or overstressed. When I crave sweets too strongly, I avoid them for three days; I eat all wholesome foods, rest, and reduce stress levels. After three days, I no longer crave sweets!

PHASE IV DIET BREAKFASTS

1. As much as possible, continue eating good breakfasts from this book. At least three to five times per week, every other day, or more often, eat the breakfasts recommended in Phases II and III.

2. Continue to use 100 percent whole grain cereals, breads, muffins, and pancakes, rather than refined products. Whole wheat can now be included (if not allergic) and some yeasted breads. (See Lunches, #4 following.) If you indulge in refined pastries and breads occasionally, do not eat them on an

empty stomach! If having eggs and pastry, eat eggs first. Toasted bread is less likely than plain bread to contain bacteria or mold that feeds Candida yeast.

3. Avoid bacon, Canadian bacon, pork in all forms, and sausages as much as possible; exclude them entirely from your diet, if you are willing. If you do eat them, limit their use to once or twice per week.

4. Milk may be drunk occasionally, but yogurt is more digestible and beneficial. If returning to coffee or caffeinated teas, use natural sweeteners and limit caffeinated beverages to two cups maximum per day. Drink tested spring water primarily now, if possible, and mainly enjoy the beverages in this book.

Phase IV Diet Lunches and Snacks

1. Continue mainly with wholesome lunches from this book. Avoid luncheon meats, cold meats, processed meats, deli meats, burgers, and hot dogs. Instead choose cooked fish, poultry, or better cuts of meat when having meat lunches. Try to eat shellfish once a week or less, twice a week maximum. A minimum of five servings of meat and/or legumes is required weekly for a well-balanced diet.

2. Hard cheeses such as mozzarella, brick, cheddar, Swiss, and others are easier to digest when eaten warm and fully cooked into other foods. A "raw" slice of cheese contains some mold and bacteria and is more of a yeast "promoter" than some meats and sweets.

3. Avoid fried foods, fast foods, and junk foods whenever possible. Choose wholesome versions of snack foods and continue to eat the ones in this book. Popcorn and rice cakes are better than potato chips. Enjoy the snack, lunch, and dessert ideas in my other books rather than refined or empty-calorie junk foods.

4. If possible, limit bread and cracker products to one to three servings per day. Include at least one serving of warm, cooked whole grains daily. Continue to avoid wheat products; if eating them, do so only every other day, or four to six days per week. Choose 100 percent whole grain breads most of the time, wheat- and yeast-free whenever possible. Toasted bread is less likely than plain bread to contain bacteria or mold that feeds Candida yeast.

5. If you eat mushrooms, eat them cooked rather than raw; bacteria and chance of Candida growth will be lessened considerably. Choose shiitake

mushrooms above other types whenever possible; they are more nutritious, higher in oxygen-rich germanium, and less likely to promote renewed Candida growth.

6. Limit mealtime beverages; follow breakfast beverage guidelines.
7. Eat lots of vegetables! Raw vegetables are more digestible earlier in the day; include them with lunches often.
8. Follow the food combining and meal and menu planning guidelines in chapter 9 for continued good health. When possible, continue with this book's recipes and diet principles.
9. Keep microwave cooking to a minimum; never use a microwave for first-time meat cooking. Never reheat leftovers over one to two days old in a microwave; use a stove or oven instead. Do not heat herbal tea water (and definitely never heat baby foods and formulas!) in a microwave. (See Phase I diet regarding microwaves.)

PHASE IV DIET SUPPERS

1. See Phase IV Diet Lunches.
2. Keep eating lots of vegetables! Three to six servings a day help keep the body healthy and prevent constipation. If you have trouble digesting vegetables, eat the easier-to-digest vegetables outlined in this book.
3. Depending on your body requirements, eat supper four hours or more before bedtime. Some individuals need food in their stomachs to sleep; if so, do not eat a heavy meal and finish one to two hours before bed, or have a filling snack one hour before bedtime.

IMPORTANT DIET TIPS FOR ALL PHASES

1. Whenever sick, lacking energy, or overstressed, return to a Phase II or III diet. This will help you through tough times and help you handle them with increased energy, stamina, and better mental, emotional, and physical strength and clarity.
2. If seriously ill with heart problems, cancer, CFS, AIDS, or other disease(s), the Phase II diet (with your doctor's modifications) is excellent for speedy healing and recovery, or for lessening a disease's advance and deterioration. (See chapter 23 for healing diet guidelines for diseases.)

3. Use this book's Phase II or III diets for many types of body cleansing programs, as these diets eliminate agitating food and focus on foods that support the body and immune system while cleansing and healing. (See chapter 23.)
4. Choose organic or natural foods when available, good quality, and reasonably priced. Avoid foods with artificial sweeteners, artificial colors or flavors, chemicals, preservatives, hormones, or other unnatural additives.

DIET QUESTIONS TO ASK YOUR DOCTOR

You may wish to photocopy this page and the next page for your doctor.

1. Should you use the Phase II or Phase III diet with Candida treatment? The main differences are that Phase III allows some tart/subacid fruits (apples, pears, grapefruit, lemon, lime, berries, and others) but no sweet fruits (bananas, mangoes, melons, grapes, and others). Phase II only allows grapefruit, lemon, lime, and cooked, plain berries. Phase II does not allow whole grain flours or products. Phase III allows some 100 percent whole grain (wheat- and yeast-free) breads, crackers, muffins, and pancakes.
2. Can you have plain, natural Acidophilus Yogurt? (Plain yogurt with a little acidophilus added to hinder bacteria)
3. Can you have occasional milk, feta, farmer's, ricotta, or quark cheese if cooked into other foods, one to four times per month or more?
4. Can you have dandelion coffee and grain substitute coffees during treatment? (These coffee substitutes may contain refined grains.)
5. Can you have soy products? This includes well-cooked tofu, tamari soy sauce simmered 20 minutes or more with other foods to kill bacteria, soybean flour, soy milk (in recipes only, not to drink), or soybeans, well cooked and mashed in burgers and casseroles.
6. Can you have well-cooked eggs? How many per week?
7. These diets are basically wheat-free and grain flour-free. Does your doctor feel that you are healthy enough to tolerate occasional 100 percent whole grain wheat products (yeast-free) like breads, muffins, pancakes, or cooked whole grain wheat breakfast cereals? Can you have whole grain flour products minus wheat and yeast?
8. Can you have whole grain corn chips (unseasoned except for salt), whole meal tortillas, popcorn, corn on the cob, or whole grain cornbread, which are very hard to digest? If so, how much, how often?

9. Are there any foods you are allergic or sensitive to that should be eliminated or limited in their use by you? Ask your doctor whether you require food allergy testing.
10. What herbal teas, digestive aids, and laxatives or laxative teas are best for you to take during Candida treatment? How should you take them?
11. Can you have citrus (lemon, lime, and grapefruit)?
12. Are there any drugs you are taking that will be affected by any foods? What foods, if any, must be totally avoided?
13. Are there any herb or natural remedies you should avoid because of drugs you are taking or special health concerns you have?
14. Can the Candida treatment your doctor prescribes for you be altered, reduced, or changed if your side effects seem too severe?

Chapter 11

SHOPPING, SHORTCUTS, SUBSTITUTIONS, AND TIPS

Most of the items you require are available in local stores unless you live in a small town, in which case you will either have to go into a larger city every two to six weeks or get special foods by mail order. Find your nearest fully stocked, natural food store, which includes natural and organic vegetables, fruits, and other foods. A health food store may sell foods but often only vitamins and supplements. Just about all the special foods you cannot find in a supermarket may be found in a natural food store. The bigger they are, usually the better they are, although there are exceptions. Some small towns have small stores that are well stocked.

You may find the foods you need in natural food stores; health food stores; specialty food stores; supermarkets; produce stores; farmers' markets; country roadside stands; Greek, Italian, and East Indian shops; and Chinese or other Asian markets. Quality foods as well as poor quality foods may be found in any of these stores. Many supermarkets today have health food sections; some health food stores sell junk foods. Examine fresh foods and carefully read labels on all packaged foods. For more on how to select vegetables, see the end of this chapter and chapter 15.

Choose foods that are natural and organic, of good quality, and reasonably priced. Avoid foods with sugar (natural or artificial); preservatives; artificial colors, flavors, or other additives; chemicals; hormones; dyes; emulsifiers;

251

stabilizers; cornstarch; MSG; hydrogenated oils; hydrolyzed plant, vegetable, or soy protein; potato starch; and oils that include corn, peanut, palm, or coconut. If you are unsure what an ingredient is, consult Ruth Winter's book *A Consumer's Dictionary of Food Additives* for a great reference that tells which items are safe. See the Book List for more books that offer shopping guidelines.

Most foods used on Candida diets are pure, simple, bulk foods; very few are packaged. The canned or bottled foods allowed must be cooked just before eating (to kill bacteria and Candida). See the Foods to Enjoy list in the Phase II (and Phase III) diet plans in chapter 10. Also, refer to the Glossary of Special Foods at the end of this book for information on what to look for in each food you purchase.

WHERE TO BUY FOODS AND INGREDIENTS

Natural Food Stores

Acidophilus powder (or capsules)

Alfalfa leaf herbal tea

Amaranth flour

Arrowroot powder

Barley green powder

Breads, whole grain rye or gluten-free and unyeasted

Butter, salted or unsalted, natural or organic

Carob pods, whole/roasted (sometimes)

Chickpea/garbanzo beans or flour

Citrus seed extract (Citricidal)

Corn chips, natural or organic, fried or baked

Corn tortillas, whole corn natural or organic

Corn-free unbuffered vitamin C crystals

Crackers, whole grain, wheat & yeast-free

Crackers, yeast-free whole grain rye

Digestive aids

Dulse, seaweed or powder

Eggs, free-range and/or organic

Egg replacers

Fish, natural/ocean, lake or stream (wild) (sometimes)

Fruits, natural or organic

Goat's milk feta cheese (get one that is mild flavored) (goat is better than cow's milk feta)

Guar gum

Grains, whole natural or organic

Greens, organic salad

Greens, exotic or wild organic

Herbal teas, organic

Herbs, fresh garden (sometimes)

Herbs and spices, natural or organic

Kelp powder (ground seaweed)

Kudzu (or kuzu) powder

Legumes, canned without sugar, natural or organic

Legumes, dried natural or organic

Milk substitutes

Nut butters (almond, filbert, sesame)

Nuts and seeds, raw natural and organic

Oils, natural cold-pressed or expeller-pressed and organic

Olive oil, extra virgin

Olives, natural or organic (black)

Popcorn, organic or natural

Poultry, natural/free-range or organic (sometimes)

Quark cheese

Raspberry leaf herbal tea, organic is best

Rice cakes

Ricotta cheese

Sea kelp, powder (ground seaweed)

Seaweeds, dried

Sesame butter

Sesame tahini

Soybeans

Soy flour (low or full fat)

Soy milk (liquid, choose unsweetened)

Soy milk powder

Spirulina powder

Sprouts

Tamari soy sauce (natural and wheat-free soy sauces)

Tapioca flour

Teas, herbal organic

Teff flour

Tofu, soft (silken) or regular/firm

Tomato paste

Vegetable juices, natural or organic

Vegetable powder

Vegetables, dried and fresh, natural or organic

Vitamin supplements, natural or organic, sometimes vegan

Yogurt, natural or organic, unsweetened, no fruit

SUPERMARKETS

Artichoke hearts, canned, packed in water

Avocados

Baking soda

Bamboo shoots, canned

Black olives, canned

Butter, salted or unsalted

Crackers, rye, yeast-free

Cream of tartar

Farmer's cheese

Feta cheese, goat or cow's

Fish, fresh wild or farmed or canned

Greens, salad (sometimes organic)

Herbal teas, natural or organic

Herbs and spices, natural (sometimes)

Legumes, canned without sugar (sometimes)

Legumes, natural dried (not usually organic)

Lotus root, canned

Milk substitutes, natural (sometimes)

Nut butters, natural or organic (sometimes)

Oils, natural cold-pressed or expeller-pressed (sometimes)

Olive oil, natural and extra virgin

Popcorn, natural

Salmon, canned and fresh wild and/or farmed

Sesame tahini, natural or organic (sometimes)

Soy milk, unsweetened (sometimes)

Tuna, canned and sometimes fresh

(continues)

(continued)

Quark cheese

Ricotta cheese

Salad greens, exotic or organic (sometimes)

Tamari soy sauce (sometimes)

Tofu, soft (silken) or regular firm

Tomato paste, canned with salt

Tomatoes, canned with salt

Vegetables, fresh, sometimes organic

Vegetable juices, natural

Water chestnuts, canned

SPECIALTY FOOD MARKETS AND ETHNIC STORES

Artichoke hearts, canned, packed in water

Bamboo shoots, canned

Black olives, canned, natural

Carob pods, whole

Cheeses, soft natural (sometimes)

Chickpea/ chana/ besan flours

Exotic foods

Fruits, fresh (sometimes organic)

Legumes, canned without sugar (sometimes)

Legumes, dried natural

Legumes, exotic

Lotus root, canned

Milk substitutes (sometimes)

Nut butters (sometimes)

Nuts, raw natural (sometimes organic)

Organic packaged foods (sometimes)

Seaweeds, dried natural (sometimes)

Sprouts, fresh

Tamari soy sauce (sometimes)

Tofu, soft (silken) or regular firm (sometimes)

Vegetables, fresh (sometimes organic)

Water chestnuts, canned

Yogurt, natural (sometimes organic)

PHARMACIES

Acidophilus powder and capsules (sometimes)

Baking powders, wheat-free

Calcium carbonate

Calcium phosphate

Corn-free unbuffered vitamin C crystals

Digestive aids (sometimes natural)

Potassium bicarbonate

Tartaric acid

Vitamin supplements, natural (sometimes organic)

BRAND NAME BUYING GUIDE

This is a partial listing. There are other good brand names. The best companies are not necessarily listed first.

Amaranth flour Nu-World Amaranth, Inc., Arrowhead Mills, Bob's Red Mill, Now Foods

Beans (canned) Eden, Westbrae, American Prairie, Progresso, Unico, Contessa, Primo, Shari Ann's, Clic, Cortina, Hain

Black olives (canned, pitted olives only) Lindsay, Townhouse, Cortina, American Prairie, Unico, Primo, Club House, Oliver, Safeway

Cranberry juice (unsweetened) Knudsen's, Sun Dew, Triple Jim's

Egg replacer Ener-G Foods, Jolly Joan

Legumes Arrowhead Mills, Bob's Red Mill, Eden, Erewhon, Lundberg's, Westbrae, Canadian Soya Industries, Shiloh Farms

Nut butters Nuts to You, Westbrae, Nature's Path, Country Fresh, Maranatha

Oils (natural and/or organic) Spectrum, Eden, Flora, Arrowhead Mills, Omega

Olive oils, extra virgin Omega, Arrowhead Mills, Spectrum, Eden, Flora (organic, not virgin), Bragg, Green House, Petrelli, Bertolli, Romanico, Colavita, San Remo, Pax Jani, Mastro, Borges, Bioitalia, Mastrodonato

Quinoa Artesian Acres, Ancient Harvest, Quinoa Corporation

Soy milk (original flavor—for cooking) So Nice (unsweetened), Provamel Natural (unsweetened), Pacific Select, Westbrae, Edensoy, Soy Dream

Specialty milk substitutes Rice Dream original, Pacific Naturally Oat Original

Tamari soy sauce (wheat-free) San-j, Eden, Amano

Teff flour Arrowhead Mills, Bob's Red Mill

Vegetable juice (Natural) Knudsen's Very Veggie, Muir Glen Organic, V-8

Whole grains Arrowhead Mills, Bob's Red Mill, Eden, Erewhon, Lundberg's, Westbrae, Canadian Soya Industries, Shiloh Farms

Yogurt (plain, natural) Olympic, Dannon, Columbo, Naja, Maya, Brown Cow, Nancy's, Mountain High, Stonyfield, Horizon, Jerseyland, Jersey Farm, Saugeen Country, Continental (Lucerne)

Yogurts, specialty (Canadian) Happy Days Goat Milk Dairy, Mountain Meadow Sheep Milk Yogurt (there are other local brands)

Yogurts, specialty (American) Redwood Hills Farm Goat Yogurt, Mystic Lake Goat Yogurt (there are other local brands)

MAIL-ORDER NATURAL FOODS

Walnut Acres
Penn's Creek, PA 17862
Call 800-433-3998, USA and Canada deliveries, for complete line of organic and natural foods and many allergy foods as well.
Internet access: www.walnutacres.com

Allergy Products Directory (send SASE)
P.O. Box 640, Menlo Park, CA 94026
Send for a listing of over 1,000 specialty food sources.

Also search under Allergies on the Internet.

ORGANIC FOODS BUYING GUIDELINES

1. Organic foods are foods grown without chemicals and pesticides, in areas where there are no concentrations of air, water, or soil pollution. No additives or preservatives are added at any time in processing and packaging. Each state and province has different rules for what conditions are necessary for a food to be labeled organic.

   Some require three years and some as many as seven years of ideal growing conditions. Check with your local Department of Agriculture for your area's requirements. Foods grown in soils and areas working toward being organic are sometimes labeled "transitional organic foods."

2. Because organic foods are grown (or raised) without growth hormones, additives, and pesticides, they often look different than other store-bought foods. Look for these differences: darker colors, smaller sizes, thicker skins, more blemishes, and stronger scent or aroma. Organic foods are naturally ripened and processed. They generally have more natural flavor and more nutrients. They are less likely to agitate and promote Candida yeast growth. Organic meats may be a little tougher and less fatty with more muscle. Organic or free-range poultry is often more flavorful.

3. Buy quality brand name organic products whenever possible. See Brand Name Buying Guide earlier in this chapter. Check with your health specialist and natural food stores for the best products.

4. When buying produce, always buy the freshest. Avoid mold, brown or rust spots, wrinkled skins, bruised or cut surfaces, over- or underripe foods, dis-

colored or misshapen produce or legumes, unhulled grains mixed with whole grains, or other signs of poor quality foods. A product is not necessarily good just because it is labeled organic! Rotten food of any kind is inedible. Do not buy damaged, spoiled, or questionable organic foods. When possible, always try to buy organic first when buying carrots, beets, and leafy greens for salads, juicing, or cooking. Even if other veggies are not organic, these are the most important ones to buy organic

MONEY-SAVING IDEAS

1. Alternate recipes with expensive ingredients with less fancy dishes to keep costs down. Most legumes, whole grains, and vegetables are low-priced. High-priced items include asparagus, artichoke hearts, wild rice, nuts and some seeds, nut butters, some organic foods, and meats and special soft cheeses.
2. Cook only as much as you can eat or store. Large batches are great money savers if you eat or freeze them before they spoil. Most grain and bean dishes keep 7 to 8 days refrigerated and about 3 months frozen.
3. Shop comparatively. Health food store prices especially may differ from store to store, as much as $1 on the same items! Stock up on storable items that are low-priced or on sale.
4. Buy foods in "bulk" or large quantities when possible. The prices are usually much cheaper. Seek out stores with bargains and do not be afraid to ask at specialty markets and health food stores for a discount on multiple items, case lots, or large quantities. Many stores offer at least 10 percent off on cases or a dozen identical items.
5. Use your own organic garden vegetables in summer and fall if possible. The garden work and fresh air will be good for you. Gardens take time but can save money.

SHORTCUTS

It is not easy learning to cook everything from scratch using totally new foods, recipes, and techniques. It is difficult for some people to cook for themselves at all, let alone when ideas are brand new; it requires study and assimilation before they can be effectively utilized. This is the hard part. Shortcuts and aids reduce learning time and speed up the time it takes to increase knowledge and apply it. This book is set up in sections with special points outlined and numbered for ease of reading and comprehension.

Read each recipe completely before buying ingredients or preparing it. Check the glossary and buying guide for extra information when required. The Substitution Chart later in this chapter can help those with food allergies or food sensitivities to substitute ingredients in recipes; most recipes offer ample alternatives.

All the main dish, soup, snack, sauce, and gravy recipes tell you how to store and reheat the foods and whether they can be frozen or not. All vegetable dishes, raw or cooked, are best if prepared fresh; occasional frozen vegetables or fruits may be used in some recipes—for example, frozen peas in main dishes and soups, or frozen berries for special treat recipes. Canned foods should be avoided (except as noted in food lists) and must be cooked before using.

Organic foods are the first choice. See Organic Foods Buying Guidelines. The pesticides, sprays, and additives in some foods aggravate Candida and can make the body predisposed to the condition.

SAVING TIME, ENERGY, AND MONEY

Certain foods are best prepared fresh. Other foods can be prepared in big batches or frozen: whole grains, legumes, tofu, some sauces, and meat dishes.

Whole grains Best if not frozen, but whole grains can be prepared in large batches and stored in the refrigerator for up to seven or eight days. Leftovers can be steamed with vegetables, added to stir-frys about halfway through cooking, added to soups, heated in a saucepan with a little water, and covered in a tasty sauce, baked into casseroles or mock meatballs, or grilled in vegetarian burgers.

Legumes (beans, peas, and lentils) May be prepared in large batches and kept up to seven or eight days refrigerated. They can be added to soups and stews, heated in a saucepan with a little water and covered in a tasty sauce, baked into casseroles or mock meatballs, or grilled in vegetarian burgers. Legumes freeze wonderfully, up to three months. Bean recipes for soups, main dishes, snacks, sauces, and gravies keep their shape, texture, and moisture when frozen and retain most of the important nutrients. Prepare double, triple, and quadruple recipes and freeze half or more in meal-size plastic containers or freezing jars if available. (See Freezing Tips, following.) Legumes can be frozen, cooked, and then frozen again.

Tofu Made from soybeans, tofu is considered a legume. Tofu may keep for up to 14 days or more refrigerated and freezes well, too (although freezing changes the texture). Use the same as Legumes. See Tofu in the glossary for more information, storage, and preparation tips.

Meats May only keep in the refrigerator for one to three days, raw or defrosted, depending on the meat. Once cooked, meats may keep two to four days refrigerated. Meats can be frozen raw for many months if wrapped properly (freezer wrap, freezer bag, or double, regular plastic bags, securely closed) to avoid freezer burn and bacteria growth. Once cooked, they can be frozen again for up to one month. However, it is better not to freeze cooked meat too often or too long as nutrients, moisture, and flavor are lost. Refreeze meat stews and gravies and avoid freezing most other precooked meats, in general.

Big Batches

It takes far less time and energy to make four batches at once than to make one batch four times! Why not prepare several meals at once? In the long run it saves money. Cooking appliances are used for shorter time periods and there is less chance of wasted leftover preparation foods with larger batches.

It is wise, however, to make only one batch of a new recipe. If you are unfamiliar with a recipe and have a failure or do not like the taste, the recipe can be changed or adapted before large amounts of it are prepared and wasted.

1. Prepare individual, small jars with the herbs and seasonings required for commonly prepared recipes so you can grab a jar in a hurry and pour the contents into a recipe rather than having to measure everything bit by bit, opening and closing various jars and containers as you go. Prepare herb and seasoning amounts for single, double, or triple batches.
2. Sort whole grains and legumes to discard distorted ones or foreign objects while sitting in front of the TV or relaxing, or when you need busy finger work, so that when you go to cook, sorting will not waste time.
3. Plan ahead. Buy ingredients for several large batch recipes at one time. If possible, buy ingredients that can be used in more than one recipe. Keep a stock of commonly used foods so that you always have a variety on hand.

4. Organize foods in the refrigerator and cupboard shelves so they are easy to find. Put certain vegetables together and arrange packaged foods in sections in the refrigerator. Keep cupboard condiments together and have separate sections for herb teas, herbs and spices, whole grains, legumes, and so on.

Tips on Making Big Batches

The best times for preparing double or triple recipes are after dinner on week nights, on weekends, or, if time permits, make a big batch for dinner and refrigerate and/or freeze leftovers.

1. Try making more than one big batch at a time. Prepare two to four different dishes. Sometimes cooking for several hours once or twice a week is better than having to cook for each meal. One can easily add a raw salad or cooked vegetables to premade main dishes.
2. Since salt or sea salt spreads further in larger batches that are cooked, do not double salt amounts when doubling a recipe! For double recipes use 1½ times the salt. For triple recipes use 2 times the salt. For quadruple recipes use 2½ (or slightly more) times the salt called for in one recipe.

   Cayenne and sea kelp spread further in big batches, and as these are usually measured in dashes, reduce amounts as desired. Other herbs and seasonings can generally be doubled, tripled, and quadrupled exactly by multiplying one batch amount by the number of batches to be prepared.
3. Keep individual servings of main dishes, sauces, appetizers, and snacks in the refrigerator and freezer. Keep these on hand so that you are less likely to cheat on your diet!
4. Store big batches of refrigerated foods in glass jars rather than plastic to avoid bacteria growth and toxins that can seep into foods from plastics. If plastic must be used, never put hot foods in plastic containers! Cool foods before storing. (Plastic is good for freezing!)
5. Label food containers with the date that food is prepared, along with the name of food if desired. For yourself, or especially if living in a shared household, reheating instructions may be added—for example, bake 20 minutes, or steam 10 minutes. Labels may also be colored-coded with colored markers or colored strips of paper taped or glued on (before chilling) for easy finding.
6. Do not cook or reheat foods in a microwave while on a Candida diet. Not all bacteria that contribute to Candida yeast are killed by average microwave cooking! This includes all foods, especially meat!

FREEZING TIPS

1. Most frozen foods keep one to three months or a bit more if properly wrapped.
2. Some frozen burgers are best wrapped in wax paper first, then placed in a plastic bag to prevent freezer burn. Do not use wax paper if you have a corn allergy! Plastic wrap or aluminum foil with the shiny side in can also be used to wrap burgers. Several wrapped burgers may be placed in one plastic bag. Use freezer bags, freezer wrap, or double-bag all bagged foods.
3. Freeze food in freezer glass jars or clean plastic. Never use plastic containers that have had laundry soap or household cleaning products in them to store edible foods! Never allow children to play with containers (or wooden spoons or boards) that you will later use for food storage (or preparation). Never allow dirty water, spoiled foods, foreign liquids, or dry powders to sit in plastic containers that you will later use for food storage. Never put hot foods into plastic containers. Do not freeze in glass containers as they do not "give" and may break easily in the freezer; use special freezer glass only. Tins may be used in the freezer, placed in a sealed plastic bag for protection from freezer burn.
4. Fill freezer containers only ¾ to ⅘ full to allow for food expansion. Food expands as it freezes. Overfilled containers will crack, break, or overflow.
5. Foods may lose flavor when frozen. Add a bit of extra seasoning to a dish before freezing or after defrosting to perk up a dish and ensure full flavor.

SUBSTITUTIONS

As many as 75 percent or more of individuals with Candida albicans also have food sensitivities (sometimes temporary) and/or food allergies. Check with your health specialist to determine if you have these problems and avoid foods that cause troublesome reactions or symptoms. Most recipes in this book offer variations and ingredient options; all the alternatives are not always given. If you have favorite recipes you would like to transform into recipes to eat on a Candida diet, the Substitution Chart that follows can make it easier. Not all substitutions work perfectly in every recipe; sometimes the flavor, nutrients, and quality of a recipe may be altered by changes. See the Glossary of Special Foods and recipes for missing items and additional tips on why and how to make substitutions. The best alternatives are listed first.

SUBSTITUTION CHART

Instead of	Use
Acidophilus powder	Bifidus powder or corn-free unbuffered vitamin C crystals; sometimes lime or lemon juice
Adzuki beans, dry	Pinto beans, kidney beans; sometimes brown lentils or mung beans
Agar-agar powder	Arrowroot powder or kudzu (use ½ as much)
Alfalfa leaves, dried	Parsley flakes or dried cilantro
Alfalfa sprouts	Simmered water chestnuts, snow peas, or grated kohlrabi or zucchini
Almonds	Filberts, pecans, pine nuts, sunflower seeds, or other seeds
Amaranth flour	Teff, chickpea, or soy flour
Apple cider or juice	Peach, pear, or apricot juice, or ¼ amount honey mixed with ¾ amount water to equal amount substituted for
Apple cider vinegar	Lemon or lime juice, or ¹⁄₁₀ amount corn-free unbuffered vitamin C
Arrowroot powder or flour	Kudzu powder in equal amounts (¹⁄₁₀ amount guar gum or equal amounts tapioca flour may sometimes be used)
Artichoke hearts, marinated	Artichoke hearts packed in water
Artichoke hearts, in water	Asparagus, broccoli, kohlrabi; sometimes avocados, water chestnuts, or brussels sprouts
Artichokes, Jerusalem	Water chestnuts, lotus root, turnips, parsnips, sometimes jicama, mung bean sprouts, or pine nuts
Asparagus	Broccoli, kohlrabi, artichoke hearts; sometimes celery or avocado
Avocados	Artichoke hearts packed in water; sometimes cooked asparagus, cooked and mashed green peas
Baking powder (store-bought, with wheat and additives)	Homemade Baking Powder recipe or Pharmacy brand
Baker's yeast	Homemade Baking Powder recipe or wheat-free Pharmacy brand
Bamboo shoots	Water chestnuts, lotus root; sometimes celery or jicama in cooking, sometimes snow peas
Barley, white pearl	Brown pot barley, millet, or quinoa

Instead of	Use
Barley, brown pot	Quinoa, millet, sometimes buckwheat or kasha
Barley green powder	Wheat grass powder, spirulina powder, chlorella powder
Basil	Oregano or dill weed, sometimes parsley
Basmati rice, white	Brown basmati rice, long grain brown rice
Basmati rice, brown	Long grain brown rice; sometimes short grain brown rice or wild rice
Beets	Carrots or radishes in salads; orange yam, winter squash, or turnips, in cooked recipes
Black beans (or turtle beans)	Kidney, pinto, or red beans; sometimes adzuki beans
Bouillon cubes (vegetable or meat)	Homemade Bouillon Cubes or Homemade Vegetable Broth Powder; sometimes simmered tamari soy sauce or Mock Tamari Soy Sauce
Broccoli	Asparagus, kohlrabi; sometimes celery, zucchini, brussels sprouts, artichoke hearts
Brown rice, long	Basmati brown rice; sometimes sweet brown rice, wehani rice, wild rice, brown pot barley, or whole oats
Brown rice, short	Sweet brown rice; sometimes long brown rice options (above)
Brussels sprouts	Cabbage, kohlrabi, broccoli, sometimes artichoke hearts
Buckwheat	Brown pot barley, alone or with a bit of whole rye
Butter	Clarified butter, natural oil
Butters, nut	Seed butters; sometimes bean paste or thick vegetables, mashed
Cabbage, white or red	Brussels sprouts, Savoy cabbage, kale, chard; sometimes broccoli or artichoke hearts, for raw—use lettuces
Carob	Carob pods
Carrots	Beets; red, orange, or yellow bell peppers, radishes (raw); turnips; parsnips; orange yams, winter squash (cooked)
Cashews	Blanched almonds or pine nuts
Cashew milk	Blanched almond milk, sesame milk, or other milks, sometimes store-bought soy milk (see Beverages)
Cauliflower	Spaghetti squash, turnips, parsnips; sometimes orange yam or other winter squash, or Jerusalem artichokes

(continues)

Instead of	Use
Cayenne	Crushed, ground chili peppers; onion, garlic, or horseradish powder (wasabi); black, pink, or white pepper
Celery	Zucchini, broccoli, kohlrabi; sometimes asparagus, fresh peas, green beans, or bamboo shoots
Cheese	Tofu cheese, feta, or ricotta cheese (cooked only)
Chickpeas (garbanzos)	Soy beans, fava beans; sometimes pintos
Chickpea flour (garbanzo, flour, besan or chana flour)	Soy flour; sometimes amaranth or teff or pinto bean flour
Chili powder	Your Own Chili Powder (see recipes)
Cilantro	Parsley; sometimes fresh alfalfa leaves
Corn	Yellow summer squash or yellow bell peppers, in raw or cooked recipes; fresh peas, cooked
Cornmeal	Chickpea flour, soybean flour, amaranth or teff flour, nut flours
Cornstarch	Arrowroot or kudzu powder, in equal amounts
Couscous	Quinoa or millet
Cucumbers	Organic cucumbers, English cucumbers, zucchini, yellow summer squash
Curry powder	Your Own Curry Powder (see recipes)
Dill weed	Basil, oregano, thyme, or a dash of rosemary
Dulse powder	Sea kelp powder, powdered seaweeds, dried vegetable powder; sometimes spirulina or chlorella powder
Eggplant	Sautéed water chestnuts, mung sprouts, long-sautéed onions; flavored, texturized, and broiled tofu
Eggs	Powdered egg replacers and water (1 tablespoon powder and ¼ cup water per egg)
Eggs, hen's	Quail, duck, or other eggs (¼ cup equivalent other eggs per 1 hen's egg)
Engevita yeast	Toasted chickpea flour (see Homemade Vegetable Broth for recipe)
Fava beans	Soybeans, chickpeas; sometimes pinto or kidney beans
Feta cheese	Ricotta cheese, farmers' cheese, or quark; sometimes tofu cheese

Instead of	Use
Filberts (hazelnuts)	Almonds or pecans; sometimes Brazil nuts or pine nuts
Flax oil	Pumpkin seed oil or fish oil, especially salmon oil
Flax seeds	Sesame seeds, sunflower seeds, or chopped pumpkin seeds
Garlic	Shallots or horseradish: powdered, prepared, or fresh; sometimes onions
Gomashio sesame salt	Toasted sunflower seeds, teff seeds, or pine nuts, with added sea salt
Grain flours	Legume or seed flours: teff, amaranth, chickpea, soy, pinto, black bean, brown lentil
Grapefruit juice	Lemon or lime juice; sometimes kiwi juice or tomato juice; apple cider vinegar may be substituted sparingly if allowed in recipes
Guar gum powder	Xanthan gum (corn derived—as thickener), slippery elm powder (to smooth or emulsify), in equal amounts, see also arrowroot and other thickeners
Herb teas	See Beverages
Herbs, fresh	See individual herbs; use vegetable powders
Horseradish	Onions, green onions, leeks, garlic, shallots, chives
Horseradish powder (wasabi)	Onion or garlic powder
Jicama	Jerusalem artichokes, water chestnuts, sometimes turnip
Jerusalem artichokes	See Artichokes, Jerusalem
Kasha	Brown pot barley, alone or mixed with a little whole grain rye (1 part rye to 3 to 6 parts barley); other whole grains mixed with Home-Roasted Nuts (1 part nuts to 6 parts grain)
Kelp, sea kelp powder	Dulse powder, dried vegetable powder, ground seaweed; sometimes spirulina or chlorella powder
Kidney beans	Pinto beans, Romano beans; sometimes adzuki or black beans
Kohlrabi	Broccoli, cabbage, brussels sprouts, mung bean sprouts; sometimes celery, zucchini, asparagus
Kudzu (kuzu)	Arrowroot powder (equal amounts); sometimes tapioca flour

(continues)

Instead of	Use
Leeks	Green onions, white onions with chives, sometimes shallots
Legumes	Nuts, seeds, or meats (as dietary substitutes)
Legume flours	Amaranth or teff flours; sometimes nut flours or meals
Lemon juice, fresh	Fresh lime juice, grapefruit juice; sometimes corn-free unbuffered vitamin C crystals or acidophilus
Lentils (green, gray, French, or brown)	Adzuki beans; sometimes dry mung beans or red lentils
Lentils, red	Small French or other lentils; sometimes orange yams
Lettuce	Spinach, exotic greens, or grated zucchini
Lime juice, fresh	Fresh lemon juice, grapefruit juice; sometimes corn-free unbuffered vitamin C crystals or acidophilus
Lotus root	Water chestnuts, Jerusalem artichokes, mung bean sprouts, bamboo shoots; sometimes snow peas
Marjoram	Savory, basil or thyme, sometimes a bit of rosemary
Milk	Milk substitutes (see recipes)
Milk powder	Soy milk powder, ½ amounts of arrowroot or kudzu; sometimes tapioca flour
Millet	Quinoa; sometimes brown pot barley or short grain brown rice
Miso	Simmered tamari soy sauce, Mock Tamari Soy Sauce, simmered Quick Sip, Liquid Aminos
Mung beans, dry	Lentils; sometimes adzuki beans
Mung bean sprouts	Water chestnuts or snow peas; sometimes lotus root or bamboo shoots or Jerusalem artichokes
Mushrooms	Long-sautéed onions (see Sweet Onion Sauce), sautéed water chestnuts, flavored/ texturized and broiled tofu
Mustard, prepared	Dry mustard powder (with water, bit of onion powder, spices)
Navy or northern beans	Chickpeas, soybeans, pinto beans
Nuts	See alternative nuts, seeds; sometimes water chestnuts, pine nuts, or sunflower seeds
Nutritional yeasts	Toasted chickpea, soybean, amaranth, or teff flours
Oats, rolled	Scotch oats, oat grits (or chopped groats)

Instead of	Use
Oats, whole	Long grain brown rice; sometimes brown pot barley or whole rye
Oil, salad	Sunflower, sesame, olive (extra virgin), flax, or pumpkin oil, all natural and expeller- or cold-pressed, organic is best
Oil, cooking	Butter, clarified butter, sunflower, sesame, olive, or canola oils, natural
Okra	Celery, green beans, sometimes zucchini
Olives, green	Black olives, cooked; sometimes long-sautéed onions or sprouted lentils, green peas
Onions, white or yellow	Leeks, green onions, shallots, horseradish: use ½ to 1 tsp. prepared horseradish per 1 small onion, 1 tsp. per medium onion, 1½ to 2 tsp. per large onion
Onions, green	Chives, horseradish, finely chopped red onion (small amounts)
Onions, red	White or yellow onions, green onions, leeks, horseradish: use ½ to 1 tsp. prepared horseradish per 1 small onion, 1 tsp. per medium onion, 1½ to 2 tsp. per large onion
Oregano	Basil, dill weed, thyme, sometimes parsley
Paprika	Cayenne (minute bits); ground, crushed red chiles
Parsley	Cilantro; sometimes fresh basil or alfalfa leaves
Parsnips	Turnips, carrots, winter squash
Peas, green	Chopped green beans, snow peas, sprouted brown/green lentils; sometimes celery or zucchini
Peas, dried	Mung beans, green lentils
Pecans	Almonds, filberts, pine nuts, sometimes Brazil nuts
Peppers, green bell	Red, orange, yellow, or purple bell peppers, celery, zucchini or yellow summer squash
Peppers, red bell	Orange, yellow, or purple bell peppers; tomatoes, radishes, grated beets
Peppers, chili or hot	Horseradish (fresh or powdered), garlic, shallots
Pine nuts (pignolias)	Brazil nuts, almonds, water chestnuts, other nuts/seeds
Pinto beans	Kidney beans, Romano beans; sometimes red, adzuki, or black beans

(continues)

Instead of	Use
Potatoes	Jerusalem artichokes, cauliflower, turnips, orange yams, winter squash; sometimes parsnips
Potatoes, yellow sweet	Turnips, orange yams, winter squash; sometimes parsnips or Jerusalem artichokes
Pumpkin seeds (pepitas)	Almonds, filberts, pine nuts, sunflower seeds
Quinoa	Millet; sometimes brown pot barley or short grain brown rice
Ricotta cheese	Feta cheese, farmer's cheese, quark, or tofu cheese (cooked)
Rolled oats or other rolled flaked whole grains	Brown rice or basmati brown rice, cooked whole oats
Romano beans	Pinto or kidney beans; sometimes adzuki or red beans
Rutabagas	Turnips, parsnips, winter squash, orange yam
Salsa	Homemade Salsa (see recipe)
Sea kelp	Dulse or ground seaweed, dried and ground vegetable powder
Sea salt	Potassium chloride (in small amounts), onion or garlic powder, salt substitutes, Gomashio (with potassium chloride)
Seaweed	Dried vegetable powder, spirulina, chlorella powder
Sesame salt	See Gomashio
Sesame seeds	Teff seeds (½ amount); sometimes chopped sunflower seeds or chopped or whole flaxseeds
Sesame tahini	Sunflower butter or other nut/seed butter
Shallots	Garlic, horseradish, leeks, red onion, white or yellow onion
Snow peas	Fresh peas, mung bean sprouts, green beans, or steamed asparagus
Soybeans	Chickpeas, fava beans; sometimes pinto or kidney beans
Soy milk	Milk substitutes (see Beneficial Beverages)
Soy sauce	See Tamari soy sauce
Spaghetti squash	Other winter squash, cauliflower, turnips
Spinach	Kale, chard, mustard greens (cooked); lettuce, exotic greens, grated zucchini (fresh)

Instead of	Use
Spirulina powder	Chlorella powder; sometimes barley or wheat grass powder
Sprouts	Water chestnuts, pine nuts, snow peas
Squash, winter	Orange yams, turnips; sometimes cauliflower or parsnips
Squash, yellow summer	Zucchini, pattypan squash, yellow bell pepper
Sugars (cane, beet, or artificial)	Natural sweeteners: honey, maple syrup, fruit juice (minute amounts) in cooking only
Sunflower seeds	Sesame seeds, chopped nuts, pine nuts, sometimes pumpkin seeds
Tahini (sesame)	Almond, filbert, or sunflower nut butter
Tamari soy sauce	Mock Tamari Soy Sauce, Quick Sip, Liquid Aminos (boil and simmer 5 minutes or more)
Tapioca flour	Soy milk powder; sometimes kudzu or arrowroot powder
Teff flour	Amaranth flour, chickpea or soy flour
Teff seeds	Sesame seeds (two to four times as many), chopped sunflower seeds (twice as many); sometimes cooked chia seeds or whole amaranth
Tempeh	Tofu; sometimes mashed beans
Thyme	Marjoram or savory; sometimes dill weed
Tofu	Legumes; feta or ricotta cheese, cooked
Tofu Cheese	Yogurt; feta or ricotta cheese, cooked
Tomatoes	Red bell peppers, grated beets, radishes
Tomato sauce	Mock Tomato Sauce (see recipe)
Turnips	Winter squash, orange yams, parsnips; sometimes cauliflower or Jerusalem artichokes
TVP (texturized vegetable protein-soy product)	Tofu, legumes
Umeboshi plum	Mashed legumes, tahini, or nut butter (any mixed with Mock Tamari Soy Sauce)
Vegetable broth powder	Homemade Vegetable Broth Powder or Homemade Vegetable Bouillon Cubes (see recipes)
Vegetable powder, dried	Sea kelp, dulse, ground seaweed

(continues)

Instead of	Use
Vinegar	Lemon or lime juice, corn-free unbuffered vitamin C crystals; sometimes acidophilus powder
Water chestnuts	Jerusalem artichokes, jicama, mung bean sprouts, lotus root, pine nuts; sometimes snow peas or bamboo shoots
Wheat: bulgur, cracked, bran, wheat germ; or other whole or cracked grains	Scotch or steel-cut oats, oat groats, chopped rye, rye grits
Xanthan gum	Guar gum (to thicken), slippery elm (to smooth or emulsify), in equal amounts (see arrowroot and thickeners)
Yams, orange	Winter squash, turnips
Yogurt	Milk substitute (3 to 4 parts blended with 1 part tofu), in cooking
Zucchini	Yellow summer squash; sometimes celery or cucumber or kohlrabi

SPECIAL COOKING TIPS

HOW TO COOK WHOLE GRAINS

1. Grains are generally cooked in 2 or more cups of water per 1 cup of grain. Those with digestive troubles should use even more water, 2½ to 4 cups per 1 cup of whole grain. See recipes.
2. Cook grains until they are no longer crunchy but not soggy or mushy. Grains should be tender and easy to chew. Improperly cooked grains are extremely hard to digest!
3. Very few grains need to be soaked before cooking. Soak wild rice (sometimes), whole oats, rye, triticale (and wheat kernels or berries).
4. Before cooking, check grains for dirt balls, gravel, husks, and other foreign particles by spreading them out thinly and fingering through them. Discard discolored, distorted grains along with unwanted particles.
5. Brown rice and quinoa are usually the only grains that need pre-washing, but wash any grain if you feel it needs it.
6. It makes little difference whether you start cooking a grain in cool or warm water. The exception is ground cereals, which get lumpy when put in warm water, unless mixed in carefully with a wire whisk.

7. To prevent grains from boiling over and to distribute heat evenly, water and grains together should never cover more than three-fourths of the cooking pot. Bring to a boil on low heat, turn to low and cover.

8. Do not add salt or oil to whole grains until the last 5 to 10 minutes of cooking, to make sure they cook properly and are more digestible.

9. Any grain in whole form will never burn during its first cooking process as long as the water does not run out, it is cooked on low heat, and the grain does not become overcooked to the point that it falls apart (this usually takes over an hour).

10. Never stir whole grains while cooking or they will stick and burn. Keep grains covered while cooking.

11. When reheating cooked whole grains, add ¼ to ⅓ cup extra water per 1 cup of grain. Cook the grain, covered, on very low heat until warmed (10 to 15 minutes). Brown rice can be reheated by steaming in a vegetable steamer.

12. One cup of dry whole grain or cereal makes about 4 servings.

13. The main dish grains can almost always be substituted one for the other in different recipes, except for wild rice, rye, and buckwheat, or kasha. Most grains are similar but differ slightly in taste.

14. Wheat, rye, triticale, barley, oats, kamut, and spelt contain gluten. Other grains contain minute amounts of gluten but are not considered gluten grains and are not usually eliminated from gluten-free diets, only from grain-free or celiac diets.

PREPARING MAIN DISH GRAINS

Buckwheat and Brown Pot Barley Use about 2 cups water per 1 cup grain. Bring the grain to a boil, then turn down the heat to a low bubble. Cover and simmer 20 to 30 minutes or until tender and no longer crunchy, adding extra water if needed. Onions can be cooked with the grain; add herbs and salt during the last 5 minutes of cooking time. (Buckwheat does not contain wheat and is essentially gluten-free.)

Kasha (toasted buckwheat, contains no wheat and essentially no gluten) Cook the same as buckwheat, but use less water and reduce the cooking time to about 20 minutes.

Whole Oats or Whole Rye See Cooked Cereals in the Breakfast chapter.

Basmati Brown Rice Cook like short or long grain brown rice, only cook for 40 to 55 minutes.

Short and Long Grain Brown Rice Put rice in a pot and fill it with water. Rub the rice together with your fingers and swish it around to remove extra starches, dirt, and stray husks. Discard all the water. If the water was very cloudy during the first washing, repeat the process once or twice until the water is relatively clear. Put 3 to 4 cups water per 1 cup rice in the pot. Bring to a boil over high heat, turn heat to low, cover, and simmer 75 to 95 minutes. When the rice is no longer crunchy but easy to chew and tender, not soggy, it is done. Onions, herbs, and spices can be added during the last 15 to 20 minutes of cooking time. Keep the pot tightly covered while cooking, but it will not hurt to peek! Cook the extra 20 minutes longer if digestion is poor. (Extra water was added to this recipe for extra tender, delicious rice that is easy to digest! Some people use 2–2½ cups water to 1 cup rice and cook about 60 minutes; however, the rice is very hard for most people to digest this way.)

Millet Cook the same as rice, but use 2½ to 3½ cups water per 1 cup dry millet. It usually does not need pre-washing. Simmer 55 to 75 minutes and use as a substitute for rice in rice dishes. This is one of the best grains, high in nutrients and very alkaline. It is especially good for delicate stomachs.

Quinoa (pronounced keen-wah) Rinse white quinoa thoroughly before cooking by rubbing the grains together well in a pot of water and changing the water. This helps remove the saponin, which may irritate digestion and allergies. Use 2 to 3 cups water to 1 cup quinoa and bring the water and quinoa to a boil on high heat. Turn low, cover and simmer 20 to 25 minutes until tender. Add sea salt, oil, or butter if desired. Use cooked quinoa in place of rice or millet in main dishes. It is especially nice when small pieces of chopped zucchini or broccoli are cooked with this grain during the entire cooking time, on top. It is delicious! See recipe in Main Dishes. (Brown quinoa cooks in only 10 to 20 minutes and needs to be rubbed vigorously under water, changing the water several times, before cooking to remove extra saponin.)

Wild Rice This is one of the few main dish grains that sometimes (rarely) requires soaking before cooking. If a brand of rice cooks easily the first time without pre-soaking, it does not need it. If the rice seems too tough after an hour of cooking, next time pre-soak it for 2 to 4 hours in 2 to 3 times as much water. Cook the rice as you would brown rice. Wild rice is rich tasting and can be expensive, so it is often mixed with 2 to 6 parts brown rice to make it stretch. Cook the two rices separately, then mix together when they are finished cooking.

Cereal Grains See Breakfasts for how to cook.

How to Cook Legumes Properly for Good Digestion (and No Gas!)

1. Measure the amount of beans required and sort through them to remove any damaged beans, gravel, dirt balls, or foreign objects.
2. Soak 1 cup of dry beans in 3 to 4 cups of cool or room temperature water for 8 or more hours, uncovered. Soak chickpeas for 12 or more hours and soybeans or fava beans for at least 24 hours.
3. Important: Throw away the water the beans soaked in! This water contains a gas released by the beans while soaking, which in turn gives you gas.
4. Rinse the beans several times, swish them around in fresh water and discard water.
5. Put the beans in a large pot so that they only fill about half the pot; add fresh water until the beans are covered by 1 inch or so of water.
6. Bring the beans and water, uncovered, to a boil on high heat.
7. When the beans are boiling, a white foam or froth will generally form on top. Scoop this off and discard it. This part is what contributes to gas.
8. Add extra water if needed so the beans are still at least 1 inch underwater and turn the heat down to very low, just low enough so the beans are barely bubbling and cover them.
9. Optional: Add 1 teaspoon ground fennel, or preferably 1 teaspoon savory to the beans during the whole cooking time. This improves digestibility.
10. Cook for 1¼ hours or more (usually under 2 hours) until the beans are very tender and the beans can easily be mashed with the tongue on the roof of your mouth.
11. Chew beans slowly; never eat them fast or when under excessive stress or fatigue.
12. If possible, have some raw foods first in a meal before eating the beans, to aid in their digestion.

13. Do not add any oil, salt, or salty ingredients like seaweed or sea kelp to beans while they are cooking. These ingredients can actually toughen the beans so that they stay hard. When they are completely tender in the cooking pot, then add these ingredients. After the beans are soft, add salt, seaweeds, and sea kelp to help them to become more digestible. If oil is used, add it at the same time as salty ingredients.

14. For those with excessive gas problems, bring dry beans to a boil when they are first added to soaking water, then let them cool down, uncovered, for 6 to 8 hours (8 to 12 hours for chickpeas; 12 to 24 hours for soybeans or fava beans) before changing the water and cooking. (In hot weather, beans must be refrigerated after the first few hours.) Another trick for extreme cases of bad digestion is to sprout the beans before cooking, but this will alter their taste and texture.

15. The easiest-to-digest beans are lentils, adzuki beans, pinto beans, black beans, and chickpeas. Those with sensitive digestion should try these first. Those with digestive problems should avoid all beans that are not blended or mashed into recipes, unless and until they adjust to them or use digestive aids as needed, especially HCL for major problems (or for those who need only a little help: plant enzymes or BEANO).

16. For extra, natural help with digestion, eat a raw salad before beans or eat the beans with yogurt and/or tomatoes (not good with citrus juices!) Do NOT eat beans and meat at the same meal!

17. One cup dry beans makes about 2½ cups soaked or cooked beans.

How to Cook Vegetables

There are five basic methods of cooking vegetables: boiling, broiling, baking, sautéing, and steaming. For a list of Vegetables to Eat Cooked, see chapter 15.

Boiling When cooking natural foods, very few vegetables are boiled as they lose vitamins and flavor. Some thick-skinned whole foods can be boiled whole without fear of losing their subtle qualities, such as whole winter squash: spaghetti, butternut, buttercup, acorn, and others. See recipes.

Broiling Broiling is a limited method of cooking; some vegetables are too hard to broil effectively unless steamed first. Broiling does add superb flavor to vegetables. Easy-to-broil vegetables: bell peppers, zucchini, yellow summer squash, edible pea pods, onions; also, grapefruit sections and tomatoes. Foods that can be broiled if partially pre-steamed (about 5 minutes or more) first:

broccoli, cauliflower, kohlrabi, carrots, turnips, parsnips, beets, asparagus, and artichoke hearts packed in water (drained). See Broiled Vegetable and Tofu Kebabs, chapter 18.

Baking Baking can be used to cook many vegetables. They can be flavorful when baked but may get dry and take a longer time to cook. Vegetables that can be baked whole: orange yams, zucchini, yellow winter squash, pattypan squash, kohlrabi, small onions, bell peppers. Tomatoes may also be baked whole. Vegetables that can be cut and baked: winter squash, carrots, beets, turnips, and parsnips, as well as all the vegetables that can be baked whole. Some are best if pre-steamed before baking. Almost all can be baked into vegetable pies, casseroles, or other dishes with multiple ingredients.

Sautéeing This method of cooking vegetables is quite flavorful. It does require a bit of oil. Some people avoid using oil and sauté with water or tamari instead, but these are not true stir-frys and actually vitamins and flavor are lost when oil (or butter) is not used for stir-frying. The oil must be very hot before any vegetables are added to a stir-fry. Then the vegetables are only lightly coated in the oil and it seals in their juices and flavors. If the oil is too cool, it gets absorbed into the vegetable and destroys nutrients while saturating the vegetables. If water or tamari are used to stir-fry, they may also permeate the vegetables, destroying valuable nutrients and flavors and the vegetables will ooze their juices while cooking, release moisture, and can become soggy. See Asian Vegetable Stir-Fry with Tofu, chapter 18, for the proper method and best vegetables to stir-fry. If you have digestive problems, sauté the vegetables for a couple of minutes longer so they are not crunchy. Bile salts can help to digest the oil if you have problems with fats (take one tablet per meal only as needed.).

Steaming This is the most popular and common method of cooking vegetables for the health-minded. The flavor is in between that of boiled and baked vegetables and the sautéed and broiled ones. Vegetables can be cooked to perfection if done properly. Buy a special steaming basket, preferably stainless steel (bamboo ones are not sanitary) and insert it in a large pot with a lid that closes completely and seals in the steam. One of the special steaming pots available at cooking shops can also be purchased. In either case, the vegetables must sit above the boiling water at all times without the water touching them or they will lose flavor and nutrients.

Method: Heat ½ inch or more of water in the pan on high heat until it comes to a rapid boil. Turn the heat to just above low, or medium-low, so that the water is still bubbling but not too frantically. Add the vegetables to the pot and steam until tender but not mushy. Cook extra tender if you have digestive troubles. Add extra water to the pot if it evaporates too fast. See One-Pot Vegetables and Brown Rice, chapter 18, for more on the method. Cooking times for steaming vary greatly, depending on the size of the vegetables, how full the steaming basket is, how hard the water is boiling, how tightly the pan lid fits, and so on. See the Vegetable Steaming Guide for an idea of how long to cook most vegetables.

VEGETABLE STEAMING GUIDE

Especially geared for those on Candida diets for best digestion, this chart gives approximate steaming times for most steamable vegetables. See Steaming, above. Cook one or more vegetables together. Put longest-cooking one in the pot first; add others later so each vegetable only cooks the basic allotted time.

Cooking Time	Whole Vegetable (or large pieces)	Cut Vegetable (1- to 1½-inch chunks, slices, or strips)
5 to 7 minutes	snow peas	bell peppers
	black olives	artichoke hearts, quarters
	bean sprouts	black olives, half
	lentil sprouts	water chestnuts, sliced
	green peas	lotus root, chopped
	garlic	
7 to 10 minutes	spinach	onions
	celery	garlic
	green onions	zucchini
	bell pepper, half	yellow summer squash
10 to 16 minutes	asparagus	cabbage
	artichoke hearts	broccoli
	onions (small)	cauliflower
	chickpea sprouts	kohlrabi
	other legume sprouts	Jerusalem artichokes
	zucchini, sliced in half	

Cooking Time	Whole Vegetable (or large pieces)	Cut Vegetable (1- to 1½-inch chunks, slices, or strips)
16 to 24 minutes	kale	carrot
	collards	turnip
	turnip greens	parsnip
	mustard greens	brussels sprouts
	beet greens	green beans
	Swiss chard	beets
	broccoli (small stalk)	orange yams
24 to 30 minutes	brussels sprouts	winter squash, 1 to 2-inch chunks
	green beans	
	kohlrabi (small)	cabbage, in large wedges
	Jerusalem artichokes	
45 minutes or more	artichokes, globe	
	cauliflower head	
	kohlrabi (large)	

SELECTION GUIDE FOR COOKING VEGETABLES

Root vegetables (carrots, beets, turnips, others)
: Choose firm, unblemished, bright-colored ones with no side roots or soft spots.

Leafy greens (kale, chard, spinach, others)
: Choose bright leaves, crisp and unwrinkled without major blemishes or holes.

Flower vegetables (broccoli, cabbage, cauliflower, asparagus, others)
: Choose firm, crisp, unblemished vegetables without yellow or black spots.

Pungent vegetables (onions, garlic, leeks, shallots)
: Choose firm ones with unwrinkled skins, avoid soft spots, black spots, yellow growing tops.

See Raw Vegetables, chapter 15, for tips on zucchini, yellow summer squash, cucumbers, celery, kohlrabi, green onions, chives, parsley, green herbs, bell peppers, avocados, radishes, lettuces, and tomatoes.

Storage Guide for Cooking Vegetables

Root vegetables	Keep 2 to 6 weeks refrigerated. Keep wrapped.
Leafy greens	Keep 3 to 7 days refrigerated. Keep wrapped.
Flower vegetables	Keep 5 to 10 days refrigerated. Keep wrapped.
Pungent vegetables	Keep 7 to 15 days or more in cupboard or on shelf. Keep out of sun and in a cool place. Do not wrap. Leave in open jar or open pot. (Refrigerate leeks up to 5–14 days.)

See chapter 15 for more on selection and storage of all raw vegetables and washing methods for vegetables. (If you cook vegetables, they may escape special washing occasionally.)

COOKWARE AND KITCHEN UTENSILS

For better health and cleanliness, less heavy-metal absorption, and reduced bacteria, it is beneficial to use certain cookware and utensils and avoid others. Cookware and utensils play an important part in creating wholesome, quality meals that complement Candida treatment.

Use:
Corningware (for electric stovetop or oven)*
Quality stainless steel
Heavy-duty enamel pots (quality, white-lined, or solid-color enamel)
Cast-iron frying pans or bean-cooking pots
Glass bakeware or Pyrex (for baking)*
Stainless steel vegetable steamer
Glass or stainless steel measuring cups and spoons, colanders, and utensils
Stainless steel spoons and ladles
Glass or wooden cutting boards
Glass or ceramic tea pots

---

*Never touch hot Corningware or glassware with wet cloths or fill with cold liquid as they may crack or break.

Do Not Use:

Aluminum pans

Copperware (includes colanders, spoons, kettles, etc.)

"Spun" stainless steel (dull-finish variety with circular rims or ribs inside pans and lids gives a metallic taste to foods)

Cheap or cracked enamel pots (or those with blue, black, or white-specked enamel, or old gray enamel which is poisonous)

Glass cookware (lead content)

Bamboo vegetable steamer (can absorb bacteria and dirt)

Aluminum measuring cups and spoons

Plastic, wood, or aluminum spoons or ladles

Acrylic, plastic, or old, dirty, or damaged cutting boards

Electric tea kettles (unsanitary and may have exposed copper coils inside)

For cleaning dishes, use:

Water as hot as you can stand it (use rubber gloves if necessary)

Antibacterial dish soap and other cleaning products

Metal scrubbers, sponges, and brushes (boil if needed)

Rinse dishes individually under hot water (not in a sink of water)

Dishwashers, for at least the heated drying cycle (helps kill bacteria on dishes). If using full cycle, add soap only for the first cycle.

For cleaning household and office, use:

Environmentally friendly and hypoallergenic cleaning products. Buy at health food stores or allergy shops (or other markets).

Clorox Bleach (diluted in water, use this bleach brand only)—buy at supermarket

To clean wooden cutting boards:

Dilute Clorox bleach: ¼ cup to 3 to 4 cups warm water.

Use a scrub brush to scour completely (do not submerge), scrub sides and back.

Rinse in very warm but not hot water, scrubbing with water first, then rinse thoroughly.

Bleach board after each 5 to 12 uses. In between, always wash boards immediately after each use.

Use diluted antibacterial dish soap and brush completely (do not
submerge); rinse thoroughly.
Drip-dry in open-air dish rack. Do not store until completely dry.

SEASONING CAST IRONWARE

Do not buy pre-seasoned ironware. Wash new ironware in warm suds and
water, rinse and dry thoroughly with paper towels or napkins. Place on a hot
stove burner or in an oven for 1 to 2 minutes to complete drying. Preheat the
oven to 300°F (150°C). Coat the pan evenly with natural cooking oil and bake
for 1 hour. Wipe off excess oil and use for cooking. Wash without heavy
scrubbing and rinse quickly right after each use. Dry as above. Do not leave
wet or submerged in water. Reseason if needed. Ironware is excellent for good
cooking, especially eggs and legumes. Do not use for cooking tomatoes, or
acid foods or light-colored creamy sauces.

OVEN TEMPERATURES

	F°	C°		F°	C°		F°	C°
Very Hot	500	260	Moderate	350	175	Very Slow	250	120
Hot	450	230	Moderately			Low	200	95
Moderately			Slow	325	165	Warming	150	65
Hot	400	205	Slow	300	150			

ABOUT MICROWAVES

BY DR. ZOLTAN P. RONA

Evidence suggests that microwaves can seriously deplete foods of their
enzymes and nutrients while creating radiation by-products that may cause
negative health effects. All heating causes loss of nutrients, but microwave
cooking produces the greatest losses. Steaming, stir-frying, and regular convec-
tion ovens are healthier alternatives.

The electromagnetic pollution of microwaves may be causing problems
with some people, especially those with a weakened immune system. Studies
indicate that extremely low frequency electromagnetic fields (EMFs) produced

by radiation from power lines, generator substations, and home appliances increase the risks for cancers, especially leukemia and brain cancers. More commonly, continuous exposure to electromagnetic fields can increase the frequency and severity of headaches, migraines, chronic fatigue, dizziness, nausea, stress, and environmental sensitivities.

One can easily test for harmful electromagnetic field radiation with a Gauss meter. Teldon makes one that can be mail-ordered by calling: 1-800-663-2212. In a widely distributed article on EMFs ("Facts on Power Line and Computer Radiation"), George S. Lechter lists the following things you can do to reduce your radiation exposure:

Measure your environment with a Gauss meter, and avoid areas where the field is above 1 mG. Measure the fields both inside and outside your home, and don't let your children play near power lines, transformers, and microwave towers.

Measure the magnetic fields from appliances, both when they are operating and when they are turned off. Magnetic fields are created only when current is flowing, but some appliances (such as TVs) are still drawing current even when they are switched off.

Don't sleep under an electric blanket or on a water bed. If you want to warm your bed before you go to sleep, when you're ready to get under the cover, unplug the electric blanket (don't just turn it off). Even though there is no magnetic field when the blanket is turned off, there may still be a high electric field.

Don't sit too close to your TV set. Distance yourself at least 6 feet, but keep in mind that EMF [electromagnetic fields] from some TV sets can be measured as far away as 10 feet or more. An ELF and VLF Gauss meter can help you decide where to sit.

Don't sit too close to your computer display. Keep at least an arm's length away from the screen, but remember that at this distance you will still be within the magnetic field. Computer monitors vary greatly in the strength of the magnetic fields that they emit, so you should check yours with an ELF and VLF meter.

Rearrange your office work area so that you and your co-workers are not exposed to EMF from the sides and backs of each other's VDTs [video display terminals].

Turn off your VDT when you are not using it.

Consider purchasing a low radiation VDT that contains an active compensating coil, or a zero radiation display based on shielded LCD technology.

Don't stand close to your microwave oven when in use. Even if your microwave oven is not leaking microwaves, it will still give off strong ELF magnetic fields.

Move your electric clock away from your pillow. Several feet away should be sufficient. Better yet, buy a battery-powered digital clock.

Keep other electric appliances away from your pillow, too. Telephones and answering machines generate EMF.

Eliminate dimmers and three-way switches; they create high fields.

Eliminate wires running under your bed.

Be wary of cordless appliances such as electric toothbrushes, which use magnetic induction to charge the battery. Such devices deliberately create a large magnetic field.

Remember that EMF passes right through walls, so check out what's on the other side. It could be a cordless electric toothbrush, or a television set, or a clock-thermostat radiating EMF into your bedroom.

If it is not possible for you to avoid the effects of EMFs, you can protect yourself by using a battery-operated electronic device called the Elmag. This device can help reduce the deleterious effects of magnetic fields on your health. (Also available from Teldon).

Chapter 12

BENEFICIAL BEVERAGES

WATER IS THE ELIXIR OF LIFE. IT IS ESSENTIAL TO THE health and well-being of every human being and animal on planet Earth. Water can bring health and vitality or virus and disease. In the contaminated age we live in, city tap water has been found to carry algae, parasites, bacteria, sewage, detergents, chlorine, lime, asbestos, sulfates, fluorine, aluminum chloride, toxic copper, and lead, as well as a multitude of other impurities. These unnecessary additives can contribute to allergies, arthritis, chronic fatigue syndrome, cancer, heart disease, senility, sterility, and a host of diseases, including Candida albicans.

Distilled water has nothing in it—no minerals, parasites, nothing. Extensive research claims that health is improved, longevity is extended, and the quality of living is enhanced by drinking distilled water on a regular, preferably exclusive, basis; however, other research warns of the possible dangers of drinking only distilled water. Some health experts have concluded that distilled water can leach minerals from the body and lead to mineral deficiencies. Distilled water can also leach out harmful contaminants in the body. Many experts do concede that distilled water can be drunk daily if a well-balanced multimineral capsule is taken twice daily and the person drinking the water is on a very high nutrient, whole foods diet. Doctors give mixed reviews as to whether these claims are true or not. (See books about water in the References.)

After more extended research, including Dr. Rona's, it is has been found that for *most* individuals, it is preferable to drink pure, tested spring water on an ongoing, day-to-day basis (as I recommend in my encyclopedic natural cookbook *For the Love of Food*) and to drink distilled (steam or demineralized) water (preferably ozonated) when cleansing and during treatments for Candida, cancer, and other major health problems only, for *limited periods of time,* preferably not more than a few weeks or a maximum of a few months. (Do not drink distilled water when fasting!)

Purchasing (spring or) distilled water in plastic 1-gallon, 2½-gallon, or 5-gallon jugs is costly and requires pick-up or deliveries that are troublesome and time-consuming. Plastic containers must be kept out of the sun or warm places (such as near heating ducts). The heat may cause vinyl chlorides and other contaminants to be leached from the plastic into the empty water, which can readily absorb it. It is possible to obtain water in glass bottles through some water companies that deliver.

A variety of water filtration systems are available, including reverse osmosis and charcoal filter models. Most of these are not effective in eliminating parasites and some are not sturdy or reliable for bacteria-free water, while higher quality models of reverse osmosis water filters provide testing kits to check water purity. A home water distiller is another option for safe drinking water only for short periods of time while cleansing. All sizes and types of water filtration systems are available: from countertop units to complete household water tanks. Choose a stainless steel model, rather than plastic, for optimum-quality drinking water.

It is also possible after filtering or distilling water to magnetize it or change/neutralize it (change the pH of the water) by adding a few tablespoons of lemon or lime juice per gallon of water. Some health experts recommend using apple cider vinegar as an alternative to lemon or lime juice. Check with your doctor to see what type of water is best for your particular body type and health concern and for how long you should use it.

BOTTLED WATER TIPS

1. Keep distilled and spring water bottles out of heat and sun. Keep cool.
2. Use sterile, covered containers to store homemade filtered or distilled water.
3. Refrigerate water if possible but drink it at room temperature. Water stores well in a basement or cool garage.

4. Drink a minimum of 4 glasses daily in cool weather, 6 or more in hot weather, as well as additional beverages such as herb tea. Drink liquids away from meals and drink slowly. Have water at meals only for sipping.
5. Never drink out of the bottle; bacteria then enters into the whole bottle. Pour water into a clean glass or pitcher. Keep fingers and children out of water containers.
6. In some areas, water that is not really distilled or spring is labeled as such and sold. Never buy water that is not in sealed containers. If you doubt the quality of any water, have it analyzed at a local laboratory or try water from another company.
7. If you are unable to obtain distilled water while at home, water can be boiled for over 5 minutes, cooled completely, and put through a hand-held water purifier like the Brita, Jamison, or Water Boy filtration systems. Be sure to use a new filter monthly. Store the water purifier in the refrigerator at all times to prevent bacteria growth and warm a glass to room temperature for 10 minutes or so before drinking. Boiling kills bacteria, and the filter removes heavy metals and other impurities. Never put warm or hot water through a water filter.
8. For very questionable water that may contain parasites—as when traveling—boil for 20 minutes, cool and filter it before drinking.
9. Add lemon or lime juice or apple cider vinegar to distilled water if doctor approved. Water can be magnetized if desired as well.

RESTAURANT BEVERAGES

If in a restaurant, choose sparkling bottled water or club soda above plain water, even if the restaurant claims to serve "filtered" water. If you are desperate for plain water, ask for lemon or lime wedges and squeeze at least 1 teaspoon of juice into your water and stir before drinking. Lemon or lime juice kills many kinds of bacteria in water that may feed yeast. Avoid ordering grapefruit juice, tomato juice, or other vegetable juices in restaurants, as the quality is often questionable. In a pinch, if sparkling bottled water or club soda is not available, order the previously mentioned juices and add 2 teaspoons (2 wedges) fresh squeezed lemon or lime juice, mixed well into the juice. Order one glass only, on rare occasions as needed.

BEVERAGES FOR BABIES

Young babies require milk or high-nutrient milk substitutes to drink even if they have Candida. More healthful substitutes for cow's milk are goat and sheep milk, as they are closer to human milk in composition, lower in fat, more digestible and less likely to contribute to Candida problems. When buying goat's milk, be sure to purchase mild-tasting varieties. (If male and female goats are kept together, the milk has a strong flavor that is offensive to most people and babies. Make sure, by calling the dairy or by tasting the milk, to only feed your baby mild-quality goat's milk.) Fifty percent of babies allergic to cow's milk can easily tolerate mild goat or sheep's milk. Soy milk is the only nondairy milk that contains enough nutrients to be used as a substitute. The problem with soy is that it is hard to digest and a baby can easily develop an allergy to it with daily consumption. It is better to rotate or alternate goat and soy milk for a healthier baby or to use just goat (or sheep's) milk by itself.

Babies with Candida should not be given fruit juices to drink. Stick with milk, water, and acceptable unsweetened herbal teas like (organic) mild mint, raspberry leaf, or catnip (for bedtime as a mild sleep aid—make sure to purchase this only in health food stores) teas. Check with your doctor on this and if some less-sweet juices are used, like apple, make sure to use *real* apple juice diluted with water, usually 1 part apple juice to 4 to 10 parts water.

TIPS FOR TREATING CANDIDA IN BABIES

1. Use glass bottles, never plastic, for formula, water, and all beverages. Make sure bottles are properly sterilized by boiling.
2. Never use a microwave on baby formulas or foods. Not all bacteria are killed that contribute to Candida, and microwaving changes the structure of foods. (See About Microwaves at the end of chapter 11.)
3. Do not feed your baby any refined foods (cereals) or sweet fruits. Check your health food store for healthful alternatives.
4. Mother may eat a clove of garlic daily or several times a week, which improves breast milk quality, fights Candida, and gets some finicky babies to drink better. Check with your holistic doctor regarding this if desired. (Do not take garlic if allergic.)

5. Give your baby ¼ to ½ teaspoon LIFE START I bifidus powder made by Natren in 3 to 4 ounces of water, on an empty stomach, one to two times daily if he or she has colic, thrush, or other symptoms of Candida.

6. If your holistic doctor allows, ¼ to ½ teaspoon 6 to 10 PPM (parts per million) colloidal silver can be given to a baby once or twice daily on an empty stomach with 1 to 2 ounces of water. (This can also be put in the ears, undiluted, for ear infections, daily until improved.)

7. Keep babies' clothing, bedding, and play areas especially clean with antibacterial cleaners that are nontoxic, to avoid extra contact with outside Candida. Keep pets away from babies with Candida.

ABOUT BEVERAGES

Water should represent 75 to 100 percent of all the beverages you consume. Other beverage options are mentioned here. Use only these, unless others are recommended by your doctor or health specialist. Most liquids are better for digestion if drunk away from meals, preferably a half-hour or more before or after a meal. Drunk this way, acidic beverages or mint teas, especially, can assist digestion. If a meal is dry or a bit of liquid is needed, try to limit beverages to 4 to 6 ounces at this time.

SPARKLING WATERS

Sparkling bottled waters like Perrier, Nanton, and others may be drunk on a Candida diet, but the minerals they contain contribute to constipation for many people. A good alternative is club soda, preferably Schweppes, which contains only carbonated water and sodium bicarbonate, or another brand that does not contain many other additives. Club soda tends to loosen the bowels and can be helpful to digestion; however, it is acidic and should not be left on the teeth at bedtime. A wedge of lemon or lime adds flavor to these drinks, and since these fruits are acidic, they are good for Candida diets and can be enjoyed often. These sparkling beverages are great drinks for parties or entertaining and can be drunk fairly often, about one to eight (maximum) 12-ounce servings per week if desired. If one has trouble drinking cold beverages because the body has trouble regulating temperatures, drink these beverages at room temperature.

Sparkling Water and Citrus

1 to 2 ounces (2 to 4 tablespoons) fresh lemon or lime juice

8 to 12 ounces club soda or sparkling bottled water, cold or room temperature

1 wedge or wheel fresh lemon or lime

Optional: ice cubes

Squeeze 2 ounces of juice from a fresh lemon or lime and add it to the water. Garnish with a citrus wedge and enjoy over ice cubes if desired. Drink as soon as possible within the hour. Do not store.

Sparkling Grapefruit Juice

6 to 8 ounces club soda or sparkling bottled water, cold or room temperature

6 to 8 ounces fresh-squeezed white grapefruit juice (not red)

Optional: ice cubes

Optional: wedge or wheel fresh lemon or lime

Optional: 1 to 2 teaspoons fresh lemon or lime juice

Mix the water and juice. Pour over ice and serve with fresh citrus if desired. If the grapefruit tastes a bit sweet, add fresh lemon or lime juice as required. Drink as soon as possible within the hour. Do not store. Enjoy a maximum of 2 to 5 glasses per week of any fresh grapefruit drinks.

HEALING HERB TEAS

Caffeinated green and black teas and coffee are not good for a Candida diet, but herb teas can be a wonderful substitute. Some health experts feel herb teas should be avoided because of possible mold content. Mold can be found on anything, including vegetables; my experience shows that herb teas are not detrimental if precautions are taken. (Consult your own health specialist for advice on this if desired.)

First, avoid tea bags. These can hide inferior teas and mold. Second, choose bulk or loose teas that are pre-packaged and sold in airtight bags or boxes. The kinds that are not pre-packaged and are found in jars or bagged in stores are more likely to pick up bacteria and dirt or become moldy in damp weather or wet store conditions. Third, inspect your teas before preparing and discard or return any that appear moldy or inferior or that have improper scents. (Get advice on teas if you are not sure how good they are.) Fourth, heat teas properly so that minor bacteria is killed in the boiling water. Use spring water for the most beneficial teas. When in doubt as to the purity of a tea, as with questionable water, serve the tea with a squirt or teaspoon of fresh lemon or lime juice. Then you can rest assured that your tea will not be affected by mold and it is as pure as any cooked food can be. The best-quality herb teas are organic and can be purchased through a local health food store. Follow the directions in the next sections for making tea and avoid all teas not mentioned here unless they are recommended by your doctor or health specialist!

Herbal Teas (enjoy often)	*Attributes*
Peppermint leaves	Good digestive aid, very mild stimulant
Spearmint leaves	Good digestive aid
Lemon grass	High in vitamin A
Raspberry leaves	High in vitamin C, good for female organs
Strawberry leaves	High in vitamin C
Fennel seeds	Good for digestion, relief of gas
Fenugreek seeds	For internal healing/intestines
Alfalfa seeds (or leaves)	High in chlorophyll, good for arthritis too
Senna leaves and flaxseed	Good laxative (not for everyday)
Slippery elm powdered bark	For sore throats, colds, flu
Taheebo or pau d'arco root	Helps kill Candida (strong), take as directed by health specialist (recipe follows)

For Medicinal Purposes

Use these teas only if your doctor or health specialist suggests (these are potent teas)!

Burdock root	Ginseng
Comfrey leaves	Eucalyptus
Ginger root	Licorice root
Goldenseal	

Avoid Completely	*Reasons*
Black, green, caffeinated teas (includes jasmine and Asian teas)	Caffeine aggravates Candida
Powdered, crushed, or whole rose hips	Parasites love mild red herbs
Uncooked chamomile, lavender, hibiscus, red clover, other flower teas	Flower teas feed Candida; some of these may also aggravate allergies
All other teas not listed here, unless recommended by your doctor or health specialist	

How to Make Herb Teas

Leaf Teas

Use 1 teaspoon of loose tea per cup. Steep only. Boiling makes leaf tea bitter and also kills valuable vitamins and enzymes. To steep: Boil the water. When it comes to a bubbling boil, remove the water from the heat (put in a tea pot if desired), add the tea to the water, stir, and cover the pot. Let it steep (sit) for 8 to 12 minutes. Strain and drink. A tea ball may be used for leaf teas only. Leftovers can be refrigerated up to 5 days and must be heated just up to boiling to serve again. Reheat only once.

Seed or Twig Teas

Use ¼ to ½ teaspoon loose tea per cup. Bring water and tea to a boil together and let it boil on just a low bubble for 5 to 10 minutes. Let it steep for another 10 minutes off the heat. Strain and drink. Leftovers can be refrigerated up to 5 days and must be heated just up to boiling to serve again. Reheat only once.

Root or Bark Tea

Use ¼ to ½ teaspoon root or bark broken or chopped into small pieces per cup. Make sure tea is broken up as much as possible. As with seed and twig tea, the water and tea should be brought to a boil together and kept at a low bubble. However, it should be on a low bubble for 15 to 20 minutes (instead of 5 to 10). Steep for 10 minutes. Strain and drink. Leftovers can be refrigerated up to 5 days and must be heated just up to boiling to serve again. Reheat only once.

Powdered Root or Powdered Bark Tea

Use ⅒ to ⅛ teaspoon powdered tea per cup (unless your health care specialist recommends differently). Mix the tea well in the water before heating. Then bring it to a boil and keep it on a low bubble for 20 to 30 minutes. No steeping or straining required. Leftovers can be refrigerated up to 7 or 8 days and must be heated up to boiling and simmered a few minutes before serving again. Reheat only once.

Herb Tea Bags

Do not use any tea bags except for taheebo tea. Follow box directions for taheebo tea bags or see recipe.

HOW TO MAKE HERB TEA COMBINATIONS

When making an herb tea combination, special care must be taken not to overcook the teas. For example, when making a combination of twig and leaf tea, one cannot boil the leaf tea with the twig tea or the tea will become bitter and lose vitamins. Leaf tea should never be boiled! The twig tea should be low-boiled by itself and the leaf tea should be added to the boiled twig tea during the steeping time only. Teas can be poured over fresh mint leaves or lemon or lime wedges. Do not use dried orange peels or other dried citrus peels, cinnamon, or other spices in teas during Candida treatment!

Sample Herb Tea Combinations

Use equal parts of each of the following:

1. Peppermint and alfalfa
2. Spearmint and strawberry or raspberry leaves
3. Peppermint, alfalfa, and lemon grass

4. Raspberry leaves and alfalfa poured over fresh lemon rounds (tastes a lot like regular caffeinated tea)
5. Fennel seeds and alfalfa leaves
6. Fenugreek seeds and mint leaves
7. Peppermint and slippery elm powder
8. Create your own combinations with no more than 2 to 4 teas.

Caution: Stick with the teas mentioned here or recommended by your doctor or health specialist. Some herb teas have strong medicinal powers and can cause stomach upset, headaches, or nausea if used incorrectly.

Taheebo or Pau d'Arco Tea

2 teaspoons Taheebo tea (measure   2½ cups water
   loose tea or tea torn out of tea bags)

Use a nonmetal pot. Any metal pot, including stainless steel, is claimed to interfere with the medicinal qualities of certain herbal teas, especially this one. Therefore, use a Corningware or uncracked, enamel pot (not glass, because of possible lead content), if possible, for simmering this tea. Avoid black or speckled enamel pots. Bring water and tea to a boil together and let it boil on just a low bubble for 25 to 30 minutes. Strain and drink. Drink about 1 cup daily or as directed by a health specialist. Keeps refrigerated for 2 days and may be reheated to serve. Purchase at health food stores or pharmacies that carry natural remedies.

JUICES

No bottled or canned juices may be drunk on a Candida diet. These may contain bacteria or mold that can feed the yeast. Absolutely no nonacid fruit or sweet, sugared, honeyed, naturally or unnaturally sweetened drinks (or foods) of any kind may be consumed. Anything sweet feeds the yeast!

Fresh citrus juice, except for orange juice (which is alkaline in the system and feeds the yeast), may be squeezed fresh and enjoyed if drunk soon after. (See recipes.) Fresh juice can be stored up to 8 hours, the same as vegetable juice, if desired. Acidic juices (lemon, lime, tomato, unsweetened cranberry) should not be swished and held in the mouth like vegetable juices, as they may damage the teeth and do not require digestive enzymes from the mouth.

Grateful for Grapefruit Juice

6 to 10 ounces fresh squeezed white
    grapefruit juice (not red)
Optional: 1 ounce lemon or lime juice,
    or lemon or lime wedge

Optional: ice cubes
Optional garnish: fresh mint leaves

Make the juice fresh just before serving. Pour over ice and garnish if desired. If grapefruit tastes a bit sweet, adding fresh lemon or lime juice as required. Drink as soon as possible within the hour. Do not store. Enjoy a maximum of 2 to 5 glasses per week of any fresh grapefruit drinks.

BE WARY OF THE GRAPEFRUIT JUICE EFFECT

BY DR. RONA

If you swallow prescription pills with grapefruit juice, there is something very important that you should know. Grapefruit juice can intensify the effects of some drugs because it can block the first phase of liver detoxification. This grapefruit juice effect is attributed to a constituent of grapefruit juice called naringenin. Naringenin inhibits an enzyme called cytochrome P450, which is found not only in the liver but also in the wall of the intestines. Naringenin gives grapefruit juice its characteristic color and flavor.

Studies by Canadians Dr. David Bailey, Dr. Malcolm Arnold, and Dr. J. David Spence indicate that the consumption of grapefruit juice may have a significant effect on raising the blood levels of certain drugs like the antihistamine terfenadine (Seldane). Seldane remains on the Canadian market despite it being implicated in at least 125 deaths. Seldane now requires a prescription. Fatal heart arrhythmias might develop in given individuals as a direct result of the sustained high blood levels of this drug. The grapefruit juice effect is variable among individuals, with drug levels being boosted anywhere from three to six times.

Besides terfenadine, other drugs affected by grapefruit juice are the calcium channel blocker nifedipine (Adalat), the anti-rejection drug cyclosporin, prescription estrogens, and the sedative triazolam (Halcion). Calcium channel blockers are used to control high blood pressure and angina. Nifedipine is one of the controversial calcium channel-blocking drugs associated with a greater risk of fatal heart attacks and cancer in several American studies. Blood levels of these drugs can jump as much as six-fold in some individuals after drinking grapefruit juice.

If you must take any of these drugs, the best advice is to avoid grapefruit juice even within 24 hours of taking the tablets or capsules. Use water or vegetable juice to help swallow the prescriptions since it will not have any significant effect on the blood levels of any of the drugs in question. It is always a good policy to consult a knowledgeable pharmacist about drug–nutrient interactions when taking any prescription or over-the-counter drug.

UNSWEETENED CRANBERRY JUICE

This juice can only be purchased at health food stores and can be quite pricey. It can be heated and cooled/chilled just like tomato juice, or if your doctor permits, it can be drunk poured right out of the bottle.

If juice quality is questionable, do heat it or add a teaspoon or two of fresh lemon or lime juice to it before drinking.

Warmed Tomato Juice

8 to 10 ounces bottled (or canned) tomato juice (no Clamato)

Optional: 2 teaspoons lemon or lime juice

Optional: few dashes cayenne

Optional: 1 stalk celery

Heat the tomato juice to boiling and simmer for 3 to 5 minutes to kill any bacteria, with the cayenne (if any). If celery is used, chop and heat it with the tomato juice, blend it raw in a blender with the juice before serving, or use as a raw stir stick. Serve hot or quick-chill in the freezer for 15 to 20 minutes. Serve immediately. Although used as a vegetable, tomatoes are actually an acidic fruit, like grapefruit, and a helpful digestive aid for meats and dairy products. This acidic drink should not be drunk alone. Eat with plain acidophilus yogurt, or, unlike other drinks, this may be enjoyed with a meat meal or nut butter appetizer/snack. Because the tomatoes have been heated, this can also be enjoyed with a whole grain/legume meal or with vegetables. If possible, add the citrus juice for extra antibacterial protection. Tomato juice, like other citrus, should not be swished in the mouth as it is too acidic and can be harmful if left on the teeth.

Warmed Mixed Vegetable Juices

8 to 10 ounces bottled (or canned) mixed vegetable juices (V-8 allowed), unsweetened without additives

Optional: 2 teaspoons lemon or lime juice

Optional: few dashes cayenne

Optional: 1 stalk celery

Prepare the same as tomato juice. Be sure not to use any juices with sweetening included in the blend!

Fresh Vegetable Juices

Most nonstarchy vegetables (starchy includes yams, winter squash, turnips, parsnips) acceptable for the Candida diet may be juiced and drunk, provided no more than 8 to 12 ounces total are enjoyed daily, five to six days per week maximum, unless your doctor suggests otherwise. (Or drink two glasses every other day, eight hours apart.) The body was not meant to "drink" dozens of vegetables in one day. Humans cannot digest too many juices. Each sip of vegetable juice should be savored. Swish the juices in the mouth so they can absorb more digestive enzymes in the saliva and drink them slowly. It should take at least 20 minutes to drink one glass of vegetable juice. Put it in a wine glass if that helps to slow your drinking down; it adds a bit of fun and elegance as well. Some raw vegetable juices like brussels sprouts, cabbage, and green peppers contribute to gas for certain people, so should be avoided. Drink sparingly or in combination with complementary vegetables that counteract flatulence (such as tomato or beet).

Only fresh-squeezed vegetable juices should be drunk; however, some bottled or canned juices can be heated (see recipes and buying guide), simmered, and quick-cooled in the freezer before drinking. (Do not freeze.) Fresh-squeezed juices that are not drunk immediately can be put in a sealed glass jar that has been run under or dipped in very hot water and cooled, filled, refrigerated immediately, and enjoyed up to four to eight hours later. Use organic vegetables (from health food stores) for juicing, always, if available. Enjoy the vegetable juice combinations as follows and see the juicer books in the Recommended Reading section for more ideas.

Carrot and Beet Juice

4 to 5 medium organic carrots, scrubbed with tips cut off

1 small or medium beet, scrubbed with tips cut off

Use chilled carrots from the refrigerator. Wash and cut the vegetables into sections that will fit into your juicer. Cold vegetables retain more vitamins while being juiced and they taste better juiced as well. If you are constipated, increase the beet to 2 small or 1 large. If your bowels are too loose, substitute the beet for celery or another green vegetable. (Maximum 5 to 6 glasses per week total for vegetable juices of any kind or combination, unless your doctor recommends.)

Vegetable Juice Combinations

1. ½ part carrot, ¼ part beet, ¼ part celery.
2. ½ part carrot, ¼ part celery, ¼ part zucchini.
3. ½ part carrot, ¼ part celery or zucchini, ¼ part red bell pepper; optional: 1 small garlic clove.
4. ¾ part green or Savoy cabbage juice, ¼ part beet; optional: 1 wedge onion.
5. ⅓ part carrot, ⅓ part broccoli or brussels sprouts, ⅓ part beet. (This combo can be gassy for some, but the beet helps make it more digestible.)
6. Create your own combinations with no more than 3 to 4 vegetables.

7. Try adding 1 to 2 tablespoons wheat grass juice or barley green juice (or ¼ to ½ teaspoon of wheat grass powder or barley powder) to any of the previous combinations if these are available and approved by your health specialist. It requires a special kind of juicer to make either of these two green juices.

Vegetable Juice and Yogurt (with Dairy)

4 to 6 ounces Acidophilus Yogurt, cold

4 to 6 ounces organic carrot juice or vegetable juice combination

Optional: 1 to 2 tablespoons wheat grass juice or barley green juice

Whiz the ingredients together lightly in a blender; drink slowly and enjoy. Do not store. (Blender will take the chill off the yogurt.)

MILK SUBSTITUTES

DAIRY-FREE MILKS

Dairy-free milk substitutes are not equally nutritious dietary substitutes for cow's milk. These dairy-free drinks or "milks" are intended to look and taste a little like dairy milk when used in recipes, for those allergic to dairy or those who need to avoid it for specific health concerns. It is beneficial to avoid milk for Candida albicans healing diets; cooked milk is okay for some individuals. (See Milk in Controversial Foods.) The following "milks" are for use in recipes only. They are not to be drunk separately unless heated up to a boil and simmered first. These milk substitutes are unsweetened and plain and are not very tasty as beverages. Lightly sweetened milk substitutes (without dried or liquid cane juice) can be made or purchased and used sparingly in recipes cooked for 20 minutes or more on a Candida diet.

> *Purchased milk substitutes for recipes only:*
> Unsweetened rice milk (or lightly sweetened)
> Unsweetened soy milk (or lightly sweetened)
> Unsweetened oat milk

Unsweetened almond milk
Unsweetened sesame or sunflower milk
Avoid all others, especially coconut milk in any form!

Blanched Almond Nut Milk (for Recipes)

1 cup water

3 to 4 tablespoons ground, raw blanched almond pieces

Blend ingredients thoroughly in a blender for several minutes, until the water becomes white. Strain if necessary and stir well before using. Keeps several days in the refrigerator or may be frozen for later use. (Grind blanched almonds alone, ¼ cup at a time, in the blender, ¾ to 1 cup at a time in a food processor, or grind in coffee mill.) Use only in cooking.

Soy Milk for Recipes

2 cups water

5 to 6 tablespoons instant soy milk powder

Blend ingredients well and stir before each use. Keeps a few days in the refrigerator. Use in cooking only. Avoid if allergic. Be sure not to overuse soy milk or soy products; they are best if rotated and used only every other day or so.

Alfalfa Milk for Recipes

1 cup alfalfa sprouts

Water

Rinse the sprouts thoroughly and cut off the brown seed hulls and the tiny root tips. Blend the sprouts in the blender with just enough water to keep the blades turning well and create a "milk." Add extra water if necessary to create the desired consistency. Straining is optional. Use immediately or within 1 to 2 hours (refrigerate until ready to use). Do not store. Use only in cooking.

Zucchini Milk for Recipes

1 cup grated small zucchini   Water

Choose firm, fresh, bright green and white zucchini. The dark or yellowish ones are bitter. Peel zucchini if desired. Blend the grated zucchini in the blender with just enough water to keep the blades turning well and create a thick, white "milk." Add extra water for desired consistency or strain if needed. Use immediately or within 1 to 2 hours (refrigerate until ready to use). Do not store. Use only in cooking.

Chapter 13

SNACKS AND MUNCHIES THAT DO NOT FEED THE YEAST

An endless array of snacks and munchies can be enjoyed on a Candida diet. Each vegetable provides many recipe options. Legumes, tofu, nuts, and seeds in various combinations can be used to create literally hundreds of possibilities. Yes, hundreds! To beat the cravings, enjoy the following taste treats and use your imagination to create many more recipes. There is no need to starve, go hungry, or suffer from insatiable cravings. Make up several of the longer-lasting snacks and keep them on hand so there is no need to cheat on your diet. Cheating creates setbacks and delays healing.

HOW TO HANDLE CONSTANT CRAVINGS

As Candida yeast die, they get hungry and disruptive. The yeast can agitate the body and contribute to stomach upset, a bit of nausea, and, of course, cravings. It helps to assume that the yeast are the ones urging you to cheat on your diet, coaxing you to want the foods you cannot have. Even if you follow the diet guidelines and eat two to three regular meals a day, a reasonable amount of snacks, and meet your nutritional needs, you still may crave more foods or undesirable foods: undesirable for a Candida diet, even if they seem desirable to your mind, memory, and taste buds!

Even when you eat enough and eat all the right foods, you may have to learn to ignore regular, even constant, cravings. A pregnant woman may crave pickles and ice cream, but that does not mean she needs them, or that they are good for her, or that they taste good together. After finishing a Candida diet, you will almost assuredly find that you dislike some foods you previously enjoyed. Your tastes (taste buds) will change and you will usually appreciate and enjoy new and different foods of higher quality. Your body will thank you with improved health, energy, and stamina.

When the cravings hit, think of them as temptation from the yeast rather than as real cravings. The yeast want you to feed them junk food—and they will try anything to get you to do it! When you refuse, they get agitated and in turn agitate you. Learn to ignore them and stick with your diet game plan. Do not give in to them. They want control of your body. Say no! Eat only enough, of the foods you require. Eating constantly, even good foods, can overload the digestive tract, possibly damage it, and slow down the healing process. Keep involved in work, household projects, hobbies, exercise, social activities, and rest as needed. Have things to do besides eat and think about food! Do hand work to resist a tendency to put food in your mouth. When you do eat, eat slowly and savor it.

Keep a supply of wholesome foods at home, in the refrigerator and the freezer. Treat yourself to a variety of foods to grab that are good for your diet. Choose these rather than those that are not beneficial for the Candida diet.

The process of cooking can actually reduce your desire to eat. As you prepare food, munch on veggies, and taste sauces and recipes, your desire to eat more food is reduced just by being around it.

Cravings are a fact of life. What you do about them makes all the difference. Learn to look behind your cravings to see what they really mean. Is the body saying you need food and nutrients? Or are dying yeast begging for goodies that make them strong and keep them alive? As healing takes place in the body, nature's real cravings will surface, sort themselves out, and you will know which foods your body really wants and needs. Until that time, trust this book's guidelines, your doctor's advice, and your own knowledge and common sense. The Candida program teaches body wisdom. Even tough situations can have fringe benefits!

SNACKS AND MUNCHIES THAT DO NOT FEED THE YEAST

LAST-MINUTE RECIPE TIPS

Not every recipe may be perfect for you. If you are allergic or sensitive to particular ingredients in these or any recipes, or your doctor recommends you avoid certain foods, see the Substitution Chart in chapter 11. Use digestive aids and laxative teas if you have trouble digesting certain foods. It is better to eat the foods and use digestion aids than to starve yourself. You need the nutrients from these good foods to heal so that some day you will not require digestive aids.

SNACK, LUNCH, APPETIZER, AND PARTY RECIPES

HOME-ROASTED NUTS

Purchased, roasted nuts are not good for those with Candida. Besides containing toxic solvent processed oils, roasting nuts in oil makes them high in calories, a great breeding ground for Candida and bacteria, destructive to the digestive tract and indigestible for many people. Buy only raw nuts and cook them yourself at home without oil.

Choose quality organic nuts if available and reasonably priced. The best choices are almonds and filberts (hazelnuts). These can be roasted whole by placing in a single layer, in a low, dry baking dish and baked in a preheated oven at 350°F for 7 to 10 minutes. After the first 3 minutes, stir or turn the nuts with a metal spatula every 2 minutes. Remove when lightly browned. Pecans and Brazil nuts are the next best choices and can be baked whole, single-layered, in a preheated oven at 325°F for 4 to 7 minutes, turning twice.

Chopped or slivered raw nuts may be roasted in a dry pan in a preheated oven at 300°F for 4 to 8 minutes, depending on the size of the nuts and how they are layered. Stir or turn every 2 minutes or so. Recipes (except for pie crusts) calling for ground nuts may use Home-Roasted Nuts (that are ground) for added flavor if desired. Home-Roasted Nuts do not need salt or flavorings. They taste delicious all by themselves.

It is best only to eat nuts when cooked into recipes. Handfuls of nuts are extremely hard to digest and may interfere with healing. Those with stronger stomachs may enjoy a well-chewed handful of freshly made Home-Roasted Nuts one to four times per month. Consult your health specialist to determine what is right for you.

HOME-ROASTED SEEDS

Like nuts, seeds can be roasted for added flavor and to help kill mold and bacteria. Toast whole (shelled) pumpkin, sunflower, and sesame seeds in a preheated 300°F oven for 6 to 10 minutes, stirring at least twice. As with nuts, toasted seeds can be used in most recipes (except pie crusts). Toasted seeds have a richer flavor than raw seeds. As with nuts, these are best eaten mainly in recipes rather than by the handful.

Tasty Tamari Nuts

1 cup nuts or hulled seeds, whole
    or lightly chopped

Optional: Few dashes cayenne

3 to 4 tablespoons tamari soy sauce
    (low-salt, wheat-free), or Mock
    Tamari Soy Sauce (page 453)

Chop the nuts lightly, if desired. In a medium frying pan, heat the tamari on medium-high heat and let simmer for 3 to 4 minutes to kill any bacteria that might feed the yeast. Some will evaporate. That is why extra tamari is used in the recipe. Use Mock Tamari Soy Sauce if you prefer to avoid soy or fermented products. Add the nuts or seeds once the tamari has simmered.

Stir constantly until the nuts absorb all the tamari. Add cayenne for a delicious, tangy accent. Cook for 4 to 7 minutes more, until hot throughout. Enjoy warm all by themselves, but chew thoroughly and eat only as a rare treat, once a week or less often.

Nut and Olive Dip

7 to 8 ounces regular tofu, cut in
    small chunks

½ cup black olives

⅓ cup Home-Roasted Nuts
    (page 302)

3 to 4 tablespoons fresh lemon juice

2 to 3 tablespoons chopped chives or
    green onion tops

1 tablespoon natural oil (toasted
    sesame or olive)

¼ teaspoon sea salt

Pre-steam the tofu and olives for 5 to 6 minutes. Combine all ingredients in a food processor until smooth. Chill and serve as a dip with raw or steamed vegetable.

Keeps for 3 to 4 days refrigerated. Must be warmed and cooled each time before eating. Do not freeze.

Nut and Artichoke Dip

Follow directions for Nut and Olive Dip. Instead of black olives, use ½ cup chopped artichoke hearts packed in water. Drain and rinse the hearts. Chop and steam for 5 to 6 minutes before using in the recipe.

Nut Butter Vegetable Dip

2½ cups asparagus, broccoli, or
    carrots, chopped, or 3 cups
    packed spinach

½ cup sesame tahini, or nut but-
    ter (sunflower, almond, or fil-
    bert)

3 to 4 teaspoons finely chopped fresh
    parsley, or 2 teaspoons dried

½ teaspoon *each* basil and dill weed
    (add ½ teaspoon tarragon for car-
    rots)

½ teaspoon sea salt

Several dashes *each* sea kelp and
cayenne

Optional: 1 small clove garlic, pressed,
    or ½ teaspoon prepared
    horseradish

Steam vegetable until tender. Heat the tahini or nut butter with the seasonings in a saucepan on low heat until hot throughout (or bake it). Combine all ingredients in a food processor until smooth. Serve with raw or steamed vegetable dippers as a snack, or use warmed, served over whole grains as a main dish.

Keeps 1 to 3 days refrigerated; must be reheated in a saucepan or baked to serve again. Do not freeze.

Spinach Tofu Dip

1 pound spinach (2 cups firmly packed)

7 to 8 ounces regular tofu, cut into small chunks

2 teaspoons tamari soy sauce, or Mock Tamari Soy Sauce

1 tablespoon fresh or dried parsley

½ to 1 teaspoon finely chopped raw onion or prepared horseradish, or ½ to 1 small clove garlic, pressed

1 teaspoon *each* dill weed and basil

½ teaspoon paprika

¼ teaspoon *each* oregano, marjoram, and thyme

Several dashes *each* sea kelp and cayenne

Optional: ½ cup Home-Roasted Nuts or Seeds, or steamed black olives

Steam the spinach alongside the tofu, 10 to 12 minutes for the spinach until tender, 6 to 8 minutes for the tofu. Bring the tamari, seasonings, and 1 to 2 teaspoons water to a boil in a tiny pan and simmer for 4 to 5 minutes. Combine the spinach, tofu, nuts (if any), and the remaining ingredients in a food processor or food mill until smooth. (A blender can be used if a few drops of water are used as needed; stop and stir the mixture several times.) Serve the dip with raw or steamed vegetables.

Leftovers keep for 1 to 2 days refrigerated but must be reheated before each serving. Do not freeze.

Carrot Tofu Dip

Follow the directions for the previous Spinach Tofu Dip, but use 2 cups chopped carrots (about 4 to 5 medium) instead of the spinach. Add 1 teaspoon tarragon.

Artichoke or Asparagus Tofu Dip

Follow directions for the previous Spinach Tofu Dip, but use 2 cups chopped asparagus or chopped artichoke hearts packed in water, drained, instead of the spinach.

Fiesta Spinach Tofu Dip

1 pound (2 cups firmly packed) spinach

7 to 8 ounces regular tofu, cut into small chunks

2 teaspoons tamari soy sauce, or Mock Tamari Soy Sauce

1 tablespoon fresh or dried parsley

½ to 1 teaspoon finely chopped raw onion or prepared horseradish

1 teaspoon *each* dill weed and basil

½ teaspoon paprika

½ teaspoon *each* oregano, marjoram, and thyme

Several dashes *each* sea kelp and cayenne

Optional: ½ cup Home-Roasted Nuts

½ cup chopped water chestnuts or mung bean sprouts

1 small red bell pepper, chopped

Optional: ¼ to ½ cup sliced olives

Steam the spinach alongside the tofu, 10 to 12 minutes for the spinach until tender, 6 to 8 minutes for the tofu. Bring tamari, seasonings, and 1 to

2 teaspoons water to a boil in a tiny pan and simmer for 4 to 5 minutes. Combine spinach, tofu, nuts (if any), and all but the last three ingredients in a food processor or food mill until smooth. (A blender can be used if a few drops of water are used as needed; stop blender and stir the mixture several times.)

Steam the water chestnuts or mung beans, and olives (if any), for 4 minutes. Cut the red pepper and steamed vegetables into small (¼- to ⅓-inch) pieces and add to spinach mixture. Serve the dip with raw or steamed vegetables.

Leftovers keep for 1 to 2 days refrigerated but must be reheated before each serving. Do not freeze.

Fiesta Carrot Tofu Dip

Follow directions for the previous Fiesta Spinach Tofu Dip, but use 2 cups chopped carrots (about 4 to 5 medium) instead of spinach. Add 1 teaspoon tarragon. Instead of the red bell pepper, use ¾ to 1 cup celery or green (or yellow) bell pepper, cut into ½- to ¾-inch pieces.

Fiesta Artichoke or Asparagus Tofu Dip

Follow directions for the previous Fiesta Spinach Tofu Dip, but use 2 cups chopped asparagus or chopped artichoke hearts packed in water, drained, instead of the spinach.

Homemade Salsa

1 to 2 tablespoons olive oil or other natural oil

1 cup (1 medium) onion, finely chopped

2 to 3 cloves garlic, minced

1 green or red bell pepper, diced

2 cups tomatoes, diced

2 tablespoons finely chopped fresh parsley or cilantro

2½ tablespoons fresh lemon juice

1 teaspoon honey or maple syrup, or 1 tablespoon apple juice (or peach, pear, or apricot)*

1 teaspoon *each* oregano and cumin powder

½ teaspoon sea salt

3 ounces (6 tablespoons) tomato paste

1 to 3 jalapeños or other hot peppers, finely chopped

Optional: Cayenne (add after simmering)

Heat the oil until hot and sauté the onions and garlic for 2 minutes. Add bell pepper and tomatoes; sauté for 3 to 4 minutes. Add the remaining ingredients and simmer for 7 to 10 minutes, covered, on medium-low heat.

Use hot in recipes or quick-chill in the freezer. Add cayenne to taste if hotter salsa is required. Keeps refrigerated for 6 to 8 days or may be frozen. Reheat and simmer for 3 to 5 minutes each time before reusing in recipes. Do not use store-bought salsas! They usually contain vinegar and sometimes marinated products.

---

*Cook at least 15 minutes, preferably 20, and Candida will not be affected.

Guacamole

1 medium ripe avocado, peeled
  and pitted

3 to 5 teaspoons fresh lemon juice

1 teaspoon minced or pressed
  onion or prepared horseradish,
  or ¼ cup finely chopped chives
  or green onion tops

2 teaspoons finely chopped fresh
  parsley or cilantro

Sea salt to taste

Few dashes *each* sea kelp and cayenne

Optional: 8 to 14 sliced black olives,
  steamed 4 to 5 minutes

Optional: ½ to 1 small clove garlic,
  pressed

Mash the avocado with the lemon juice and seasonings; add the olives if desired. Chill and serve with raw or steamed vegetable dippers. Consume within 12 to 24 hours. Keep refrigerated in between.

Cauliflower Curry Dip

1 cup chopped cauliflower

¼ cup milk substitute

1 small clove garlic, minced

1 teaspoon curry powder

¼ teaspoon finely chopped onion

¼ teaspoon *each* sea salt and cumin

Few dashes ginger

Couple dashes cayenne

Optional: ¼ teaspoon turmeric for yellow color

Steam the cauliflower until tender. Heat the milk substitute and seasonings and simmer for 3 to 4 minutes (to kill bacteria). Combine all the ingredients in a food processor until smooth. Stop and stir if required. Serve warm, or chill for 30 to 60 minutes, covered. Enjoy with raw or steamed vegetable dippers.

Best eaten in one sitting; however, it can be stored for up to 2 to 3 days and baked to reheat. Note: Optional added turmeric can be agitating to some individuals, especially those with allergies. However, it may be healing for certain health problems as well.

Sweet Orange Yam Dip

2 cups chopped orange yams (peeled
or unpeeled), rinsed 2 to 3 times

Flavorings #1

¼ to ½ teaspoon cinnamon

1 to 3 teaspoons butter or natural oil

Couple dashes nutmeg

Couple dashes allspice or cloves

Sea salt to taste

Optional: 2 to 4 tablespoons ground
Home-Roasted Nuts or
Seeds

Flavorings #2

½ cup finely chopped onion, sautéed
in 1 to 2 teaspoons butter or natural
oil

1 tablespoon simmered tamari soy
sauce, or substitute

Cayenne and sea salt to taste

Optional: 2 to 4 tablespoons ground
Home-Roasted Nuts or
Seeds

Rinse the cut orange yam thoroughly and steam until very tender, almost mushy. Use a food processor or small-holed hand masher to mix all the ingredients in Flavorings #1 or #2 with the steamed yam. Serve hot and enjoy with raw or steamed vegetable dippers. Keeps for 3 to 5 days refrigerated. Do not freeze. Can be reheated in a saucepan, or baked.

Black Bean Dip

1 cup dried black beans, soaked*

1 cup (1 medium) chopped onion

2 to 4 cloves garlic, minced

3 tablespoons finely chopped fresh parsley, or 1 tablespoon dried

½ cup Brown Bean Juice, from the black beans (page 380)

½ to ¾ teaspoon sea salt

½ teaspoon ground cumin (cominos)

Several dashes sea kelp

Cayenne to taste

Optional: 2 to 3 teaspoons finely chopped jalapeños or other hot peppers

Optional: 1 cup chopped tomatoes or Homemade Salsa

Optional: 1 to 2 scallions, chopped very fine

Optional: 1 red bell pepper, diced

Cook the soaked beans until tender. Add the onion and garlic and cook with the beans, 20 minutes or more. Drain; save all but the ½ cup bean juice for other recipes. Use a food processor to combine all the main ingredients and jalapeños or hot peppers (if any). Process until smooth; thin with extra bean juice for thinner dip if you choose. Serve the dip topped with one or more of the optional ingredients and guacamole, if desired. Eat with raw or steamed vegetable dippers. Try, occasionally, with Chickpea Chapatis (page 455).

Keeps for 6 to 7 days refrigerated and freezes well (without toppings). Bake to reheat before each serving. Add 1 to 2 teaspoons water when reheating if too dry.

---

* Pinto, kidney, adzuki, or red beans can be substituted.

Fat-Reduced Falafel Spread

1 cup dried chickpeas, soaked

¼ cup sesame tahini (drain oil before measuring)

2 to 3 cloves garlic, pressed or minced

2 to 3 teaspoons very finely chopped or pressed onion

3 to 5 teaspoons simmered tamari soy sauce or Mock Tamari Soy Sauce

2 to 3 tablespoons fresh chopped parsley or 2 to 3 teaspoons dried

1 teaspoon cumin seeds

1 teaspoon chili powder, or 1 teaspoon Your Own Chili Powder (page 449)

½ to ¾ teaspoon sea salt

¼ teaspoon *each* sea kelp, celery seed, and cumin powder

Several dashes cayenne, to taste

Cook the chickpeas until very tender; drain and save the liquid. While the chickpeas are still quite hot, mash them with the remaining ingredients. Add ½ to 1 cup of the reserved cooking liquid as needed to make a spreading consistency and adjust herbs and spices to taste.

Traditionally, falafel balls are deep-fried, but this is an unnecessary addition of fats to the diet. Sesame tahini is also oily and the oil is poured off here and the typical tahini amount cut in half. The falafel retains a special flavor with added seasonings.

This spread is delicious as a hot side dish for meals with vegetables and whole grains. It can be stuffed into celery or small tomatoes for a tasty appetizer or served with raw or steamed vegetable dippers. It can be baked to reheat and should be eaten warm. Keeps for 6 to 8 days refrigerated and freezes well. Falafel is a variation of hummus, excluded from this book as beans and lemon juice are not a good food combination and are difficult to digest.

Toasted Sunflower Paté

Dry ingredients

1½ cups raw ground sunflower seeds

½ cup amaranth or teff flour

3 to 4 teaspoons dried parsley flakes, crushed

1½ teaspoons dried basil, crushed

1 teaspoon sea salt

1 teaspoon dry ground mustard

1 teaspoon thyme, crushed

½ teaspoon sage leaves, well crushed, or ⅓ teaspoon powdered sage

¼ teaspoon sea kelp (important to flavor)

Several dashes cayenne

Optional: 1 tablespoon arrowroot powder

Wet ingredients

2¼ cups water, milk substitute, broth, or bouillon (unsalted)

⅓ cup natural oil

3 tablespoons tamari soy sauce or substitute, or 2 vegetable bouillon cubes with ¼ cup water

4 to 5 teaspoons prepared horseradish

1 tablespoon toasted sesame oil

1 cup finely grated carrot or orange yam (rinse yam 2 to 3 times)

Preheat the oven to 350°F. Mix dry ingredients together in a bowl. Mix all the wet ingredients together well and then mix in the carrot or yam. (If bouillon cubes are used, mash or blend them with the liquid first.) Add the dry ingredients to the wet and mix thoroughly. Oil a 9-inch glass pie plate and scoop in the paté mixture. Bake for 35 to 40 minutes until set and browned. Let cool for 1 to 2 hours, then chill thoroughly to set completely before serving. It is tastiest when served at room temperature.

Enjoy the paté as an appetizer, snack, or protein main dish. May be served alone or with a green salad and/or cooked vegetables with whole grains to make a complete meal. Great for picnics, lunches, or parties. Keeps for 6 to 7 days refrigerated or may be frozen in pie wedges. Unless coming from the freezer, paté must be reheated in the oven until hot throughout before serving again.

Toasted Almond or Filbert Paté

Follow directions for the Toasted Sunflower Paté. Substitute 1½ cups ground, raw almonds or filberts (hazelnuts) instead of the sunflower seeds. The grated vegetable can be the same or use 1 cup finely grated parsnip or small white and purple turnip.

Roasted Garlic

4 to 12 bulbs of regular garlic, preferably organic

Extra virgin olive oil

⅛ teaspoon parsley flakes, dried

⅛ teaspoon rosemary, crushed

⅛ teaspoon oregano

⅛ teaspoon basil

Pinch dill weed

Peel the extra layers of garlic skin off each bulb leaving each bulb in one piece. (Leave the skins on each individual clove within each bulb.) Slice the top tips, about ¼ inch or less, off each of the garlic cloves in each bulb and place the bulbs in a 2-inch deep baking dish, cut side up. Pour olive oil generously over each bulb, using at least 2 tablespoons on each bulb. Sprinkle each bulb generously with dried parsley flakes. Crush ⅛ tsp. rosemary over each bulb. Then sprinkle about ⅛ tsp. *each* of oregano and basil over each one. Add a pinch of dill weed on each, cover the baking dish tightly with aluminum foil, and bake in a pre-heated oven about 300 to 350°F for about one hour or until the garlic is completely tender and the aroma of the herbs fills the air.

Use this soft, mellow-tasting garlic as a spread instead of butter on flatbreads, on vegetables, and in all kinds of recipes for special flavor. Make a large batch and keep leftovers refrigerated. Reheat with a recipe or by baking alone in foil. This recipe is a delicious, nutritious addition to foods that gently discourages Candida.

Yogurt Nut Dip

½ cup plain yogurt

⅓ cup tahini or nut butter (sunflower, pumpkin seed, almond,
or filbert), heated and cooled

2 to 3 tablespoons fresh lemon juice

1½ tablespoons fresh chopped
parsley, or 1 teaspoon dried

1 small clove garlic, pressed

½ teaspoon dill

¼ teaspoon ground cumin

Several dashes cayenne

Acidophilus Yogurt is not necessary in this recipe because of the lemon juice; however, it may be used if desired. (See recipe below.) Mix all ingredients together well with a fork or wire whisk. Enjoy with raw or steamed vegetable dippers. This recipe cannot be reheated so try to eat it in one sitting, or add 1 to 2 teaspoons extra lemon juice or 1/16 teaspoon acidophilus powder to recipe before serving a second time. (Do not eat after second serving.) Keeps fresh, refrigerated, for 1 to 2 days. Do not freeze.

A. Yogurt / Acidophilus Yogurt

6 to 8 ounces quality plain yogurt

1/16 teaspoon acidophilus powder

Mix acidophilus powder into yogurt just before serving.

NOTE: Yogurt is the only dairy product besides butter that can be eaten raw on a Candida diet. However, it must be mixed with acidophilus powder, garlic or fresh lemon juice before consuming raw. This recipe will ensure that no unwanted bacteria in the yogurt survive when the yogurt is eaten. Enjoy Acidophilus "A. Yogurt" by itself or in all uncooked recipes calling for fresh, raw yogurt.

Yogurt and Carrot Juice Delight

3 to 4 ounces fresh organic carrot
   juice (or homemade refrigerated juice made within 12
   hours)

6 to 8 ounces Acidophilus Yogurt
   (page 315)

Optional: ¼ part of the carrot juice can
   be beet juice

Pour juice over yogurt and create a delicious snack or treat. Enjoy this lovely yogurt with a large spoon. This recipe makes one serving and should be eaten immediately once prepared. For better digestion, substitute ¼ part of the carrot juice with beet juice. Tastes naturally sweet.

Orange Yogurt Surprise

½ to ⅔ cup yams, butternut or buttercup squash, or carrots

2 to 3 dashes cinnamon

Optional: Sea salt to taste

8 ounces Acidophilus Yogurt
   (page 315)

Peel the yams or squash and rinse several times before steaming. Organic carrots do not need peeling or extra rinsing, just scrubbing. Steam the orange vegetable until very tender, then mash with cinnamon and/or sea salt. Scoop the yogurt over the hot mashed vegetable and enjoy. This recipe makes one serving and should be eaten immediately once prepared.

MORE SNACK RECIPES

Chapter 14

BREAKFASTS THAT ENERGIZE

SHOULD YOU EAT BREAKFAST? FOR DECADES, BREAKFAST has been proclaimed "the most important meal of the day." It has been said that breakfast should be "the largest meal of the day." This statement was made so long ago; at the time many people were laborers or farmers and worked 10-hour days. Today, people often work 8 hours a day or less and their jobs are sedentary office or clerical work. People no longer "put in a few good hours' work before breakfast." (There are some exceptions.)

These statements are not an attempt to discredit breakfast; it is an important meal. However, we must change with the times: Breakfast just is not what it used to be. Steak and eggs with pancakes for an early breakfast would put most people to sleep or weigh them down so much that they would not get much work done. Such a breakfast is far from energizing. Digestion takes a great deal of energy and that energy would be better spent on healing.

Big breakfasts are out for most individuals. A moderately sized, substantial, not-too-easy or difficult-to-digest meal is required. In our modern society, many people skip breakfast altogether. This works well for some but is impossible for others, who cannot function without morning sustenance. A wholesome healing diet requires two to three full meals daily and one or more snacks for most Americans and Canadians. (Different cultures and climates have specific needs that vary.)

Breakfast may be missed if this works better for your body type and individual health needs. My professional experience shows that most people with

Candida function and heal better and faster if breakfast is eaten. If breakfast is excluded, lunch must be eaten by noon each day for optimum health. At least one meal must be eaten daily by twelve o'clock (breakfast or lunch) for optimum health and healing! (This is if you sleep regular hours and are not a day sleeper/night worker. Then the rule changes to: Eat one meal within four to five hours after rising.)

If you eat fairly regular, proper, wholesome meals two to three times daily (and one to four snacks), you should not be starving when you wake up and your energy levels will be more consistent and stable and healing time will be faster.

A traditional breakfast such as coffee, pastry/Danish, dry sugared cereals, pancakes with syrup, and bacon or sausage is out! What is left to eat? There are actually many options. Many of them are not what you expect or are accustomed to. Difficult times require versatile measures.

The menus provided here are innovative, delicious, and nourishing breakfast alternatives.

BREAKFASTS FOR CANDIDA TREATMENT DIETS

During Candida treatments, the most wholesome breakfasts are:

1. Wholesome whole grain cereals with delicious vegetable or nut sauces. (See #6, for sauce options.)
2. Well-cooked eggs or tofu.
3. Special seed or whole grain pancakes, eaten alone or with unsweetened fruit sauces or cooked fruits. (Depends on Phase Diet.)
4. Special main dishes: Orange Yam Pie; Confetti Carrot Pie; Festival Vegetable Rice Pie; mock meatballs and burgers, with or without sauces; and other recipes that have morning appeal.
5. Soups and stews that are hearty, made with whole grains and are not too spicy or not mainly bean-based: Digest-Aid-Meal-in-a-Soup, Wild Rice Celery Soup, Broccoli Wild Rice Soup, Orange Yam or Carrot Soup, Rainbow Barley Soup.
6. Plates of starchy vegetables: cauliflower, spaghetti squash, butternut or buttercup squash, other winter squash or carrots, eaten alone with butter, sea salt, and seasonings, or with special sauces: Sesame Tahini and Ginger Sauce, Toasted Sesame Seed Sauce, Toasted Almond or Filbert Sauce,

Toasted Nut and Vegetable Sauce, Amorous Avocado Tofu Sauce, Orange Yam Sauce, Green Herb and Orange Yam Sauce, Savory Sweet Onion Sauce, Homemade Tomato Sauce, Mock Tomato Sauce.

Try these wholesome, tasty recipes for breakfast (or snacks) and watch your energy levels stabilize while your endurance levels rise. Healing is greatly assisted with these special morning breakfasts. Enjoy.

WHOLE GRAIN BREAKFAST CEREALS

Read How to Cook Whole Grains in chapter 11 before making any of these cereals if you want to have tasty, properly prepared cereals that are as nutritious as possible.

Tips for Preparing Breakfast Cereals

1. Do not mix too many different whole grain cereals together for each breakfast. This makes digestion more difficult. Have only one grain per meal, except on rare occasions when two may be mixed together. (Five-, seven-, and nine-grain cereals or breads are not really beneficial!)

2. Add 1 to 2 teaspoons ground seeds to breakfast cereals for added nutrients and flavor. Ground seeds can be Home Roasted or cooked into a cereal for at least 10 minutes. Add ground seeds or "meals" to cereals 1 to 5 times per week as desired. Flax meal is a helpful, mild digestive aid, high in many nutrients and healing omega-3 and -6 fatty acids. Ground sesame seeds add very high iron and high calcium, phosphorus, and good amounts of magnesium and vitamin A. Ground sunflower seeds add extra vitamins A and D, high iron and calcium, and very high phosphorus and potassium. Ground pumpkin seeds are a great antiparasite/antifungal food and are especially high in magnesium, phosphorus, and zinc with good amounts of vitamin A. (Pumpkin seeds and oil are also very beneficial for prostrate problems.)

3. Enjoy most whole grains with butter and sea salt or one of the tasty sauces recommended earlier.

Cooked Cereals

Amaranth Amaranth grain can be cooked as a breakfast cereal, but it is not that tasty. It is better to use the flour in recipes or to cook the amaranth with another grain. If desired, cook it in 2 times as much water for a rice-like texture, and 2½ to 3 times as much water for cereal or to add it to breads. Cook until tender, 15 to 20 minutes.

Quinoa (pronounced keen-wah) For brown quinoa, rinse thoroughly before cooking by rubbing the grains together well in a pot of water and changing the water 2 to 4 times. For white quinoa, one rubbing and rinsing is enough as this kind is already dry brushed to clean it. This helps to remove the saponin, which may irritate digestion or allergies. Once rinsed, this is a highly nutritious, very digestible, healing grain. (Some say it is actually a seed, yet experts still disagree on this.) For white quinoa, bring 2½ to 3½ cups water per 1 cup quinoa to a boil together on high heat, reduce the heat to low, and cook for 20 to 30 minutes, covered, until very tender for a porridge-like consistency. For brown quinoa, use 2½ cups water and cook for 10 to 15 minutes. See Quinoa with Zucchini or Broccoli, chapter 18, for detailed quinoa cooking information. Reheat quinoa like millet (see next entry).

Millet For a soft, cereal-like texture, use 3 to 4 cups water per 1 cup millet. (Washing the grain is optional.) Bring water and millet to a boil together. Turn down the heat and simmer, covered, for 55 to 65 minutes, until the millet breaks down and is very soft and mushy. To reheat millet, break it up gently with a fork and add a bit of extra water, heat on low for 10 to 15 minutes until hot throughout, and add flavorings.

Whole oats or whole rye Soak in 2½ cups water per 1 cup grain for several hours or overnight. Change the water and cook 1½ cups water to 1 cup grain for 45 to 60 minutes. The grains are usually a little bit chewy when done. Cook until fairly tender for the best digestion. Cook only one or two different grains together. Rye is rather heavy and is best mixed with another grain or seed. These grains reheat easily in a bit of water and do not stick. Use a food processor to blend cooked grains for easier digestion if needed.

Scotch oats or steel-cut oats For larger chunks of oat pieces, soak the oats in 2 times as much water for 2 to 4 hours. Drain the water and use 1¼ cups water per 1 cup Scotch oats. For tiny, well-chopped oat pieces, skip the pre-soaking and cook 1 cup oats in 1½ to 2 cups water. Heat up to a boil on high heat and reduce to low. Simmer for 20 minutes or until tender and no longer crunchy. Add a bit of extra water as needed to cook to perfection. Reheat like millet.

Sweet brown rice Cook and serve like brown rice (as follows), but use 2½ to 3½ cups water per 1 cup rice and cook it for 60 to 90 minutes, until tender. This short grain rice is naturally a little sweeter than other rices and makes a tasty breakfast grain. It reheats especially well.

Brown rice Short grain is tastier, but long grain may be used. Put the rice in a pot of water and rub it together with your fingers and swish it around to remove extra starch, dirt, and stray husks. Discard the water. If the water was very cloudy during the first washing, repeat the process once or twice until the water is relatively clear. Heat 3 to 4 cups water per 1 cup rice and bring it to a boil over high heat, then reduce heat to low, cover, and simmer for 75 to 90 minutes. When the rice is no longer crunchy but easy to chew and tender, not soggy, it is done. Extra water is used for breakfast rice along with extra cooking time. (Make a big batch ahead of time and reheat a serving for each meal.) Avoid most supermarket brown rices that cook quicker because some of the rice polish layers are removed.

Teff Bring ½ cup teff seed and 2 cups water to a boil, then turn down heat and simmer for 15 to 20 minutes, or until all the water is absorbed. Mix with another grain if desired for added flavor and texture; it is not especially tasty alone, like amaranth.

PANCAKE, TOFU, AND EGG BREAKFASTS

Amaranth or Teff Pancakes

Serves 2

For All Phases if doctor allows. Once weekly only for Phase II diets.

RECIPE 1. With Eggs

Wet Ingredients

2 tablespoons plus ½ teaspoon simmered apple, pear, or peach juice

3 large eggs, well beaten

⅔ cup water

1 tablespoon natural oil (like canola or sunflower)

Dry Ingredients

1½ cups amaranth or teff flour

¼ cup tapioca flour (or instant soy milk powder)

¼ cup arrowroot powder (or kudzu powder)

1 teaspoon Homemade Baking Powder (recipe follows)

¼ teaspoon sea salt

Optional: ¼ teaspoon cinnamon

RECIPE 2. Without Eggs

Wet Ingredients

3 tablespoons plus 1 teaspoon simmered apple, pear, or peach juice

1¼ cups water

1 tablespoon natural oil (like canola or sunflower)

Dry Ingredients

1½ cups amaranth or teff flour

¼ cup tapioca flour (or instant soy milk powder)

¼ cup arrowroot powder (or kudzu powder)

4 teaspoons Homemade Baking Powder (recipe follows)

¼ teaspoon sea salt

(Do not use cinnamon or rising may be hindered)

The juice must be simmered for 2 to 3 minutes and quick-chilled in the freezer for 5 to 10 minutes before using in this recipe. The juice has a bit extra added to make up for evaporation. Mix the wet ingredients together. In a separate bowl, mix the dry ingredients together.

Oil a frying pan and bring it quickly to medium-high heat. Add the dry ingredients to the wet and mix well. Add a bit of extra water or arrowroot powder if the batter is too thin or thick. Use a wire whisk to mix well.

Start making the pancakes immediately after the batter is mixed. Cook small pancakes for 60 to 90 seconds until the edges dry up a bit and large bubbles form, dissolve, and leave pockets in the batter. (Watch the heat or the pancakes will cook too fast and burn.) Turn over and cook another for 20 to 40 seconds or until well browned underneath. Do not flatten the pancakes when turning them! Turn again to check for readiness, then flatten if desired.

(continues)

Re-oil the frying pan generously before starting each new batch. Enjoy these pancakes with butter or Berry Berry Sauce or cooked fruit if allowed. Recipe makes about 18 to 20 pancakes. Keeps for 2 to 4 days refrigerated; may be reheated in an oven or toaster oven. Always eat warmed. May be frozen but are best fresh.

Whole Grain Pancakes
Phases I, III, and IV only

Use the Amaranth or Teff Pancakes recipe; instead of the amaranth or teff flour use 1½ cups of oat, buckwheat, millet, quinoa, or barley flour, or a combination of any two of these flours, ¾ cup each.

Homemade Baking Powder

2 tablespoons baking soda, potassium bicarbonate, or calcium bicarbonate

4 tablespoons arrowroot powder, tapioca flour, or kudzu powder

4 tablespoons cream of tartar, tartaric acid, or calcium phosphate (monobasic)

Put the ingredients in a clean flour sifter in the order given. Sift 4 to 5 times, into bowls, until thoroughly mixed. Place in a clean, dry glass jar with a metal lid and store in a cool, dry cupboard. Make sure the jar is tightly closed and avoid prolonged air exposure. Too much air (or moisture) can spoil the powder. Use within 2 months. Supermarket brands may contain white wheat flour, potato starch, and aluminum. Some holistic pharmacies prepare and sell acceptable baking powder brands.

Herb-Scrambled Tofu with Vegetables

Serves 2 to 3

14 to 16 ounces regular tofu, cut into chunks

2 tablespoons natural oil (sunflower or canola are best)

3 to 4 green onions, diced

½ cup finely chopped red bell pepper or finely grated carrot

½ cup finely chopped asparagus, broccoli, or zucchini

1 tablespoon simmered tamari soy sauce or substitute, or 1 Homemade Vegetable Bouillon Cube, broken up in skillet

3 to 4 teaspoons finely chopped fresh parsley

1 teaspoon finely chopped fresh basil or dill weed

½ teaspoon sea salt

½ teaspoon curry powder, or ¼ teaspoon cumin powder plus ¼ teaspoon paprika

Several dashes cayenne to taste

Steam the tofu for 4 to 5 minutes before using in this recipe so it is partially cooked. The sautéeing process alone is not always enough to cook it completely and ensure that it is safe for a Candida diet. After steaming, mash the tofu until very small and crumbled.

In an iron skillet or metal frying pan, heat the oil on medium-high heat and sauté the onions and vegetables for about 2 minutes. Add the tofu and remaining ingredients and sauté for several minutes more (4 to 6 minutes), until the flavors mingle and the mixture is hot throughout. Serve immediately, alone or with other vegetables. Delicious topped with a sauce or Homemade Salsa (page 308) Keeps for 2 to 4 days refrigerated; may be baked to reheat. Do not freeze.

Herb-Scrambled Eggs with Vegetables

Serves 2

3 to 4 teaspoons natural oil or butter

  1 finely chopped green onion, or 1 teaspoon finely chopped onion

  ½ red bell pepper, chopped small, or snow peas, chopped small

8 to 10 stalks asparagus, chopped small, or 1 small stalk broccoli, chopped

Optional: ¼ cup mung bean sprouts, or 8 water chestnuts, chopped

4 large eggs

4 tablespoons water

2 teaspoons finely chopped fresh parsley, or 1 teaspoon dried parsley, crushed

⅛ teaspoon *each* basil, paprika, and dill weed

Several dashes *each* sea salt, sea kelp, and cayenne

Heat half the oil or butter in a skillet or frying pan on high heat and when hot, add the onion and other vegetables. Sauté for 2 minutes or more, stirring constantly until the vegetables are tender but not soft. Remove the vegetables from the heat and place them in a bowl. Wipe out the pan, add the remaining oil, and heat on medium-high heat. Beat the eggs and water well with a wire whisk and add all the seasonings. When the oil sizzles in the pan, add the eggs.

Let the eggs sizzle for 30 to 45 seconds and then stir. Stir occasionally for 3 to 4 minutes over the heat until the eggs are set and firm, yet still tender. They should not be runny if they were well beaten. Overcooked, they get rubbery. When the eggs are cooked fully and hot throughout, serve immediately. Eat at once alone or with other protein or vegetable dishes. Delicious topped with a sauce, Homemade Salsa, or Acidophilus Yogurt. Do not store.

Avocado Omelet

Serves 2

4 large eggs

¼ cup water

2 to 3 teaspoons finely chopped fresh parsley, or 1 teaspoon dried

⅛ teaspoon *each* sea salt, paprika, and basil, crushed

Several dashes cayenne

2 to 3 teaspoons natural oil or butter (or mixture of the two)

1 medium ripe avocado, sliced

Optional: Several dashes onion and/or garlic powder

Optional: 12 to 18 black olives, sliced in half lengthwise

Optional: 2 tablespoons feta cheese, crumbled (if allowed)

Beat the eggs, water, and all the seasonings with a wire whisk, a hand mixer, or in a blender until light and foamy. Preheat the oven broiler on high and place a rack 4 to 5 inches below. Heat the oil and/or butter in an all-metal, large stainless steel or iron frying pan on medium-high heat. When hot, pour in the egg mixture and cook (do not stir) on medium heat until brown underneath. Check under the edges by lifting with a spatula. It is okay to let some of the runny egg mixture from the top of the omelet run under it. When lightly browned underneath, place the avocado slices artistically on top, followed by the olives; sprinkle with feta cheese if used. Place the pan in the hot oven so the top of the omelet can cook. When the top is "set" or solidified (2 to 5 minutes) and the cheese is browned, the omelet is ready. Use a spatula or "turner" to scoop up one-half of the omelet and fold it over the other, forming a half moon with the vegetables inside. Serve immediately and enjoy. Serve plain or with a sauce, Homemade Salsa, or Acidophilus Yogurt. Keeps refrigerated for 12 to 36 hours and may be baked to reheat. Do not freeze.

VARIATION: Instead of avocados, top the omelet with separately sautéed vegetables like red bell pepper, broccoli, asparagus, zucchini, green onions, mung bean sprouts, and/or water chestnuts.

Zucchini Frittata

Serves 2

4 large eggs, well beaten until foamy

1 tablespoon finely chopped fresh parsley

1 teaspoon finely chopped fresh basil or dill weed, or ¼ teaspoon dried

¼ teaspoon *each* paprika and oregano

⅛ teaspoon sea salt

Several dashes cayenne

2 cups grated small zucchini

⅓ cup finely chopped chives or green onion tops, green part only

1 tablespoon natural oil or butter (or mixture of both)

Preheat the oven broiler and place a rack 4 to 5 inches below it. Beat the eggs and seasonings together well and stir in the zucchini and chives or green onions. Heat the butter or oil on high heat in a large all-metal skillet or cast-iron frying pan. When the oil is hot, pour/scoop in the well-mixed zucchini and egg mixture. Reduce the heat to medium and cook like an omelet, using a spatula to lift the edges of the frittata. As it cooks, let the liquid egg run underneath to be cooked. When the frittata is fully cooked and browned underneath when lifted up, remove from the heat and place under the broiler for 2 to 5 minutes, until the top is firm and set. Serve immediately and enjoy. Serve plain or with a sauce, Homemade Salsa or Acidophilus Yogurt. Keeps refrigerated for 12 to 36 hours and may be baked to reheat. Do not freeze.

VARIATION: Use steamed, tender yellow crookneck squash, bell peppers, grated kohlrabi or Jerusalem artichokes, avocado, asparagus or other acceptable vegetables instead if desired.

Omelet Soufflé or Frittata Soufflé

Use the Omelet or Frittata recipe but instead of using well-beaten eggs, separate the whites and yolks. Use a hand mixer to beat the egg whites until stiff peaks form. Beat the yolks separately. Gently fold the beaten yolks into the fluffy egg whites and continue with the recipe as usual for light, fluffy eggs.

Chapter 15

SUPER SALADS AND HOMEMADE DRESSINGS

Everything You Need to Know About Raw Vegetables

V EGETABLES ARE AMONG THE FEW FOODS THAT CAN be eaten raw on a Candida diet. Nutrients and enzymes from raw foods are essential to healing; however, many individuals with Candida yeast have food allergies and/or digestive problems as well and cannot tolerate too many raw foods or certain types of raw foods. Some cannot tolerate any raw vegetables, except for vegetable juices. For these individuals, raw vegetable juices can be an essential part of the healing diet, and five to six glasses per week should generally be drunk. (See Beneficial Beverages.) Four to six servings of cooked vegetables should be eaten each day by those who have trouble digesting raw vegetables. Enjoy three to five servings of cooked vegetables daily if one to two servings of raw vegetables are eaten. Eating vegetables can help to reduce or eliminate constipation!

Some vegetables are harder to digest because they are a bit toxic, such as those found in the deadly nightshade family: potatoes, yellow sweet potatoes, tomatoes, eggplant, and peppers, hot or bell. This does not mean that these foods cannot be eaten at all, only that they must be reduced in the diet as they are not the best foods for the body. In the case of potatoes and yellow sweet potatoes, neither should be eaten on a Candida diet; they are too starchy and the yeast like them. Tomatoes can be eaten occasionally: one to two servings every two to three days because they are acidic, and acidic foods agitate the yeast and fight them (as with lemons/limes). Green bell peppers are unripe peppers. Eating them is like eating green tomatoes. They are less nutritious, as well as harder to digest, and they can cause gas. Keep their use to a minimum or exclude them. Other colored peppers such as yellow, purple, orange, and especially the red bell peppers are ripe and easier to digest. These may be enjoyed, one to two servings every other day or so, as long as they are tolerated. Cayenne pepper may be eaten five to six days a week in small amounts if not allergic.

ROTATION DIETS

It helps digestion and allergies to rotate foods that may be somewhat agitating. Rotating means to eat one to two servings of a certain food only every other day or every third or fourth day to give the body a rest from handling a food that is difficult for it to assimilate. This helps minimize allergic reactions and digestive discomforts. Anyone with severe digestive problems should rotate all foods in their diet. Easier-to-tolerate foods can be eaten five to six days per week. No food should be eaten every day of the week. Sensitive people can easily become allergic to foods eaten daily. Those with severe allergies may need to rotate foods according to food families. See my book *All Natural Allergy Cookbook* for food families and ask your doctor if you need to rotate foods by food families.

RAW VEGETABLES AND CANDIDA

Some individuals with very mild cases of Candida will have no problems digesting vegetables, but they should stay away from starchy ones like potatoes, yellow sweet potatoes, and corn, and exclude aggravating vegetables like mushrooms, eggplants, and raw sprouts that feed the yeast.

Raw sprouts must totally be avoided because they contain high mold and bacteria amounts. (Cooked sprouts are okay.) Avoid eating raw edible flowers as their pollen may agitate Candida and allergies.

Fresh green leafy herbs like parsley, basil, chives, dill weed, oregano, mint, and thyme are full of nutrients like chlorophyll, iron, and iodine. They are generally easy to digest and there is less chance of fresh herbs than dried herbs containing mold. The only problem with fresh herbs is that some individuals may have a "healing reaction" to these greens, especially if they are not used to eating them. Therefore, if fresh herbs are new to your diet, do not overindulge. Fresh herbs are best for salads and raw dishes on a Candida diet. The dried herbs are best used in cooking. Avocados, although a fruit, are often and easily eaten alone or with other vegetables. They are high in fat content compared to other vegetables (no cholesterol) but nutritious and easy to digest for most individuals. One to two may be enjoyed weekly, unless allergic.

"Gassy" vegetables (those that cause gas for many individuals) should be reduced or eliminated in the diets of those who have trouble digesting them. These include raw cauliflower, cabbage, broccoli, brussels sprouts, and cucumbers. The first four are best if cooked. (These may be juiced for some individuals.) Choose English cucumbers or organic regular cucumbers for easier digestion. If even these are troublesome, zucchini can be chopped or grated like cucumber and makes a wonderful, even more nutritious substitute for cucumbers. Grated zucchini can even be used instead of lettuce in some recipes.

Head lettuce or iceberg lettuce is actually one of the hardest foods to digest. Allergy doctors take patients off of this vegetable almost immediately. In restaurants, iceberg lettuce may be sulfured, which aggravates the liver and kidneys with poisons. At home, one may avoid the sulfur but not the fibrous white veins that can clog the digestive tract. Even with romaine lettuce, the white, thick stalks should be discarded and not eaten if there is even a hint of digestive troubles or constipation. Choose leafy, bright green lettuces if these are tolerated, or use spinach or the exotic green mixtures available in most markets these days. Enjoy Boston, bibb, leaf, and red lettuces if tolerated. Discard white or thick, fibrous parts around the stalks of all lettuces. Endive, escarole, radicchio, and dandelion leaves are harder to digest and may prove troublesome for some. Other exotic greens may be enjoyed often.

Other raw vegetables that are harder to digest and should be minimized or excluded for some individuals include radicchio, fresh peas, green beans, snow peas (edible pea pods), kale, asparagus, green onions, onions, rutabagas, turnips and parsnips, sometimes radishes, and/or celery. Celery is more digestible if the veins are peeled back and removed.

Hard vegetables like carrots, beets, and peeled kohlrabi are especially good for Candida diets and should be grated very finely and chewed well. It is best to buy organic carrots and beets from a natural (health) food store. If organic, do not peel, just use a good scrub brush on carrots and beets. Buy fresh organic vegetables whenever possible, as pesticides and other chemicals on some vegetables may assist Candida yeast growth. (See Organic Foods Buying Guidelines.)

Chew all raw vegetables and salads extremely well to ensure the best digestion. The more you chew, the more saliva mixes with the vegetables to help them break down better in the small intestines. Acidic fruits like tomatoes, lemons, limes, and grapefruit, and also plain yogurt, help to break down salads for easier digestion. (Use Acidophilus Yogurt, unless lemon or lime juice is added. See recipes.) Eat these foods with raw vegetables or add them to dressings for improved digestion. Those who have difficulty breaking down raw vegetables or salads in their systems will find they are easier to digest when eaten at lunchtime or before 3 or 4 P.M. Avoid eating more than five to seven different raw vegetables at a single meal.

Digestive aids and supplements may be taken to help break down raw vegetables. These can include one or more of the following: papaya enzymes (papain), pineapple enzymes (bromelain), plant enzymes, HCL, Beano, beet powder, and vitamin C. (Bile salts may be taken if oil dressings are hard to assimilate. See Digestive Aids.) Specially purchased digestive teas and mint teas can also be drunk 30 to 60 minutes before or after a meal to assist digestion on occasion. A few fresh mint leaves can be chewed alone or added to salads once in a while. Fennel seeds can be chewed and then discarded as an alternative digestive aid. Consult your health specialist for advice on digestive aids.

FAST FACTS ABOUT RAW VEGETABLES

1. Eat one to three servings of raw vegetables daily. Drink one serving of raw vegetable juices five to six days per week if raw vegetables are not tolerated. See the Beneficial Beverages chapter for "how" to prepare and drink these.
2. Exclude these vegetables (raw or cooked) on the Candida diet: mushrooms, potatoes, yellow sweet potatoes, eggplant, corn, rutabagas, green olives, endive, escarole, radicchio, dandelion leaves, edible flowers, and head or iceberg lettuce. Exclude these vegetables (raw only) on a Candida diet: sprouts, artichoke hearts, black olives, cabbage, usually broccoli and cauliflower, or any vegetables that are too "gassy" for you.
3. Easier-to-digest raw vegetables: red (yellow, purple, and orange) bell peppers, zucchini, English cucumbers or regular organic cucumbers, spinach,

green leafy lettuces, chives, parsley, other fresh green herbs, grated carrots, grated beets, and peeled, grated kohlrabi. Avocados are also easy to digest and may be eaten with these vegetables.

4. Rotate vegetables/foods if you have trouble digesting them. Avoid and exclude any vegetables/foods you are allergic to.

5. Buy good-quality organic vegetables whenever possible, especially carrots, beets, green lettuces, and leafy green vegetables.

6. Use at least one of the following (if possible) with a salad or in the dressing to assist digestion: lemon or lime juice, tomatoes, grapefruit juice or sections, or Acidophilus Yogurt.

7. Avoid eating more than five to seven different raw vegetables at a single meal. Try to eat raw vegetables earlier in the day and take digestive aids if needed to help break down raw foods.

8. For some specific types of parasites and for some very chronic Candida cases, most red vegetables and fruits have to be excluded from the diet for a while as these interfere with treatment. Let your doctor decide if and how long this may be necessary for you. The red foods include: red bell peppers, sometimes hot red peppers, sometimes cayenne red pepper, tomatoes, watermelon, red berries, pink and red grapefruit (and as always any red herbal teas).

SELECTING VEGETABLES

Organic vegetables are always the first choice if they are fresh and firm. Some stores sell spoiled, heavily blemished, even rotten and moldy organic and/or regular vegetables. Never buy vegetables in this condition. If they are spoiled, it doesn't matter if they are organic or cheap, do not buy them! Make sure organic vegetables come from reliable, honest farmers and dealers. Produce can be mislabeled, so check your sources.

If you grow your own vegetables or get them from a roadside stand, do not eat them if they are grown too near the road or there is a chance of pesticide, soil, water, or air pollution. Have your soil tested before planting a garden to assure the right mineral balance and avoid contaminated soil. Seasonal produce usually has the best flavors; however, most of these raw salad options are in season year-round.

VEGETABLE BUYING GUIDELINES

Artichokes, Jerusalem (Sunchokes) These look like ginger, only smaller and with white and brown ribbing instead of just brown like ginger. They are usually organic. These are excellent for Candida because they are the very best source of FOSs, which feed friendly bacteria and inhibit Candida yeast! Also, they are wonderful for low blood sugar and diabetes. They help balance the blood sugar. Choose firm, unblemished roots with uniform color and avoid red spots. Refrigerate.

Avocados Soft ones must not be wrinkled, be spotted white, have indentations, or have very soft spots. Hard ones cannot be too hard or they may never ripen. Very hard black ones may have softened and then hardened again and are spoiled. Press lightly to feel an ever-so-slight softness beneath the skin. Store on a countertop until slight pressing indicates complete softness inside (a learned ability). Refrigerate when ripe.

Beets, carrots, radishes Must have clear, unblemished skin. Pinch them all along their surfaces to avoid any with soft or soggy skin. They should be firm, crisp, smooth, and bright-colored with no signs of mold, no cuts, and no "basement smell." Avoid old, musty storage beets. Discard split radishes as they may absorb bacteria and are not cookable.

Celery Choose firm, unblemished stalks. The whiter they are, the better. If too green, they may have been picked too soon and will be quite stringy and harder to digest.

Cucumbers Choose firm ones from end to end. Also, unblemished ones that are bright green with a slightly white undertone. Avoid cucumbers that are yellowish or too dark as they are usually old and bitter, often overripe and soft.

Greens, spinach, lettuces Choose crispy, bright-green leaves without lots of holes in them, yellow patches, rust spots (dark, reddish, dotlike, or spotty blemishes) or those with dark, spoiled edges. Leaves should be firm, not wilted or dry.

Kohlrabi Choose pale-green bulbs, firm, unblemished, and not too large.

Onions, garlic (if tolerated, raw) Choose very firm, unwrinkled ones with clear, smooth skins. Avoid dark spots, soft spots, or those with bits of yellow or pale green tops growing from their heads.

Parsley, chives, green onions, other fresh green herbs These nutritious, tasty additions to salads and dressings are best when bright-green, unblemished, and a little bit crisp. Avoid yellow leaves, black spots, and limp or withered leaves or stems.

Peppers, hot and bell Choose smooth, unblemished, very firm, and crispy peppers with no dark or soft spots. Avoid those with waxy- or "greasy-" feeling skin.

Tomatoes Choose soft but not mushy red tomatoes in the summer. Avoid ones with blemishes, spots, or any that are too soft or spoiled. Avoid pinkish or yellowish ones with a visible, almost web-like underskin. These taste pulpy and flavorless. In the winter, the Roma tomatoes are the best bet. Choose pale-red winter tomatoes and ripen them in a plastic bag (see Storage). With this ripening technique, red ripe tomatoes may be enjoyed all winter. As with peppers, avoid those with waxy- or "greasy-" feeling skin.

Zucchini, yellow summer squash As with cucumbers, these must be firm all along the surface, with no soft spots, unblemished, and bright in color. Zucchini cannot have a yellow tinge or dark color or they will be bitter.

VEGETABLE STORAGE TIPS

Store vegetables in clean plastic bags, preferably in the crisper section of your refrigerator, or use plastic containers kept out of the crisper section. Bag ends may be left a bit open for air flow. Plastic storage bags for vegetables can be reused if desired (if okayed by your health specialist), if washed with suds and hot water and hung to dry. Do not worry about minor bacteria in bags, as vegetables will be washed before eating.

Do not leave vegetables unwrapped in the refrigerator; they absorb and spread even more bacteria when unprotected by wraps or containers. Unwrapped, they wilt and spoil almost twice as fast and they pick up or contribute to refrigerator odors, which denote high levels of bacteria.

Larger-size glass or tin storage containers can be purchased if one wants or needs to avoid plastic wraps or containers. Check vegetables every 1 to 3 days to trim and discard those that are not fresh enough for use. One moldy vegetable left with fresher ones will spoil them more quickly if not discarded.

Vegetable Storage Times and Techniques

Artichokes, Jerusalem (Sunchokes) It is best not to peel them, just use a good scrub brush on them. Refrigerate in a plastic bag in your crisper section for up to 3 and sometimes even 4 weeks if purchased very fresh. Use raw only when fairly fresh; otherwise, cook them as you would a potato or turnip.

Avocados Keep on counter until ripened, up to 1 week. Refrigerate when ripe. Whole, ripe avocados keep 3 to 7 days. Halves, with the pits, keep 12 to 36 hours if wrapped, less without pits. Discard blackened parts and scrape off cut edges before using.

Beets, carrots, radishes Refrigerate for 1 to 4 weeks if wrapped. They keep longer if very fresh when purchased. Do not use old ones raw that sprout top growth or little white side roots during storage. (These parts can be scraped off and the vegetables used for cooking if not too overripe.) If the beets have green leaves on them, twist these off and store them separately (eat greens as a cooked veggie) from the red beet bottoms. Discard radish greens before storing. Carrot greens may be stored separately and used in soups, if desired.

Celery Keep refrigerated for 1 to 2 weeks or more. If slightly wilted, revive by cutting ¼ inch off stem end and placing it in warm water to make it drink. If the celery does not drink and stays wilted, discard it or use in cooking if quality is not too poor.

Cucumbers Keep refrigerated for 4 to 12 days until soft. Keep cut cucumbers wrapped. Discard if soft or mushy.

Greens, spinach, lettuces Keep for 3 to 10 days, depending on freshness when purchased. Some bunch lettuces can be revived like celery. Discard when soft, heavily blemished, or wrinkled.

Kohlrabi Refrigerate for 4 to 12 days. Discard if soft, discolored, or heavily blemished. Kolhrabi is always peeled before using in any recipe.

Onions, garlic Store in dark, open jar on counter or in pot under the sink. Keep under sink or in cool basement or garage in warm weather. Don't refrigerate. Discard when soft, moldy, blemished, or withered. Keep for 1 to 4 weeks.

Parsley, chives, green onions, other fresh green herbs Keep refrigerated for 4 to 14 days. Do not wash until ready to use. If the green herbs get limp, revive them in cold water. Store green onions and chives in a separate plastic bag without holes, sealed with a twist tie so their stronger scents do not affect the flavors of other foods. (If using only the green onion tops, in salad and dressing recipes, save the white parts for cooked recipes.)

Peppers, hot or bell Keep refrigerated for 5 to 12 days until eaten or discard if soft, wrinkled, blemished, or spoiled. If only small parts are spoiled, cut those off and use the rest of the pepper in cooking, not raw.

Tomatoes If ripe, refrigerate for 3 to 8 days. If not ripe, ripen them in a plastic bag with holes in it on a countertop (a sunny counter in winter) for 3 to 7 days. Check daily and refrigerate when ripe. Stored this way, red ripe tomatoes may be enjoyed all winter.

Zucchini, yellow summer squash Keep refrigerated for 4 to 12 days until soft. Soft parts can be removed and the rest used raw, if firm and fresh enough. Discard all mushy or moldy ones.

Preparation of Raw Vegetables

To reduce bacteria, wash vegetables with one of these solutions. All vegetables that are to be eaten raw must be washed with one of the following. Amounts are for a sinkful: approximately 2 gallons of water. Reduce amounts if less water is used. Swish the solution well in water and let vegetables soak in water/solution 15 minutes or so, unless package says otherwise. Soak vegetables just before cutting and using.

1. Hydrogen peroxide: ¼ cup 3 percent solution or 1 teaspoon 35 percent solution. (No fumes.)
2. Aerobic oxygen: 40 to 50 drops or 1 teaspoon. (No fumes.)
3. Citricidal: 20 to 25 drops or ½ teaspoon. Dissolve drops in very warm water and add to soaking water. Let sit in water 20 minutes, swish, and put vegetables in. Rinse after with distilled water. (No fumes. Slight taste.)
4. Aromatherapy: 1 pure concentrated drop of tea tree oil and 1 pure concentrated drop of thyme oil (No fumes. Slight taste.)
5. Clorox bleach (No bleach substitutes!): 1 teaspoon. Rinse vegetables well with distilled water after. (Some fumes.)
6. Baking soda: 1 tablespoon well mixed in water. Rinse vegetables after with distilled water. (No fumes.)

7. Specially purchased vegetable cleaners that are safe and reduce bacteria (Use products recommended by health specialists.): Follow directions on package. (Example: Para-Wash by Organica)
8. Two to three tablespoons apple cider vinegar, if doctor allows.

Preparing Vegetables for Salads

Wash all vegetables just before preparing, rather than in advance as they may rot, mold, and blemish faster when stored wet. Cut vegetables as directed in recipes for optimum digestion and flavor. See Vegetables to Enjoy Raw, further on, for specific vegetables that may be used in salads if you are creating your own recipes. Cut a slice off the stem end or recut previously cut edges off any vegetable before cutting for a new salad.

Use regularly bleached wooden cutting boards or glass cutting boards to keep bacteria from growing and spreading; use well-cleaned utensils. (See Cookware and Kitchen Utensils in chapter 11.) Most salad dressings must be made fresh for salads for Candida diets to prevent bacteria growth; see recipe directions. It is best not to eat leftover salads, so make only enough for one meal or give leftovers to a family member without Candida yeast problems.

Fast Facts for Fantastic Salads

1. Wash all raw vegetables (except for those that are steamed), in one of the previously recommended antibacterial cleaners. Wash thoroughly. Salad greens should be spun dry in a salad spinner.
2. Tear lettuce and spinach leaves into bite-sized pieces. They are easier to tackle with a fork and fit the mouth better. Do not twist or squeeze the greens when tearing or they will be bruised and turn dark and wilt. Tear gently. Avoid cutting salad greens as they will not stay fresh as long. Discard thick, white fibrous parts of lettuce.
3. Prepare salads just before eating to preserve nutrients and discourage bacteria growth.
4. Avoid making salads from hard-to-digest or "gassy" vegetables. Stick with the vegetables recommended here unless your digestion is quite good. Include several colors in a salad for eye appeal and a variety of nutrients.
5. Eat salad before a vegetarian meal and after meat in a meat meal. Digestive enzymes are strongest at the beginning of a meal; hardest-to-digest food should be eaten first.

6. Follow the salad tips in these recipes and use the dressings given here. If creating your own dressings, stick with the Candida diet requirements. Do not drown the salad in dressing. Too much dressing makes a salad wilt and may hinder digestion, especially if it is oil-based dressing.

7. Try to use tomatoes, lemon or lime juice, white grapefruit juice, vitamin C crystals, or Acidophilus Yogurt with a salad to aid digestion. These acidic or high-enzyme foods help digestion. Use digestive aids if needed! (See Digestive Aids.) It is better to get help digesting than avoid high-nutrient foods that can help speed healing.

8. Peel kohlrabi before grating or chopping for salads and all recipes. Remove celery strings for easier digestion. Use a good scrub brush on all root veggies like carrots, parsnips, beets, and Jerusalem artichokes. Do not peel root vegetables if they are organic, unless they are not very fresh.

Vegetables to Enjoy Raw (If tolerated and not allergic)

artichokes, Jerusalem, peeled or unpeeled, grated or sliced thin
avocados (fruit that eats like a veggie)
basil leaves
beets, fresh grated
bell peppers (red, orange, yellow or purple)
carrots, grated or sliced thin
celery, deveined
chives, chopped
cucumber, organic regular or English
garlic
ginger (sometimes)
green onions, chopped
greens, exotic salad and wild
kohlrabi, peeled and chopped small or grated
lettuce, Boston, bibb, red, leaf, green parts of romaine
mint leaves
parsley, fresh
radishes
spinach, all types
tomato, ripe
yellow summer squash, chopped or grated
zucchini, chopped or grated

Vegetables to Eat Cooked (If tolerated and not allergic)

artichoke hearts (packed in water)
artichokes, globe
artichokes, Jerusalem
asparagus
beans, green
beets
bell peppers (red, orange, yellow and purple)
broccoli
brussels sprouts
cabbage
carrots
cauliflower
celery
chard, Swiss
collards
garlic
ginger
greens, beet or mustard
kale
kohlrabi (peeled)
leeks
onions
parsnips
peas and pea pods
shallots
snow peas
spinach
sprouts
squash, summer or winter
tomatoes
turnips
yams, orange
zucchini

Great Green Salad

Serves 2

8 to 10 large lettuce leaves (leaf, red, bibb or Boston), torn

1 small or medium tomato, cut in thin wedges, or 6 to 8 radishes, sliced in thin rounds

¼ organic or English cucumber, sliced in ¼-inch rounds, or ¼ small zucchini, sliced in ¼-inch rounds

Optional: ½ bell pepper (red, yellow, purple, orange, or green), cut in thin strips

Optional: 2 to 3 teaspoons loosely chopped fresh parsley, chives, or green onion tops, green part only

Optional: 8 to 10 spinach leaves, torn

Wash and tear the greens into bite-sized pieces. Toss everything together and mix with any favorite dressing acceptable for a Candida diet. Eat fresh. Do not store.

Spinach Sunshine Salad

Serves 2 to 4

1 small bunch spinach, leaves only, stems removed, torn

½ small or medium avocado, chopped; or 2 stalks celery, chopped in ¼-inch half moons; or ½ cup steamed asparagus, chopped and quick-chilled in freezer 5 to 10 minutes

1 cup quartered and chopped zucchini chunks

2 small carrots, finely grated

Toss the spinach and green vegetables together. Garnish each serving with half or a quarter of the grated carrot for a "sunny" topping and serve with any appropriate oil-based or creamy dressing. Eat fresh. Do not store.

Sweet Beet Salad

Serves 2

8 to 10 large lettuce leaves (leaf, red, bibb, Boston), torn

1 bell pepper (red, yellow, purple, orange, or green), cut in thin strips

½ avocado, chopped; or ½ cup chopped artichoke hearts (packed in water, drained), steamed 4 to 5 minutes

2 small or 1 medium fresh beet, finely grated

1 fresh lemon (or lime)

Optional: 1 to 2 Jerusalem artichokes, finely grated

Toss together the lettuce, bell pepper, artichoke, and avocado or artichoke hearts. Dish out the salad and spread the beets over the top. (Adding beet to the mixture will dye the whole salad red.) Squeeze 1 to 2 teaspoons of lemon juice over the beets on each salad and serve with a suitable oil-based or creamy dressing. Eat fresh. Do not store.

Zucchini Salad

Serves 2

1 small zucchini, regular grated

1 medium tomato, cut in small chunks, or 1 red or orange bell pepper, cut in ¾-inch chunks, or 6 to 8 radishes, sliced in thin rounds

2 stalks celery, chopped in ¼-inch half moons

8 to 12 spinach leaves, torn small

Toss all ingredients gently together and serve with any suitable dressing. Eat fresh. Do not store.

Rainbow Grated Salad

Serves 2

8 large leaves leaf or romaine lettuce (stalks/spines removed), thinly chopped or shredded

½ small zucchini or ½ kohlrabi, regular grated

1 large carrot, finely grated

1 small fresh beet, finely grated

Optional: 4 to 6 radishes, finely grated

Optional: ¼ to ½ yellow summer squash, grated regular

Optional: 1 to 2 Jerusalem artichokes, finely grated

Toss all the ingredients together except for the beet, which can be sprinkled on top or around the inner edge of the salad bowl. Serve with a creamy vegetable, tofu, or yogurt dressing. Eat fresh. Do not store.

Confetti Salad

Serves 2

1 bell pepper (red, yellow, purple, or orange, not green), diced

1 cup diced zucchini or yellow summer squash

1 cup diced celery (or substitute)

1 medium tomato, seeded and diced

Optional: 2 cups chopped spinach or lettuce

Mix the diced vegetables together and toss them with an oil-based dressing. Serve on a bed of chopped spinach or lettuce if desired and enjoy. Eat fresh. Do not store.

Kohlrabi Coleslaw

Serves 2

1½ to 2 cups regular grated, peeled
  kohlrabi

½ cup finely grated carrot

½ cup regular grated red bell
  pepper, or ½ cup finely grated
  fresh beet

Optional: 2 to 3 teaspoons finely
  chopped chives or green
  onion tops, green part only

Optional: ½ cup regular grated small
  zucchini, organic cucumber,
  or English cucumber

Optional: 1 to 2 Jerusalem artichokes,
  finely grated

Mix the kohlrabi with everything but the beet and arrange on two plates or bowls. Top with grated beet, if used. (Adding beet to the mixture will dye the whole salad red.) Choose a creamy vegetable, tofu, or yogurt dressing. Eat fresh. Do not store.

Exotic Greens Salad

Serves 2

3 cups exotic mixed greens (minus
  endive, escarole, and radicchio),
  torn slightly or left whole

1 medium tomato, cut in thin wedges,
  or 1 medium red bell pepper, cut in
  thin strips

4 artichoke hearts (packed in water,
  drained), quartered and steamed

4 to 5 minutes, or 8 to 12 black
  olives, sliced in half lengthwise and
  steamed 3 to 4 minutes, or ½ avocado, cut in thin slices

Optional: 2 to 3 teaspoons loosely
  chopped fresh parsley

Arrange the greens artistically on a small or medium plate and arrange other ingredients on top. Dribble a creamy tofu, yogurt, or creamy nut or vegetable dressing over your artwork and enjoy. Eat fresh. Do not store.

Mediterranean Salad

Serves 2

4 to 6 artichoke hearts (packed in water, drained), cut in quarters or eighths

10 to 14 black olives, cut in half lengthwise

1 cup quartered and chopped organic cucumber, English cucumber, or zucchini

1 small or medium tomato, cut in 1-inch chunks

1 small bell pepper (red, yellow, purple, orange, or green), cut in 1-inch chunks

Optional: 1 to 2 tablespoons chopped red onion, or 1 to 2 green onions, chopped

Steam the artichoke hearts and olives for 4 minutes and quick-chill them in an open bowl in the freezer for 20 minutes or so, until cool. While these vegetables are chilling, prepare the rest of the salad and mix it with the chilled vegetables when ready. Serve with one of the oil-based dressings or a creamy dressing as desired. Eat fresh. Do not store.

Avocado Boat Treat

Serves 2

1 medium avocado, peeled or unpeeled

¼ organic or English cucumber, quartered and cut in ¼-inch chunks

6 to 8 cherry tomatoes, quartered, or 1 small tomato, chopped small

6 to 10 spinach leaves, chopped small

Optional: 2 cups chopped lettuce, spinach, or exotic mixed greens

Cut the avocado in half lengthwise and remove the pit. It is best to peel back the skin, in strips, and remove it. Cut a thin slice off the bottom of each avocado half so it sits on a plate without rolling over. Place it on a small plate,

(continues)

on a bed of greens (1 cup each), if desired. Mix the remaining ingredients together and heap them into and overflowing the avocado boat. Top with creamy vegetable, tofu, yogurt, or nut dressing. Eat fresh. Do not store.

Zucchini Ribbon and Red Pepper Salad
Serves 2

1 small zucchini

2 cups chopped exotic mixed greens or spinach (no endive, escarole, or radicchio)

2 small or 1 large red bell pepper, cut in 1-inch chunks

Optional: 1 to 2 Jerusalem artichokes, finely grated

Cut the ends off the zucchini and use a potato peeler to cut thin strips of ribbons from one end of the zucchini to the other. Arrange the salad greens on a small plate and top them artistically with the zucchini ribbons. Sprinkle on the red bell pepper chunks. Surround with artichokes if desired. Dribble a creamy vegetable, tofu, yogurt, or creamy nut dressing onto each salad and enjoy. Eat fresh. Do not store.

Stuffed Tomato Salad
Serves 2

⅓ cup diced artichoke hearts (packed in water, drained)

2 large tomatoes, left whole

⅓ cup diced celery

⅓ cup diced yellow, purple, orange, or red bell pepper

⅓ cup diced organic or English cucumber

1 to 2 tablespoons lightly chopped fresh parsley

Optional: 4 to 6 finely chopped fresh mint or basil leaves

Optional: 1 to 2 tablespoons chopped chives or green onion tops, green part only

Steam the artichoke hearts for 4 to 5 minutes and quick-chill them in an open bowl in the freezer for 20 minutes or so, until cool. Core the tomatoes and remove 4 to 5 tablespoons of the inner pulp so they can be stuffed. Mix the chilled artichoke with all the other vegetables and stuff them into the tomatoes. The stuffed tomatoes can be eaten raw or broiled, then topped with dressing. Serve with a creamy vegetable, tofu, yogurt, or nut dressing. Use a knife and fork to enjoy. Eat fresh. Do not store unless you wish to broil the tomatoes within 12 hours of preparation; then refrigerate until broiling.

Layered Vegetable Salad

Serves 4

Layer 1: 1 large bunch spinach, chopped

Layer 2: 2 large tomatoes, cut in small chunks, or 2 medium red bell peppers, cut in ½- to ⅔-inch chunks

Layer 3: 2 cups quartered and chopped zucchini, or organic or English cucumber

Layer 4: 2 to 3 medium carrots, finely grated

Layer 5: 8 to 12 large lettuce leaves (leaf, red, bibb or Boston), chopped

Layer 6: 1 small beet, finely grated

Optional: 1 tablespoon fresh lemon or lime juice

Use a glass bowl that is evenly deep so you can see the different layers through the bowl, if desired. Place the spinach layer in the bowl first and add all the remaining layers until you come to the beet. Toss the beet in the citrus juice if desired and sprinkle the beet over the top of the salad. Serve with any suitable dressing and enjoy. Eat fresh. Do not store.

NOTE: When using the following dressings for non-Candida diets, larger batches may be prepared and stored (refrigerated) if desired.

SALAD DRESSING RECIPES

Fresh Herbs and Oil Dressing
Makes ¾ cup

½ cup natural oil (olive, canola, sun-flower, or sesame are best)

2 tablespoons fresh lemon or lime juice, or ½ teaspoon corn-free, unbuffered vitamin C crystals

1 tablespoon finely chopped fresh parsley

2 teaspoons finely chopped fresh mint and/or fresh basil leaves

1 teaspoon chopped fresh dill weed or other fresh, green herb of choice

¼ to ½ teaspoon sea salt

Several dashes cayenne

Optional: 2 to 3 teaspoons flaxseed oil or pumpkin seed oil

Optional: ½ teaspoon Gomashio/ Sesame Salt (use only ¼ tea-spoon sea salt)

Optional: 1 clove garlic, pressed, or 2 teaspoons finely chopped chives or green onion tops, green part only

Beat all the ingredients together with a fork in a jar. Chill for at least 1 hour so flavors can mingle before serving. This is one of the few dressings that can be kept refrigerated and reused for up to 2 days.

Italian Herbs and Oil Dressing

Makes ¾ cup

½ cup natural oil (olive, canola, sunflower, or sesame are best)

2 tablespoons fresh lemon or lime juice, or ½ teaspoon corn-free, unbuffered vitamin C crystals

1 tablespoon finely chopped fresh parsley

2 to 3 teaspoons finely chopped chives or green onion tops, green part only, and/or 1 clove garlic, pressed

2 teaspoons finely chopped fresh basil leaves

2 teaspoons finely chopped fresh oregano leaves

¼ to ½ teaspoon sea salt

⅛ to ¼ teaspoon fennel seed, freshly ground

Several dashes cayenne

Optional: 2 to 3 teaspoons flaxseed oil or pumpkin seed oil

Beat all the ingredients together with a fork in a jar. Chill for at least 1 hour so flavors can mingle before serving. This is one of the few dressings that can be kept refrigerated and reused for up to 2 days.

Dilly Cucumber Dressing

Makes ⅔ cup

½ medium organic cucumber, peeled and seeded, or ¼ large English cucumber, peeled

2 teaspoons fresh chopped dill weed

¼ cup natural oil (olive, canola, sunflower, or sesame are best)

Sea salt to taste

Several dashes cayenne

Optional: 1 small clove garlic, pressed

Optional: 1 to 2 teaspoons toasted sesame oil

Blend all the ingredients in a blender until smooth and serve immediately, or chill, covered, for up to 1 hour in the refrigerator before serving. Eat fresh. Do not store.

Emerald Dressing

Makes about 1 cup

1 medium avocado, peeled and
 pitted

2 to 3 tablespoons natural oil (olive,
 canola, sunflower, or sesame
 are best)

1 to 2 tablespoons fresh lime or
 lemon juice, or ½ teaspoon
 corn-free, unbuffered vitamin C
 crystals

1 to 2 tablespoons chopped chives or
 green onion tops, green part
 only

1 tablespoon finely chopped fresh
 parsley

Sea salt to taste

Few dashes cayenne

Optional: 1 small clove garlic, pressed

Optional: 2 tablespoons freshly made
 Home-Roasted Nuts or
 Seeds

Use a blender or food processor to blend all ingredients until smooth.
Fast-chill the dressing in the freezer before using or chill, covered, for up to
1 hour and serve. Eat fresh within 4 to 6 hours.

Garlic French Dressing

Makes ½ cup

⅓ cup natural oil (olive, canola,
 sunflower, or sesame are best)

2 tablespoons fresh Homemade
 Ketchup

2 to 3 teaspoons fresh lemon or lime
 juice, or ½ teaspoon corn-free,
 unbuffered vitamin C crystals

2 cloves garlic, pressed

¼ teaspoon sea salt, or to taste

Several dashes cayenne

Blend or beat all ingredients together. Quick-chill in the freezer or refrigerate, covered, for up to 1 hour and serve. Eat fresh. Do not store.

Grapefruit Juice Dressing

Makes ½ cup

½ cup fresh white grapefruit juice

1 to 2 cloves garlic, pressed

Sea salt to taste

Optional: 1 tablespoon fresh lemon or lime juice, or ½ teaspoon corn-free, unbuffered vitamin C crystals

Blend or beat all ingredients together and serve immediately or chill for 1 hour, covered, in the refrigerator. Eat fresh or use within 4 to 6 hours.

Green Onion and Garlic Dressing

Makes ⅓ cup

1 green onion (white and green parts), chopped

1 to 2 cloves garlic, minced

1 tablespoon fresh lemon or lime juice, or ½ teaspoon corn-free, unbuffered vitamin C crystals

3 tablespoons natural oil (olive, canola, sunflower, or sesame are best)

Sea salt to taste

Few dashes cayenne

Optional: ¼ to ½ teaspoon Gomashio/ Sesame Salt

Use a blender to combine all ingredients until smooth. Serve immediately or chill first. Can be refrigerated for up to 2 to 3 days.

Velvet Vegetable Dressing

Makes about 1 cup

1 cup chopped carrots, broccoli, orange yam, packed spinach, asparagus, artichoke hearts (packed in water, drained), or butternut or buttercup squash

¼ cup chopped chives or green onion tops, green part only

1 to 2 cloves garlic, pressed

Sea salt to taste

Few dashes cayenne

Optional: 2 tablespoons freshly made Home-Roasted Nuts or Seeds, ground

Optional: 2 tablespoons finely chopped fresh parsley

Optional: 1 tablespoon melted butter or natural oil (canola, sunflower, or sesame are best)

Steam one type of vegetable until very tender. Use a food processor to combine all ingredients. Quick-chill in the freezer and serve generously over almost any salad. This dressing can be refrigerated for up to 2 to 4 days but must be reheated in a saucepan or baked and quick-chilled again before serving.

Tomato and Herb Dressing

Makes about 1 cup

⅔ cup chopped tomatoes, seeded, peeled if desired

¼ cup olive oil (or natural canola, sunflower, or sesame oil)

¼ cup chopped chives or green onion tops, green part only

1 to 2 cloves garlic, pressed

1 tablespoon fresh lemon or lime juice, or ½ teaspoon corn-free, unbuffered vitamin C crystals

1 to 2 tablespoons finely chopped fresh parsley

2 teaspoons finely chopped fresh basil and/or oregano leaves

Sea salt to taste

Few dashes cayenne

Optional: 1 to 2 teaspoons fresh dill weed

Use a blender to blend all ingredients together lightly for a chunky-style dressing, or blend until smooth if desired. Eat immediately, quick-chill in the freezer, or chill for up to 1 hour, covered. Keeps for 4 to 6 hours refrigerated or may be kept for 2 to 3 days if heated in a saucepan and quick-chilled before serving.

Tahini Dressing

Makes ¾ cup

2 ounces (¼ cup) regular tofu, or ⅓ cup cauliflower

2 to 3 tablespoons sesame tahini (can pour off oil if desired), or other nut butter if preferred

2 tablespoons natural oil (flax, pumpkin, sunflower, or sesame are best)

1 tablespoon water

1 to 2 tablespoons fresh lemon or lime juice, or ½ teaspoon corn-free, unbuffered vitamin C crystals

2 tablespoons chopped chives or green onion tops, green part only

2 teaspoons finely chopped fresh parsley

1 clove garlic, pressed

Sea salt or Gomashio/Sesame Salt to taste

Few dashes cayenne

Cut the tofu (or chop cauliflower) into 3 or 4 pieces and steam for 8 to 10 minutes. The tahini must be heated in a small saucepan and simmered for 2 to 3 minutes or baked until hot throughout. Use a blender or food processor to combine all ingredients until smooth. Correct seasonings to taste. Quick-chill in the freezer or refrigerate for up to 1 hour. Eat fresh. Do not store.

Onion and Oil Dressing

Makes ¾ cup

3 ounces (6 tablespoons) regular tofu, or ⅓ cup cauliflower

½ cup finely chopped green onion tops, green part only

¼ cup natural oil (olive, canola, sunflower, or sesame are best)

1 to 2 tablespoons fresh lemon or lime juice, or ½ teaspoon corn-free, unbuffered vitamin C crystals

2 tablespoons chopped chives or green onion tops, green part only

2 tablespoons finely chopped fresh parsley

1 to 2 cloves garlic, pressed

Sea salt or Gomashio/Sesame Salt to taste

Few dashes cayenne

Optional: 4 to 6 finely chopped fresh basil or oregano leaves

Cut the tofu (or chop cauliflower) into 3 or 4 pieces and steam for 8 to 10 minutes. Use a blender or food processor to combine all ingredients until smooth. Correct seasonings to taste. Quick-chill in the freezer or refrigerate for up to 1 hour. Eat fresh. Do not store.

Parsley Nut Dressing

Makes about 1 cup

⅓ cup freshly made Home-Roasted Nuts or Seeds (almonds, filberts, pecans, pine nuts, or sunflower seeds are best), ground

¼ cup finely chopped fresh parsley

3 to 4 tablespoons natural oil (olive, canola, sunflower, or sesame are best)

2 tablespoons fresh lemon or lime juice, or ½ teaspoon corn-free, unbuffered vitamin C crystals

2 tablespoons chopped chives or green onion tops, green part only

1 clove garlic, pressed

Sea salt or Gomashio/Sesame Salt to taste

Few dashes cayenne

Optional: 2 to 4 finely chopped fresh

Use a food processor or blender to combine all ingredients thoroughly. (If vitamin C is used, extra oil or distilled water may be required if a blender is used.) Correct seasonings to taste. Serve immediately or quick-chill in the freezer or chill for up to 1 hour in the refrigerator. Eat fresh. Do not store.

Yogurt Garlic Dressing (with Dairy)

Makes 1 cup

1 cup plain yogurt

1 to 2 cloves garlic, pressed

1 to 2 tablespoons fresh lemon or lime juice, or ½ teaspoon corn-free, unbuffered vitamin C crystals

Optional: few dashes cayenne

Optional: few dashes sea salt

Mix all ingredients together very well with a fork. Do not blend. Can quick-chill or refrigerate for up to 1 hour before serving. Use generously on salads. Keeps for 4 to 6 hours refrigerated. (If citrus juice is not used, Acidophilus Yogurt must be used.)

Yogurt Cucumber Dressing (with Dairy)

Makes about 1 cup

½ cup plain yogurt

½ cup grated organic or English cucumber

2 to 3 teaspoons finely chopped fresh parsley, chives, or green onion tops, green part only

1 to 2 cloves garlic, pressed

Few dashes cayenne

Sea salt to taste

Optional: 1 tablespoon fresh lemon or lime juice, or ½ teaspoon corn-free, unbuffered vitamin C crystals

Mix all ingredients together very well with a fork. Do not blend. Can quick-chill or refrigerate for up to 1 hour before serving. Use generously on salads. Keeps for 4 to 6 hours refrigerated. (If citrus juice is not used, Acidophilus Yogurt must be used.)

Yogurt Dill Dressing (with Dairy)

Makes about 1 cup

1 cup plain yogurt

3 to 4 teaspoons finely chopped fresh dill weed

Few dashes cayenne and/or sea salt

Optional: 1 to 2 cloves garlic, pressed

Optional: 1 to 2 tablespoons chives or green onion tops, green part only, finely chopped

Optional: 1 tablespoon fresh lemon or lime juice, or ½ teaspoon corn-free, unbuffered vitamin C crystals

Mix all ingredients together very well with a fork. Do not blend. Can quick-chill or refrigerate for up to 1 hour before serving. Use generously on salads. Keeps for 4 to 6 hours refrigerated. (If citrus juice is not used, Acidophilus Yogurt must be used.)

Yogurt Chive or Green Onion Dressing (with Dairy)

Makes 1 cup

¾ cup Acidophilus Yogurt

⅓ cup chives or green onion tops, green part only, chopped

2 to 3 teaspoons fresh parsley, chopped

3 to 4 finely chopped fresh basil and/or mint leaves

Optional: sea salt to taste

Mix all ingredients together very well with a fork. Do not blend. Can quick-chill or refrigerate for up to 1 hour before serving. Use generously on salads. Keeps for 4 to 6 hours refrigerated.

EASY SALAD DRESSING OPTIONS

Use one of the following on a salad instead of dressing:

1. 2 to 3 teaspoons fresh lemon or lime juice
2. 3 to 5 teaspoons fresh white grapefruit juice with or without grapefruit chunks added
3. 4 to 6 tablespoons Acidophilus Yogurt

Chapter 16

SOUPS FOR ALL SEASONS

THESE DELECTABLE SOUPS ARE A CORNUCOPIA OF ingredients, textures, and flavors that will excite the taste buds, nourish the body, and stimulate good health. Some are side dishes and some can be a meal in themselves. Serving suggestions are given at the end of each recipe. Dairy is an option for some recipes, but they can all be prepared without dairy. It is okay to use dairy milk or a bit of sweetener, provided they are cooked into the recipe for 15 to 20 minutes or more. Minute amounts of milk sugar and sweetening do not feed the yeast when cooked this long and mixed with many other ingredients. (See Honey and Sweeteners in Controversial Foods.)

Do not worry about minute amounts of mold on herbs for the same reasons. However, avoid using herbs, vegetables, or any foods that appear moldy, overripe, or not completely fresh. When in doubt, throw it out!

Be sure to look at chapter 19 for special recipes for Homemade Ketchup, Gomashio Sea Salt, Homemade Vegetable Broth Powder, Homemade Vegetable Bouillon Cubes, Oven-Dehydrated Vegetables, Your Own Chili or Curry Powders, Mock Tamari Soy Sauce, and exciting new recipes that add exceptional flavor to soups. See chapter 13 for Home-Roasted Nuts and Seeds and Homemade Salsa.

These recipes were made to taste delicious; even those that call for milk substitutes will amaze you with their rich, full, yet delicate flavors. Try to make the recipe as written the first time (unless you have allergies, then see the Substitution Chart, chapter 11). After the first try, you can alter the recipes to suit your personal style and delete or include special foods.

Regardless of how you use these recipes, you are sure to love them and continue to use them even after Candida has been healed. Use your own vegetable stock or meat stock or try the following:

HOW TO MAKE VEGETABLE SOUP STOCK

To make your own vegetable stock, choose one of these three methods:

1. Use leftover water from steaming vegetables as stock.
2. Odd leftover vegetables, especially broccoli, cauliflower, zucchini, kohlrabi, greens, celery, carrots, turnips, parsnips, squash, yams, and cabbage, can be covered in water, brought to a boil on high heat, and simmered on low heat for 20 to 60 minutes. After simmering, cool and strain the mixture. Save the liquid for stock. Avoid using beets or tomatoes for stock. These may dye the water and alter the color of the soup. (Do not use potatoes, yellow sweet potatoes, corn, mushrooms, or any other vegetables that may aggravate Candida. See chapter 15 for accepted vegetable lists, for both raw and cooked recipes, to be used during Candida treatment.)
3. Leftover cooked vegetables, such as the ones suggested above, can be blended or put in a food processor with water, puréed, and used as stock. Use 1 cup vegetables for every 5 to 6 cups water.

Digest-Aid-Meal-in-a-Soup

Serves 1

½ cup cooked legumes/beans: brown, red, or black beans (adzuki, pinto, romano, chickpeas, kidney, red beans, black beans)

½ cup cooked whole grains (brown rice, wild rice, buckwheat, kasha, brown pot barley, and especially quinoa or millet)

½ cup green vegetables (asparagus, artichoke hearts packed in water, broccoli, kohlrabi, zucchini, kale, chard, spinach, or other cookable green leafy vegetables)

½ cup white, orange, or yellow vegetable (cauliflower, small white and purple turnip, carrots, orange yam, winter squash, yellow summer squash, Jerusalem artichokes, and occasionally parsnips)

1½ cups liquid (Brown Bean Juice, stock, broth, water, milk substitute, and only occasionally tomato juice, yogurt, or milk

Seasonings #1

1 to 2 chopped green onions, or 2 cloves garlic, minced, or ¼ to 1 teaspoon prepared horseradish

2 to 3 teaspoons butter or natural oil, or 3 to 4 teaspoons simmered tamari soy sauce or substitute

Sea salt or salt substitute and cayenne to taste

Seasonings #2

2 to 3 teaspoons finely chopped onion and 1 small clove garlic, or ¼ to 1 teaspoon prepared horseradish

1 tablespoon finely chopped fresh parsley, or 1 teaspoon dried parsley

½ teaspoon *each* basil and dill weed

¼ teaspoon *each* thyme and marjoram

2 to 3 teaspoons butter or natural oil

Sea salt or potassium chloride or another salt substitute to taste

Few dashes *each* sea kelp and cayenne

Seasonings #3

2 to 3 teaspoons finely chopped onion and 1 small clove garlic, or ½ to 1 teaspoon prepared horseradish

3 to 4 teaspoons simmered tamari soy sauce or substitute

1 teaspoon Homemade Vegetable Broth Powder, or ½ to 1 Homemade Vegetable Bouillon Cube

Sea salt or potassium chloride or another salt substitute to taste

Few dashes *each* sea kelp and cayenne

Optional: 1 to 2 teaspoons ground flaxseeds, or 1 to 2 teaspoons Gomashio

Seasonings #4

¼ cup chives or green onion tops (green part only), chopped

1 teaspoon Homemade Vegetable Broth Powder, or ½ to 1 Homemade Vegetable Bouillon Cube

1 tablespoon finely chopped fresh parsley, or 1 teaspoon dried parsley

½ to 1 teaspoon basil or dill weed

¼ teaspoon *each* thyme and marjoram

2 to 3 teaspoons butter or natural oil

Sea salt or potassium chloride or another salt substitute to taste

Few dashes *each* sea kelp and cayenne

Use pre-made beans and whole grains with fresh vegetables steamed together. Use a blender to blend the beans, whole grains, vegetables, and liquid with one of the three seasoning recipes, or create your own seasoning mixture according to your taste and diet requirements. Bring the mixture up to a boil on medium heat then simmer on low for 20 to 25 minutes, or until the sharp edge is off the pungent vegetables, it is hot throughout, and the flavors mingle.

Correct seasonings as desired. This soup can be made quickly and simply and adjusted for those with digestive troubles or food allergies. This is a complete meal in itself. Keeps for 3 to 5 days refrigerated and may be frozen.

Wild Rice Celery Soup

Serves 4 to 6

2 cups cooked wild rice (½ to ⅔ cup dry)

2 cups chopped celery

3½ cups milk, or 3¼ cups milk substitute and 2 ounces (¼ cup) tofu

2 to 3 tablespoons simmered tamari soy sauce or substitute

2 tablespoons finely chopped onion

1 small or medium clove garlic

3 tablespoons chopped, fresh parsley, or 4 to 5 teaspoons dried parsley

1 teaspoon Homemade Vegetable Broth Powder, or ½ to 1 Vegetable Bouillon Cube

½ teaspoon sea salt

½ teaspoon paprika, or 2 pinches saffron

Few dashes *each* sea kelp and cayenne

Optional: 1 to 2 tablespoons butter, or 1 tablespoon natural oil

Garnishes: ¼ cup chopped chives or green onion tops (green part only), or Gomashio

Cook the wild rice if not already cooked. Steam the celery (and tofu, if any) until tender. Blend all the ingredients, except for the garnishes and ¼ to ⅓ cup of the wild rice, together in a blender until smooth. Heat the blended mixture with the whole wild rice in a covered saucepan on medium heat until it comes to a low boil. Turn the heat to low and simmer for 20 to 30 minutes, until the flavors blend and the edge is off the onions and garlic. Stir occasionally. Serve hot with a green vegetable or a salad with optional legume dish. Keeps for 3 to 5 days refrigerated. Best if not frozen.

Broccoli Wild Rice Soup

Serves 2 to 3

1 cup cooked wild rice (about ⅓ cup dry)

3 to 3½ cups broccoli, chopped

1½ cups milk substitute, milk, thick bouillon, thick broth, or Brown Bean Juice

2 teaspoons finely chopped onion, or ½ to 1 teaspoon prepared horseradish

1 small clove garlic, minced, or ¼ teaspoon extra horseradish

4 to 5 teaspoons simmered tamari soy sauce or substitute, or 1 Homemade Vegetable Bouillon Cube

3 tablespoons finely chopped fresh parsley, or 4 teaspoons dried parsley

½ teaspoon *each* basil, dill weed, and vegetable broth powder

¼ teaspoon sea salt

Several dashes *each* sea kelp and cayenne

Optional topping: 2 to 4 teaspoons Home-Roasted Nuts (ground almonds or filberts), or Gomashio

If the rice has not been pre-cooked, cook it first for 1 hour plus. Steam the broccoli until tender. Use a blender to blend all ingredients except for the rice and topping. Blend until smooth, then place the blended mixture and rice in a saucepan and simmer on medium-low heat for 15 minutes, until the flavors mingle and refine. If desired, top with fresh, ground Home-Roasted Nuts and enjoy. Serve with a legume dish or other main dish and an optional salad. Keeps for 1 to 3 days refrigerated. Do not freeze.

Garlic Spinach Soup

Serves 4

2 tablespoons butter or natural oil

12 medium-large cloves garlic, sliced

4 cups water, stock, bouillon, or broth (unsalted)

6 medium cloves garlic, pressed

7 to 8 green onion tops (green part only), finely chopped

1 large bunch spinach leaves, lightly chopped

¼ cup tomato juice, or ¼ cup fresh lemon juice

¼ cup fresh finely chopped parsley

1 Homemade Vegetable Bouillon Cube, or 1 teaspoon Home-made Vegetable Broth Powder

½ to ¾ teaspoon sea salt

1 teaspoon *each* basil and oregano

½ teaspoon sea kelp

3 tablespoons simmered tamari soy sauce or substitute

Heat the butter or oil on low to medium heat and sauté the garlic slices in the oil or butter until thoroughly browned (more than 10 minutes), stirring frequently. Remove and discard the garlic. Add the liquid and the remaining ingredients to the garlic butter or oil. Simmer covered for 20 to 25 minutes. This robust yet light soup is very healing and strengthening. Besides being good for Candida diets, it is especially good for flu, colds, and infections. Best eaten within 2 to 4 days. Do not freeze.

Great Greens Soup

Serves 2 to 3

4 to 5 bunches mixed greens:
spinach, beet greens, chard,
kale, and/or mustard greens (3
to 3½ cups cooked)

2 to 3 green onions, chopped small

1 small clove garlic, minced

1 cup Brown Bean Juice, milk
substitute, or milk

1 teaspoon *each* basil and dill
weed

½ to ¾ teaspoon sea salt

½ teaspoon *each* marjoram and
thyme

2 teaspoons Homemade Veg-
etable Broth Powder, or 1
Homemade Vegetable Bouillon
Cube

2 to 3 dashes powdered ginger, or ¼
teaspoon fresh squeezed ginger
juice

Several dashes sea kelp and cayenne

Choose firm bright or dark green leaves. Remove any blemishes. Wash
the greens and chop lightly. Steam the greens until tender. Blend the cooked
greens with all the remaining ingredients. Simmer on medium-low heat for 15
to 20 minutes until hot throughout and the flavors mingle. Enjoy hot with
whole grains and/or legumes. A salad is optional. This hearty soup is rich in
iron and minerals. Keeps for 1 to 2 days refrigerated. Do not freeze.

Orange Yam or Carrot Soup

Serves 4

4 cups orange yams, chopped and rinsed 2 to 3 times (peeled or unpeeled), or 4 cups chopped carrots

1¾ to 2 cups milk substitute, stock, or broth (unsalted)

2 to 3 tablespoons butter, or 1 to 2 tablespoons natural oil

2 Homemade Vegetable Bouillon Cubes, or 2 tablespoons simmered tamari soy sauce or substitute

2 teaspoons finely chopped onion

4 teaspoons finely chopped fresh parsley, or 2 teaspoons dried parsley

2 teaspoons dill weed or tarragon, crushed

½ teaspoon sea salt

Several dashes sea kelp

Cayenne to taste

Optional: ¼ to ½ teaspoon crushed, dried mint leaves

Garnish: chopped chives or green onion tops (green part only), or chopped, fresh parsley

Steam the orange vegetable until tender. Liquefy all ingredients until smooth in a blender or food processor. Heat the soup in a saucepan on low to medium heat just up to boiling and simmer for 10 minutes. Do not boil. Serve hot, garnished with chopped chives, green onions, or chopped fresh parsley if desired. Serve with a salad and/or green vegetable with whole grains and legumes or other main dishes. Keeps refrigerated for 2 to 5 days. Do not freeze.

Rainbow Barley Soup

Serves 6 to 8

2 cups water, stock, or broth (unsalted)

2 cups Brown Bean Juice or thick bouillon (unsalted)

½ to ¾ cup brown pot barley

5 to 6 large tomatoes, chopped small, or 1 (28-ounce, 796-ml) can tomatoes, cored and chopped with the juice

1 medium onion (about 1 cup), chopped small

1 cup (2 to 3 medium) carrots, cut in ¼-inchrounds

1 cup celery, chopped in ¼-inch moons

1 cup broccoli, chopped in ½- to ¾-inch chunks

1 cup zucchini or yellow summer squash

2 Homemade Vegetable Bouillon Cubes, or 2 to 3 tablespoons simmered tamari soy sauce or substitute

2 teaspoons Homemade Vegetable Broth Powder

¼ cup fresh chopped parsley, or 2 tablespoons dried parsley

¾ to 1 teaspoon sea salt

1 teaspoon *each* basil and dill weed

¼ teaspoon sea kelp

Several dashes cayenne

Optional: 1 cup fresh or frozen green peas

Optional: 2 to 3 Jerusalem artichokes, chopped

Optional: 1 to 2 teaspoons honey or other sweetener, to balance flavors (cook at least 15 minutes and Candida will not be affected)

Optional topping: Gomashio

Bring the liquids, barley, and vegetables (except the peas, if any) up to boil on heat, then turn down to low and simmer for 40 minutes. Add the remaining ingredients/seasonings and simmer for another 20 to 30 minutes so the flavors can mingle and develop. Enjoy hot for a meal in itself or serve with a green salad prelude and/or a bean dish accompaniment. Keeps for 5 to 7 days refrigerated. Best if not frozen.

Brown Bean and Broccoli Soup

Serves 10 to 12

2 cups dry pinto or adzuki beans, soaked 6 to 8 hours

12 cups water, stock, broth, or bouillon (unsalted)

1 large onion (about 2 cups), finely chopped

3 to 4 cups chopped broccoli

3 to 4 tablespoons simmered tamari soy sauce or substitute

⅓ cup finely chopped fresh parsley, or 3 tablespoons dried parsley

2 tablespoons natural oil or butter

4 teaspoons Homemade Vegetable Broth Powder

2 Homemade Vegetable Bouillon Cubes

1 teaspoon basil

½ to 1 teaspoon sea salt

½ teaspoon cumin powder or paprika

¼ teaspoon sea kelp

Cayenne to taste

Optional: 1 to 2 teaspoons honey or other sweetener, to balance flavors (cook at least 15 minutes and Candida will not be affected)

Optional topping: Gomashio

Cook the beans until very tender. After cooking, add enough water or stock to total 12 cups of liquid. Add the onion and broccoli and cook on low to medium heat for 20 minutes. Then add the remaining ingredients and cook for another 20 minutes on medium heat.

Take 4 cups of beans and liquid from the soup, use a blender or food processor to liquefy it, then re-add it to the soup. Serve hot and enjoy. Serve with whole grains and an optional salad. This easy-to-digest and nutritious soup is high in calcium and protein. Keeps for 5 to 7 days refrigerated and may be frozen.

Taco Bean Soup

Serves 4

- 1 cup dry beans (pinto, kidney, red, or black beans), soaked 8 hours
- 1 medium (about 1 cup) onion, chopped small
- 2 to 3 cloves garlic, minced
- 3 cups bean cooking liquid (with added water if needed)
- 3 tablespoons finely chopped fresh parsley, or 1 tablespoon dried parsley
- 2 teaspoons chili powder, or Your Own Chili Powder
- 1 teaspoon sea salt
- 1 Homemade Vegetable Bouillon Cube, or 1 teaspoon Homemade Vegetable Broth Powder
- 2 to 3 teaspoons finely chopped jalapeño or other fresh, hot pepper, or 1 teaspoon dried, crushed red chili peppers
- Several dashes *each* sea kelp and cayenne to taste

Cook the beans until tender. Add the onions and garlic and cook for 20 to 30 minutes more until they are completely tender. Drain and measure the liquid from the beans and take away or add enough water to total 3 cups. Blend half the bean liquid and half the beans in a blender with all the remaining ingredients. Add these back to the rest of the soup and simmer everything together for another 15 to 20 minutes, or until the flavors mingle and the soup is completely hot throughout. Serve and enjoy.

Can serve with flatbreads or chapatis and Homemade Salsa simmered 4 to 5 minutes, if desired. Include a salad and/or cooked vegetables with a whole grain dish for a complete meal. One-half cup of pre-cooked, hot whole grain can also be added to each serving of soup rather than served on the side. Keeps for 7 to 8 days refrigerated and freezes very well.

Healing Vegetable Soup

Serves 8

2 cups chopped cauliflower, small white and purple turnips, or unpeeled Jerusalem artichokes, cut into ½- to ¾-inch chunks

4 medium carrots, cut in ¼-inch slices, or 2 cups chopped orange yams

1 cup chopped asparagus, or 1 large stalk broccoli, chopped small

1 to 2 tablespoons natural oil

1 large onion (about 2 cups), chopped small

8 cups water, stock, broth, or bouillon (unsalted)

4 stalks celery, chopped in ¼-inchmoons

1 small zucchini or yellow summer squash, quartered and cut in ¼-inch chunks

Optional: 1 cup fresh or frozen green peas, or ¾ cup chopped green beans

Optional: 2 to 4 Jerusalem artichokes, chopped

1 tablespoon simmered tamari soy sauce or substitute

4 teaspoons Homemade Vegetable Broth Powder, or 3 Homemade Vegetable Bouillon Cubes

¼ cup fresh chopped parsley, or 3 teaspoons dried parsley

1 to 1½ teaspoons sea salt

1 teaspoon *each* basil and oregano

½ teaspoon sea kelp

Several dashes cayenne

Optional: 1 to 2 teaspoons honey or other sweetener, to balance flavors (cook at least 15 minutes and Candida will not be affected)

Steam the white vegetables, carrots or yams, and asparagus or broccoli for 8 minutes before making the soup. Heat the oil and sauté the onions in the oil in a large pot until the onions are slightly tender, about 2 minutes. Then add the water, steamed vegetables, and all the rest of the ingredients. Cook the soup on low to medium heat for 35 to 50 minutes until all the vegetables are tender but not soggy and the flavors develop. Take 3 to 4 cups of the liquid and vegetables from the soup and use a blender to liquefy it. Add it back into the soup. This adds flavor and depth and gives the soup a natural thickness.

Correct the soup's spices according to personal taste. Serve with whole grains and/or legumes and an optional salad. Keeps refrigerated for 5 to 7 days. Do not freeze.

Lentil Vegetable Pottage

Serves 5 to 6

1 cup dry brown/green lentils

5 cups water, stock, broth, or bouillon (unsalted)

6 stalks celery, chopped in ⅓-inch moons

3 to 4 medium carrots, sliced in ¼-inch rounds

1 large onion, chopped small

2 cloves garlic, minced

2 tablespoons butter or natural oil

2 Homemade Vegetable Bouillon Cubes, or 2 tablespoons simmered tamari soy sauce or substitute

¼ cup finely chopped fresh parsley, or 3 teaspoons dried parsley

1 teaspoon *each* sea salt, basil, and Homemade Vegetable Broth Powder

½ teaspoon *each* dill weed, oregano, and thyme

⅛ teaspoon cayenne

Several dashes sea kelp

Optional: 1 medium or large red bell pepper, chopped small

Optional topping: Gomashio

Bring the dry lentils, liquid, and vegetables (except for the red bell pepper) to a boil on high heat, then simmer for 1 hour on low heat, or until the lentils are very tender. Add the remaining ingredients and simmer another 15 to 25 minutes, stirring occasionally, until the flavors mingle. If desired, blend 1 to 2 cups of the soup and return it to the pot for a richer, fuller flavor and added body. Correct spices according to taste. Serve hot and enjoy. This is a full meal alone or serve with a whole grain and optional salad. Keeps for 5 to 7 days in the refrigerator or may be frozen.

Perfect Parsley Soup

Serves 4 to 6

4 cups chopped cauliflower (or small white and purple turnips)

1 large bunch spinach leaves

1 cup water, stock, broth, or bouillon (unsalted)

1½ cups milk substitute

1 packed cup coarsely chopped fresh parsley

1 to 2 tablespoons natural oil or butter

2 Homemade Vegetable Bouillon Cubes, or 3 teaspoons Homemade Vegetable Broth Powder

2 to 3 tablespoons simmered tamari soy sauce or substitute

3 teaspoons finely chopped onion

1 small clove garlic, minced

1 teaspoon *each* paprika and basil

Sea salt and cayenne to taste

1 cup very finely chopped parsley (chopped 2 to 3 times as fine)

Steam the cauliflower or turnips for 4 minutes over 1 cup of water or stock. Add the washed spinach leaves on top of them and continue cooking for another 6 to 8 minutes, until both are very tender. Blend the simmered vegetables and any liquid with all the other ingredients except the 1 cup finely chopped parsley. Put the blended soup mixture in a medium saucepan and stir in the finely chopped parsley. Bring the mixture just up to a boil and let it simmer on low heat for 14 to 18 minutes as the flavors mingle. Correct the seasonings as desired. Serve garnished with extra sprigs of parsley or chopped green onion tops (green part only). Serve with legumes and/or whole grains and optional salad. Keeps fresh for 3 to 6 days refrigerated. Do not freeze.

Blended Black Turtle Bean Soup

Serves 8 to 10

2 to 2¼ cups dry black beans, soaked 8 to 12 hours

2 cups carrots or orange yams, rinsed well and chopped small

2½ to 3½ cups bean cooking liquid

1 large onion, chopped*

2 cloves garlic, or 1½ teaspoons garlic powder*

3 Homemade Vegetable Bouillon Cubes, or 3 teaspoons Homemade Vegetable Broth Powder

⅓ to ½ cup finely chopped fresh parsley, or 2 to 3 tablespoons dried parsley

1 teaspoon *each* sea salt, paprika, and basil

½ teaspoon sea kelp

Cayenne to taste

Optional: 2 to 3 Jerusalem artichokes, chopped

Optional topping: Gomashio

Cook the beans. Steam the carrots or yams until tender. When the beans are completely soft, add the fresh onion and garlic, if any, and cook for another 15 to 20 minutes until they are tender. Blend the beans and vegetables in a blender with only 2½ to 3½ cups of the bean cooking liquid. (Drain the rest, if any, and use in other recipes or add water if needed.) Add all the remaining ingredients and blend until smooth. Just use enough liquid to make the blender work easily to make a thick soup, or thin with a bit of extra liquid and seasonings. Heat the blended soup and simmer on medium-low heat for 20 to 25 minutes so the flavors can mingle. Serve hot, or store. Serve with green vegetable or salad and optional whole grain. Keeps for 7 to 8 days refrigerated and freezes well.

---

*Instead of onions and garlic, 1 to 3 teaspoons of prepared horseradish may be added to the blender.

Blended Three Bean Tomato Soup

Serves 10 to 12

⅔ cup adzuki, pinto, or Romano beans, soaked

⅔ cup kidney or red beans, soaked

⅔ cup black beans, soaked (or instead of above beans: 2 cups of any 1 bean, soaked)

1 cup asparagus, artichoke hearts packed in water (drained), or kohlrabi, chopped small

7 cups water or stock

5 to 6 large tomatoes, or 1 (28-ounce, 796-ml) can tomatoes, cored and chopped with the juice

½ cup chopped water chestnuts or mung bean sprouts

1 large onion (about 1½ cups), chopped*

2 cloves garlic, minced*

¼ cup fresh chopped parsley, or 4 to 5 teaspoons dried parsley

2 Homemade Vegetable Bouillon Cubes

3 teaspoons Homemade Vegetable Broth Powder

1 to 2 tablespoons natural oil or butter

2 tablespoons simmered tamari soy sauce or substitute

1 teaspoon *each* sea salt, dill weed, and basil

½ teaspoon oregano

¼ teaspoon sea kelp

Cayenne to taste

Optional: 2 to 3 Jerusalem artichokes, chopped

Optional topping: Gomashio

All the beans can be soaked together. Use any one or two types of beans alone if desired. Cook the beans until very tender. Steam the green vegetable for 5 to 6 minutes until semi-tender. Then measure the water and add or subtract water as required. Add all the remaining ingredients to the pot and cook on low heat for 25 to 35 minutes until everything is tender. Then blend the soup bit by bit until thoroughly liquefied. Return the soup to the pot and simmer again for 10 minutes or so until flavors have completely mingled. Serve hot and garnish with chopped parsley, chives, or green onion tops (green part only). This is a very thick, rich soup. Do not eat more than 2 bowls at a sitting and include salad, vegetables, or other light foods to round off this lovely, filling soup. Keeps for 4 to 6 days refrigerated, or may be frozen.

* Instead of onions and garlic, 1 to 3 teaspoons of prepared horseradish may be added to the blender.

Harvest Red Lentil Soup

Serves 8 to 12

2½ to 3 cups chopped yam (1 large or 2 small), rinsed 2 to 3 times

3 large carrots (about 1 cup or bit more), chopped

10 cups water, stock, broth, or bouillon (unsalted)

1½ cups red lentils

4 stalks celery, chopped

1 medium to large stalk broccoli, chopped small

1 small zucchini, cut in half moon slices

1 large onion (1½ to 2 cups), chopped*

3 cloves garlic, minced*

2 tablespoons natural oil

3 tablespoons simmered tamari soy sauce or substitute

½ cup finely chopped fresh parsley, or 3 tablespoons dried

3 Homemade Vegetable Bouillon Cubes, or 4 teaspoons Homemade Vegetable Broth Powder

1½ to 2 teaspoons sea salt

1 teaspoon *each* basil, paprika, and oregano

¼ teaspoon sea kelp

8 to 10 dashes cayenne to taste

Optional: 2 to 3 Jerusalem artichokes, chopped

Optional: 1 to 2 teaspoons honey or other sweetening, to balance flavors (cook at least 15 minutes and Candida will not be affected)

Optional topping: Gomashio

Steam the yams with the carrots until semi-tender. Bring the water to a boil with the lentils and all the remaining vegetables in it. Sauté the onion and garlic in the oil.* After 30 to 45 minutes, add the steamed vegetables, onion (or horseradish), and all the remaining ingredients to the soup pot. Simmer everything for 20 to 25 minutes more so flavors can mingle. Serve hot and enjoy. This soup is a meal in itself but may be served with salad and whole grains and/or other legumes. Keeps for 5 to 7 days refrigerated. May be frozen, but is better fresh.

---

*Or use 1 to 3 teaspoons prepared horseradish added to the soup with the last ingredients instead of onions and garlic if desired.

Marvelous Minestrone Soup

Serves 10 to 12

⅔ cup dry kidney or red beans, soaked and cooked

⅔ cup dry chickpeas, soaked and cooked

2 tablespoons olive oil or natural oil

1 large onion (1½ to 2 cups), chopped

8 cups water, stock, broth, or light bouillon (unsalted)

8 to 9 large tomatoes, chopped, or 2 (21-ounce, 598-ml) cans tomatoes, cored and chopped with the juice

2 cups celery, chopped in ¼-inch moons

3 medium carrots, diced very small

2 to 3 cloves garlic, pressed

3 tablespoons simmered tamari soy sauce or substitute

2 Homemade Vegetable Bouillon Cubes, or 3 teaspoons Homemade Vegetable Broth Powder

3 tablespoons finely chopped fresh parsley, or 2 tablespoons dried

1½ to 2 teaspoons sea salt

1 teaspoon *each* oregano and basil

Cayenne to taste

Soak and cook the beans together until tender. Heat the oil in a large soup pot and sauté the onion for 2 to 3 minutes. Add the liquid and all the vegetables and simmer for about 40 minutes, or until the vegetables are fairly tender. Add the pre-cooked, drained beans and the remaining ingredients, and simmer for another 20 to 25 minutes so the flavors mingle and the soup is hot throughout. Serve with whole grains and salad for a complete meal. Keeps for 7 to 8 days refrigerated. May be frozen but is better fresh.

Quick and Easy Artichoke Heart Soup

Serves 3 to 4

1 cup artichoke hearts packed in water, drained and chopped

2 cups milk, or 1¾ cups milk substitute and 2 ounces (¼ cup) tofu, steamed

2 tablespoons finely chopped fresh parsley, or 1 tablespoon dried

1 tablespoon finely chopped raw onion*

2 Homemade Vegetable Bouillon Cubes, or 1 to 2 tablespoons simmered tamari soy sauce or substitute

1 small clove garlic, minced*

1 teaspoon basil

½ teaspoon *each* sea salt and dill weed

Couple dashes nutmeg or allspice

Several dashes *each* sea kelp and cayenne to taste

Optional: 1 tablespoon butter or natural oil

Optional: ½ bunch spinach, steamed until tender

Blend all the ingredients in a blender until smooth. Try to use one or both of the optional ingredients if milk substitute is used. Heat the soup on medium heat until it comes up to a boil. Turn the heat to low and simmer 25 to 30 minutes, or until the flavors balance and the sharp edge is off the onion and garlic. Serve hot and enjoy with a whole grain and/or legume dish with a salad if desired. Keeps for 3 to 5 days refrigerated. Do not freeze.

---

*Onion and garlic in this recipe can be substituted with ½ to 1 teaspoon prepared horseradish.

Asparagus Ambrosia Soup

Serves 4

3 to 3½ cups chopped asparagus, bottom ¼ to ⅓ of stalks removed

2 cups milk, or 1½ cups milk substitute and 4 ounces (½ cup) tofu

¼ cup chives or green onion tops (green part only)

1 medium clove garlic, minced

1 teaspoon Homemade Vegetable Broth Powder, or 2 teaspoons simmered tamari soy sauce or substitute

1 tablespoon finely chopped fresh parsley, or 1 teaspoon dried

1 teaspoon basil

½ teaspoon thyme

Few dashes sea kelp

Sea salt and cayenne to taste

Optional: 2 tablespoons butter or 1 tablespoon natural oil

Optional: ¼ cup chopped water chestnuts

The bottom green parts of the asparagus can be peeled and steamed with the tops. Steam the chopped asparagus tops and peeled bottoms (and tofu, if any) until tender. Blend all the ingredients together until smooth. Try to use one or both of the optional ingredients if milk substitute is used. Heat the mixture on medium heat just up to a boil, then simmer on low heat for 20 to 30 minutes until the edge is off the garlic, the flavors blend, and the soup is hot throughout. Enjoy this tasty soup with whole grains and legumes with or without a salad. Keeps for 3 to 5 days refrigerated. Do not freeze.

Spinach Surprise Soup

Serves 3 to 4

4 large bunches spinach, steamed until tender

2 cups milk, or 1½ cups milk substitute and 4 ounces (½ cup) tofu

¼ cup chives or green onion tops (green part only), chopped

1 medium clove garlic, minced

1 teaspoon Homemade Vegetable Broth Powder, or 2 to 3 teaspoons simmered tamari soy sauce or substitute

1 tablespoon finely chopped fresh parsley, or 1 teaspoon dried

1 teaspoon basil

½ teaspoon dill weed

Few dashes sea kelp

Sea salt and cayenne to taste

Optional: 2 tablespoons butter or 1 tablespoon natural oil

½ cup almonds, Home-Roasted and finely chopped or slivered (or filberts, pine nuts, or pecans), or ½ cup chopped water chestnuts

Steam the spinach (and tofu, if any) until tender. Blend all the ingredients together until smooth except for the nuts. Add the nuts and heat the mixture on medium heat just up to a boil, then simmer on low heat for 20 to 30 minutes until the edge is off the garlic, the flavors blend, and the soup is hot throughout. Enjoy this tasty soup with whole grains and legumes with or without a salad. Keeps for 2 to 4 days refrigerated. Do not freeze.

Chapter 17

SASSY SAUCES AND GRAVIES

Wʜᴇɴ ʏᴏᴜ ᴀʀᴇ ᴛᴏᴏ ᴛɪʀᴇᴅ ᴛᴏ ɢᴇᴛ ꜰᴀɴᴄʏ ᴏʀ sᴘᴇɴᴅ a lot of time cooking, a sauce or gravy can add zest, flavor, color, and quality to simple steamed vegetables, plain cooked whole grains, and unadorned legumes. The vegetables must be prepared fresh, the whole grains can be prepared within the week, but the legumes and the sauce can be frozen for convenient and quick meals. These sauces and gravies, added to vegetables, whole grains, or legumes, create whole new main dish treats and bring a rainbow of variety to wholesome, common staples, adding a special touch to any meal. There is nothing average about these lovely flavors. Enjoy sauces and gravies often. Make big batches and freeze some. These recipes are rich in vitamins and nutrients and aim to bring good taste to wholesome foods. When a main dish recipe seems like too much work, try these delicious alternatives.

Brown Bean Juice (for Recipes)

Makes 4 to 6 cups

2 cups pinto, kidney, or adzuki
   beans,* soaked

8 to 10 cups water

---

*Red and black beans can also be used to make this juice; however, black beans make a black juice that only works well in some recipes.

Cook the beans with water until very tender. Strain the beans with a colander or strainer, drain, and save the liquid. Freeze or use the beans for another recipe. This wholesome brown juice adds flavor and nutrients to sauces, gravies, soups, stews, and main dishes. Many recipes in this book call for Brown Bean Juice. The thicker and "muddier" it is, the better. Keeps for 6 to 7 days refrigerated or may be frozen.

Mock Meat Gravy

Makes 2½ cups

2 cups Brown Bean Juice

2 tablespoons simmered tamari soy sauce or substitute, or ½ to 2 Homemade Vegetable Bouillon Cubes

1 to 2 tablespoons butter or natural oil

¼ cup amaranth, teff, or chick-pea flour (soy may also be used, as a last choice)

1½ to 2 tablespoons arrowroot powder or kudzu*

½ teaspoon chili powder, vegetable broth powder, or curry powder, or ¼ teaspoon basil with ¼ teaspoon cumin powder

¼ teaspoon sea salt or substitute

¼ teaspoon sea kelp

Several dashes cayenne or to taste

Use a wire whisk or blender to combine the Brown Bean Juice with all the remaining ingredients. Stir over medium-low heat until thickened. Correct or alter the seasonings to taste, and serve the gravy on brown rice, whole grains, vegetables, mock meatballs and mock meat loaves, burgers, casseroles, and other main dishes.

---

*⅔ cup steamed, mashed cauliflower, winter squash, or orange yam may be blended into everything instead of the arrowroot or kudzu.

Sesame Tahini and Ginger Sauce

Makes 2½ cups

2 to 3 tablespoons natural oil

1 medium (1 cup) onion, chopped small

1½ to 2 cups Brown Bean Juice, water, broth, or stock (unsalted)

1 cup sesame tahini (can pour off oil if desired)

2 tablespoons ground nuts or seeds (almonds, filberts, sunflower, pumpkin, or sesame seeds)

2 Homemade Vegetable Bouillon Cubes, or 2 to 3 tablespoons simmered tamari soy sauce or substitute

3 to 4 teaspoons peeled, finely grated ginger

1 teaspoon honey or maple syrup or 1 tablespoon apple, peach, or pear juice*

1 teaspoon sea salt

Several dashes *each* nutmeg and ground ginger

Cayenne to taste

Optional: 1 tablespoon fresh lemon or lime juice

Heat the oil on high heat and sauté the onion until tender. Add the remaining ingredients and simmer everything on low heat for about 30 minutes, stirring regularly. Serve hot over steamed vegetables and whole grains. Keeps refrigerated for 6 to 8 days or may be frozen.

---

*Cook at least 15, preferably 20, minutes or more, and Candida will not be affected.

Toasted Sesame Seed Sauce

Makes about 3½ cups

1 cup sesame tahini

1 cup Home-Roasted Seeds, hulled white sesame seeds, ground

2 cups Brown Bean Juice, broth, stock, or bouillon (unsalted)

2 tablespoons arrowroot powder

2 tablespoons finely chopped onion

1 to 2 cloves garlic, crushed

1 tablespoon simmered tamari soy sauce or substitute, or 2 teaspoons Homemade Vegetable Broth Powder

1 Homemade Vegetable Bouillon Cube

1 tablespoon fresh lemon or lime juice

½ teaspoon paprika

Sea salt to taste

Few dashes cayenne to taste

Place all the ingredients in a blender and liquefy. Heat in a saucepan on medium-low heat, stirring regularly, until thickened and hot throughout, about 20 minutes. Serve on vegetables, whole grains, burgers, or casseroles. Keeps for 6 to 8 days refrigerated or may be frozen.

Saffron Sesame Seed Sauce

Makes about 3½ cups

1 cup sesame tahini

1 cup Home-Roasted Seeds, hulled white sesame seeds, ground

1¾ cups milk substitute with 2 ounces (¼ cup) tofu, or 2 cups milk

2 tablespoons arrowroot powder

2 to 3 tablespoons finely chopped onion

2 cloves garlic, crushed

1 tablespoon simmered tamari soy sauce or substitute, or 2 teaspoons Homemade Vegetable Broth Powder

1 Homemade Vegetable Bouillon Cube

½ teaspoon powdered saffron or 1 g saffron strands

½ teaspoon paprika

Sea salt to taste

Several dashes cayenne to taste

Optional: squeeze of ginger juice

Optional: 1 teaspoon honey or maple syrup or 1 tablespoon apple, peach, or pear juice*

Place all the ingredients in a blender and liquefy. Heat in a saucepan on medium-low heat, stirring regularly, until thickened and hot throughout, about 20 minutes. Serve on vegetables, whole grains, burgers, or casseroles. Keeps for 4 to 6 days refrigerated or may be frozen.

---

*Cook at least 15, preferably 20, minutes or more, and Candida will not be affected.

Toasted Almond or Filbert Sauce

Makes 3 cups

1½ cups Home-Roasted Nuts, almonds, or filberts, ground

2 cups milk substitute or Brown Bean Juice

2 tablespoons arrowroot powder or kudzu

2 tablespoons finely chopped onion

1 to 2 cloves garlic, pressed or minced

1 tablespoon simmered tamari soy sauce or substitute, or 1 Homemade Vegetable Bouillon Cube

3 to 4 teaspoons peeled, finely grated ginger

1 to 2 teaspoons lemon or lime juice, or ½ to 1 teaspoon squeezed ginger juice

Few dashes cayenne to taste

Sea salt to taste

Use a blender to blend all ingredients until smooth. Heat the mixture on medium-low heat and keep it just under a boil. Simmer for 15 to 20 minutes, stirring regularly, until thickened and hot throughout. Serve over vegetables, spaghetti squash, or whole grains. Keeps for 6 to 8 days refrigerated or may be frozen.

Toasted Nut and Vegetable Sauce

Makes 3½ cups

1 cup chopped carrots, broccoli, asparagus, orange yam, well-packed spinach, or peeled, seeded tomatoes

¾ to 1 cup Home-Roasted Nuts, almonds or filberts, ground

2 cups milk substitute or Brown Bean Juice

2 tablespoons arrowroot powder or kudzu

2 to 3 tablespoons finely chopped onion

2 cloves garlic, pressed or minced

1 tablespoon finely chopped fresh parsley or 1 teaspoon dried

1 tablespoon simmered tamari soy sauce or substitute, or 1 Homemade Vegetable Bouillon Cube

3 to 4 teaspoons peeled, finely grated ginger

1 to 2 teaspoons lemon or lime juice or ½ to 1 teaspoon squeezed ginger juice

1 teaspoon basil or dill weed

Few dashes cayenne to taste

Sea salt to taste

Steam the vegetable until tender. Use a blender to blend it with all ingredients until smooth. Heat the mixture on medium-low heat and keep it just under a boil. Simmer for 15 to 20 minutes, stirring regularly, until thickened and hot throughout. Serve over vegetables, spaghetti squash, or whole grains. Keeps for 6 to 8 days refrigerated or may be frozen.

Amorous Avocado Tofu Sauce

Makes 3 to 3½ cups

1 to 2 teaspoons butter or natural oil

¼ cup finely chopped chives or green onion tops (green part only)

1 small clove garlic, minced or ¼ to ½ teaspoon prepared horseradish

14 to 16 ounces soft or regular tofu, steamed 7 to 9 minutes

2 medium avocados, ripe, peeled and pitted

¼ to ½ cup milk substitute, broth, or stock

2 teaspoons fresh lemon or lime juice

2 Homemade Vegetable Bouillon Cubes, or 1 to 2 tablespoons simmered tamari soy sauce or substitute

Few dashes sea kelp

Sea salt and cayenne to taste

Optional: 2 tablespoons finely chopped fresh parsley

Heat the butter or oil and sauté the chives and garlic until tender. (Do not sauté horseradish.) Use a food processor to combine all ingredients thoroughly. Heat on very low heat until hot throughout. Stir regularly. Serve hot over vegetables, legumes, or whole grains. Keeps for 1 to 2 days refrigerated. Do not freeze.

Orange Yam Sauce

Makes about 3 cups

4 cups chopped, orange yams, peeled (about 2 large yams)

⅓ to ½ cup milk substitute or milk

1 tablespoon simmered tamari soy sauce or substitute, or 1 Homemade Vegetable Bouillon Cube

2 teaspoons finely chopped onion

¾ to 1 teaspoon curry powder

¼ to ½ teaspoon sea salt

Several dashes of cayenne or to taste

Optional: several dashes sea kelp

Optional: ¼ teaspoon prepared horse-radish, or 1 small clove garlic, pressed or finely chopped

Rinse the cut yam several times and steam until tender. Use a food processor or masher to mix all the ingredients thoroughly until smooth. Heat the sauce on low heat in a covered saucepan or double-boiler if desired until hot throughout, about 15 minutes or more. Stir regularly. Serve hot on vegetables or over whole grains. Keeps for 3 to 5 days refrigerated. May be frozen but is best fresh.

Green Herb and Orange Yam Sauce

Makes about 3 cups

4 cups chopped, orange yams, peeled (about 2 large yams)

⅓ to ½ cup milk substitute or milk

1 Homemade Vegetable Bouillon Cube, or 1 teaspoon Home-made Vegetable Broth Powder

¼ cup finely chopped chives or green onion tops (green part only)

2 to 3 tablespoons finely chopped fresh parsley

1 teaspoon finely chopped, fresh basil, or ¼ teaspoon dried basil or dried dill weed

¼ to ½ teaspoon sea salt

¼ teaspoon oregano or thyme

Several dashes of cayenne to taste

Optional: several dashes sea kelp

Optional: ¼ teaspoon prepared horse-radish, or 1 small clove garlic, pressed or finely chopped

Rinse the cut yam several times and steam until tender. Use a food processor or masher to mix all the ingredients thoroughly until smooth. Heat the sauce on low heat in a covered saucepan or double-boiler if desired, until hot throughout, about 15 minutes or more. Stir regularly. Serve hot on vegetables or over whole grains. Keeps for 3 to 5 days refrigerated. May be frozen but is best fresh.

Green Garlic Sauce

Makes 1½ cups

1 large bunch spinach, lightly chopped

1 cup Brown Bean Juice, broth, stock, milk substitute, or bouillon (unsalted)

¼ cup natural oil or butter

¼ cup chives or green onion tops (green part only)

8 to 10 cloves garlic, minced

1 Homemade Vegetable Bouillon Cube, or 1 tablespoon simmered tamari soy sauce or substitute

1 tablespoon finely chopped fresh parsley or 1 teaspoon dried

1 teaspoon paprika

½ teaspoon *each* basil and thyme

¼ to ½ teaspoon sea salt

Several dashes *each* sea kelp and cayenne

Steam the spinach until tender. Blend it with all the remaining ingredients and put in a saucepan. Bring to a boil on medium heat, covered, then turn down to low and simmer for 20 minutes or so, until the sharp edge is off the garlic and the flavors mingle. Stir regularly. Serve over vegetables, spaghetti squash, or whole grains. Keeps for 3 to 6 days refrigerated. May be frozen but is best fresh.

Nutty Garlic Sauce

Makes 2 cups

½ cup Home-Roasted Nuts, or blanched almonds, or filberts, ground

1¼ cups milk substitute, light broth, or stock (unsalted)

¼ cup natural oil or butter

8 to 10 cloves garlic, minced

1 Homemade Vegetable Bouillon Cube, or 1 tablespoon simmered tamari soy sauce or substitute

1 tablespoon finely chopped fresh parsley or 1 teaspoon dried

1 teaspoon paprika

½ teaspoon *each* basil and thyme

¼ to ½ teaspoon sea salt

Several dashes *each* sea kelp and cayenne

Blend all the ingredients and put in a saucepan. Bring to a boil on medium heat, covered, then turn down to low and simmer for 20 minutes or so, until the sharp edge is off the garlic and the flavors mingle. Stir regularly. Serve over vegetables, spaghetti squash, or whole grains. Keeps for 3 to 6 days refrigerated. May be frozen but is best fresh.

Savory Sweet Onion Sauce (Naturally Sweet)

Makes 2 to 3 cups

1 to 2 tablespoons natural oil or butter

4 cups finely chopped onions (or cut in strips or slice in thin rings if preferred)

⅓ to ½ cup Brown Bean Juice, broth, or bouillon (unsalted)

2 to 4 tablespoons simmered tamari soy sauce or substitute, or 2 Homemade Vegetable Bouillon Cubes

Heat the oil or butter on high heat and sauté the onion for 2 to 3 minutes or so until tender, stirring constantly. Add the liquid, tamari soy sauce, or broken-up bouillon cubes and simmer, covered, on medium-low heat for 1 hour. Serve hot over whole grains and/or vegetables, or as a gravy or topping for casseroles or burgers. The onions turn deliciously sweet during the long simmering process. Keeps for 7 to 10 days refrigerated. May be frozen but is best fresh. This recipe may be used as a mushroom substitute in some recipes.

Homemade Tomato Sauce

Makes 4 to 5 cups

1 to 2 tablespoons natural oil (can use olive)

1 large (about 1½ cups) onion, chopped small

4 cloves garlic, minced

5 to 6 large tomatoes or 1 (28-ounce, 796-ml) can tomatoes, cored and chopped with juice

1 (14-ounce, 398-ml) can tomato paste

1 to 1½ cups water, broth, or stock (unsalted)

3 bay leaves

1 to 2 tablespoons tamari soy sauce or substitute, or 2 Homemade Vegetable Bouillon Cubes

1 teaspoon honey or maple syrup or 1 tablespoon apple, peach, or pear juice*

3 to 4 tablespoons finely chopped, fresh parsley, or 3 teaspoons dried

4 teaspoons finely chopped fresh basil or 1½ teaspoons dried

1 teaspoon oregano

¾ to 1 teaspoon sea salt

½ teaspoon *each* marjoram, thyme, and rosemary, crushed

¼ teaspoon sea kelp

Optional: 1 cup chopped red or green bell pepper

Optional: ½ cup chopped water chestnuts or whole pine nuts

(continues)

---

*Cook at least 15, preferably 20, minutes or more, and Candida will not be affected.

Heat the oil in a large pot on high heat. When the oil is hot, sauté the onion and garlic for 2 minutes. Add the chopped tomatoes and reduce the heat to low. Cook covered for 15 to 20 minutes, until the tomatoes turn to liquid. Add the remaining ingredients and simmer on low heat for 40 to 60 minutes, covered, stirring occasionally. A little extra liquid may be added for thinner consistency. Correct the herbs and spices as desired. Remove bay leaves when the sauce is finished. This recipe can be doubled or tripled for large batches, but be sure to reduce the salt when increasing it. Keeps for 6 to 8 days refrigerated and freezes well.

Mock Tomato Sauce (Without Vinegar)

Makes 10 to 12 cups

7 cups peeled, chopped orange yams or peeled butternut or buttercup squash

1 cup chopped, fresh beets (about 2 large)

1 tablespoon natural oil or butter (can use olive oil)

1 cup (1 medium) chopped onion

3 cloves garlic, minced

6 cups water, stock or broth

3 Homemade Vegetable Bouillon Cubes, or 3 tablespoons simmered tamari soy sauce or substitute

1 strip of wakame or kombu seaweed, washed and minced

3 tablespoons finely chopped fresh parsley or 3 teaspoons dried

1 teaspoon *each* basil and oregano

¼ teaspoon *each* sea kelp, thyme, and rosemary, crushed

2 to 3 bay leaves

1 teaspoon honey or maple syrup or 1 tablespoon apple, peach, or pear juice (cook at least 15 minutes and Candida will not be affected)

1 to 2 teaspoons fresh lemon or lime juice

Steam the yams or squash and beets until tender. Heat the oil on high heat and sauté the onions until transparent. Blend all the ingredients except bay leaves until smooth. Add bay leaves and heat in a saucepan until hot throughout and the flavors mingle, 25 to 30 minutes or more. Remove bay leaves. Serve hot in place of tomato sauce over vegetables, steamed turnips or cauliflower, spaghetti squash, whole grains, beans, burgers, and casseroles. Keeps for 5 to 6 days refrigerated or may be frozen.

Chapter 18

MAGNIFICENT MAIN DISHES

THESE MAIN DISH MARVELS ARE BRAND-NEW, specially designed recipes meant to thrill the taste buds and make you forget you are on a Candida diet. Indeed, some of these dishes may make you thankful that you have Candida; otherwise, you might never have discovered how delicious wholesome natural cooking can be! On a Candida diet, snacks and goodies are limited, but main dishes can be eaten to your heart's content. (Within reason!) Do avoid foods to which you are allergic or sensitive. Dairy products are an option in a few of these recipes, but all can be prepared without dairy. (Special recipes using dairy, fish, and poultry are at the end of the chapter.) You will notice many options for each item in all the recipes; see the Substitution Chart in chapter 11 for additional information.

You can enjoy two or three of these tantalizing recipes per day without guilt or setbacks. The soup chapter contains recipes that are complete in one meal (chapter 16). The sauce recipes (chapter 17) can be served over whole grains and legumes to make more simple, quick and easy, exciting main dishes. Some of the appetizer, salad, and breakfast recipes are also great as main dishes. There are over 45 alternative main dishes to choose from in this chapter and over 75 main dishes altogether throughout this book. See chapter 9 for more on meal planning and menus, and note the serving suggestions at the end of each main dish and soup recipe.

If you are concerned about occasional, minute use of sweeteners, tamari soy sauce, milk, soy products, herbs, or bouillon cubes in some of these recipes, don't be! See the Glossary, Controversial Foods, or individual recipes for notes on how these foods can be tolerated without affecting Candida growth if proper precautions are taken or by using substitutes or Mock version recipes.

Have fun preparing these easy-to-follow, kitchen-tested recipes. If you can follow directions, you can create tasty, successful recipes every time!

VEGETARIAN MAIN DISHES

Herb and Veggie Burgers

Serves 2 to 4

½ cup finely chopped carrot, yam, or winter squash, in ¼-inch chunks

½ cup finely chopped broccoli, asparagus, kohlrabi, celery, or green bell pepper, in ¼-inch chunks

1 cup cooked brown rice or other, cooked, somewhat firm whole grain; or 1 cup regular tofu, finely crumbled

⅓ cup amaranth or teff flour

¼ cup finely chopped onion

2 tablespoons arrowroot powder

1 tablespoon dried parsley, crushed, or 2 tablespoons finely chopped fresh parsley

2 teaspoons Brown Bean Juice, milk substitute, milk, tomato juice, stock, or water

1 teaspoon natural oil

1 clove garlic, minced

1 teaspoon basil

½ teaspoon *each* sea salt and dill weed

¼ teaspoon *each* marjoram and thyme

Several dashes *each* sea kelp and cayenne

Steam the orange and green vegetables together until very tender. Using a fork, mix them with the grain or tofu and all the remaining ingredients. Mix well but do not mash the burger ingredients. Heat a very large skillet or griddle (a cast-iron pan works wonderfully) on high heat. While the pan is heating, shape the veggie mixture into 4 medium burgers. Reduce the heat to medium, oil the pan generously, and place the burgers side by side. If the pan is not big enough, cook 2 to 3 at a time. Use a metal spatula to press the burgers flat and let them cook 5 to 6 minutes on the first side, 4 to 5 minutes on the other side. Do not cover while cooking; press the burgers down occasionally so they flatten more and are more easily cooked in the center. Enjoy hot with Homemade Ketchup, a dressing or sauce, and tomato slices if desired. Serve with a salad or other vegetables on the side. If whole grain is used in this recipe, a bean side dish is suggested. If tofu is used, serve a whole grain side dish. Keeps for 2 to 4 days refrigerated and may be reheated by baking. Best if not frozen.

Vital Vegetable Nut Burgers

Serves 8

⅔ cup carrots, chopped small

⅔ cup celery or zucchini, chopped small

1¼ cups amaranth or teff flour

1 cup ground raw almonds, filberts, pecans, or sunflower seeds

1 tablespoon ground pumpkin seeds or sesame seeds

2 tablespoons chickpea or brown lentil flour (soy can be used, as a last choice)

⅔ cup finely chopped onion

½ cup milk substitute, milk, bouillon, or broth (unsalted)

3 to 4 tablespoons natural oil

3 teaspoons dried parsley, or 2 tablespoons fresh chopped parsley

½ teaspoon *each* sea salt, basil, oregano, and thyme

Optional: 1 to 2 cloves garlic, chopped

Steam the carrots and green vegetable until very tender, then mash them and add to the remaining ingredients. Use a fork to mix well. Oil a large skillet or flat grill and cook on medium-low heat. Form the mixture into 8 to 12 burgers and lightly coat each one with extra flour. Cook them for several minutes on each side until nicely browned. Serve with Homemade Ketchup, a dressing or sauce, or a gravy alongside whole grains and other vegetables for a complete meal. Cooked burgers keep for 3 to 5 days refrigerated or may be frozen. They reheat best by baking. ⅓ cup Jerusalem artichokes can be substituted for ⅓ cup of the carrots if desired.

Best Bean Burgers

Serves 6 to 12

1 cup dry chickpeas or soybeans, soaked 24 hours

1 cup Scotch oats, soaked 4 to 8 hours

½ cup ground raw sunflower or sesame seeds, or ground raw nuts

½ cup amaranth or teff flour

1 medium onion, finely chopped

2 tablespoons simmered tamari soy sauce or substitute, or 2 Homemade

Vegetable Bouillon Cubes

2 tablespoons natural oil

2 teaspoons sea salt

Optional: 1 to 2 teaspoons ground or whole flaxseeds

Optional: 1 to 2 well-beaten large eggs or 2 to 3 teaspoons arrow-root powder

Rinse the soaked chickpeas or beans carefully by swishing them in fresh water and draining several times. Put the washed, drained beans through a hand (meat) grinder, food processor, homogenizing juicer, or other appliance that will grind them into a coarse consistency. Drain the cracked Scotch oats and add them to the ground beans. Add the remaining ingredients and mix everything together well. If the mixture seems too dry, add a little water.

Tear off 12 square sheets of wax paper. (Use plastic wrap or aluminum foil, shiny side in if corn-allergic.) Divide the bean mixture equally onto the 12 sheets. Shape and press the mixture into burgers and fold them up individually and securely in the paper or wrap. Place the burgers flat in a plastic bag for freshness and protection from freezer burn. Freeze solid before cooking.

Cook the bean burgers as you would regular burgers. Heat a lightly oiled fry pan or skillet on medium heat. Take burgers directly from the freezer, unwrap them, and put them in the hot pan. Cook for about 15 to 20 minutes on the first side and 8 to 12 minutes on the second side. Keep covered while cooking and cook until browned and firm. Serve with Homemade Ketchup, a dressing or sauce, or gravy with vegetable side dishes or salad. Add other whole grains or legumes if desired. Burgers keep for 2 to 3 months frozen. Cooked burgers will keep for 3 to 6 days refrigerated.

Super Sunflower-Bean Burgers (Oil-Free)

Serves 3 to 6

1 cup cooked, mashed beans (pinto, kidney, adzuki, or black beans)

1 cup vegetable pulp from a juicer, or finely chopped steamed vegetables (carrots, celery, peppers, broccoli)

½ cup ground raw sunflower seeds

1 tablespoon ground raw pumpkin seeds or sunflower seeds

½ to ¾ cup amaranth or teff flour

½ cup finely chopped onion

3 teaspoons dried parsley

2 to 3 teaspoons simmered tamari soy sauce or substitute, or ½ Homemade Vegetable Bouillon Cube

½ teaspoon *each* basil and dill weed

¼ to ½ teaspoon sea salt

Several dashes cayenne

Optional: 1 teaspoon ground or whole flaxseeds

Precook and mash the beans. Mix all the ingredients together well; use extra amaranth or teff flour if mixture is too wet. Shape the mixture into 6 medium burgers about ½ inch thick and 4 inches in diameter. The burgers can be broiled on a wire grill or oiled, flat surface for 8 to 10 minutes on the first side and 5 to 8 minutes on the other side, or the burgers can be baked at about 375°F for 25 to 30 minutes. Serve with Homemade Ketchup, a dressing or sauce, or a gravy alongside whole grains and other vegetables for a complete meal. Cooked burgers keep for 3 to 5 days refrigerated or may be frozen.

Mexi Burgers (Oil-Free)

Serves 3 to 6

1 cup cooked, mashed beans (pinto, kidney, red, or black beans)

½ cup steamed, finely chopped red, yellow, orange, purple, or green bell peppers

½ cup steamed, finely chopped celery or zucchini

½ cup ground raw sunflower seeds

1 tablespoon ground pumpkin seeds or extra ground sunflower seeds

½ to ¾ cup amaranth or teff flour

½ cup finely chopped onion

2 tablespoons finely chopped, fresh parsley or cilantro

1 to 2 teaspoons finely chopped jalapeño or hot peppers

2 to 3 teaspoons simmered tamari soy sauce or substitute, or ½ Homemade Vegetable Bouillon Cube

½ teaspoon *each* basil and dill weed

¼ to ½ teaspoon sea salt

Several dashes cayenne

Optional: 1 cup Homemade Salsa, heated, simmered, and served warm or hot

Optional: ½ cup chopped black olives, heated with the salsa

Optional: Guacamole

Follow the previous directions for the Super Sunflower-Bean Burgers. Top each burger with the heated salsa/olive mixture and/or Guacamole if desired.

Mock Meatballs I

Serves 4 to 6

Use the Super Sunflower-Bean Burgers or the Mexi Burgers recipe and form the bean mixture into 24 1-inch balls. Broil them on an oiled, flat pan about 1 inch apart for 10 to 12 minutes, until browned and firm. Serve mixed in 3 to 4 cups hot tomato sauce, Mock Tomato Sauce, or brown gravy over cooked whole grains, steamed spaghetti squash, or steamed cauliflower.

Mock Meatballs II

Serves 4

2 tablespoons natural oil

1 large onion, finely chopped

1 cup broccoli or asparagus, chopped small (½ inch or less)

1 cup carrots or orange yams, chopped small (rinse yams if used)

1 cup celery or bell pepper, chopped small

½ cup water chestnuts, almonds or pecans, chopped small

½ cup black olives, chopped small, or artichoke hearts packed in water, drained, and chopped small

2 to 3 cloves garlic, minced or pressed

2 tablespoons Homemade Vegetable Broth Powder, or 2 Homemade Vegetable Bouillon Cubes

2 to 3 teaspoons simmered tamari soy sauce or substitute

3 to 4 tablespoons fresh chopped parsley, or 4 teaspoons dried

1 teaspoon *each* basil, paprika, and dill weed

½ teaspoon *each* marjoram and thyme

¼ teaspoon sea salt

2 cups crumbled regular tofu, or 2 cups cooked whole grain (brown rice, millet, brown pot barley, kasha, or quinoa)

½ cup ground raw almonds, filberts, pecans, or sunflower seeds

2 tablespoons soy, chickpea, or brown lentil flour

Preheat the oven to 400°F. Heat the oil until hot and sauté the onion for 1 minute, stirring regularly. Add the broccoli/asparagus and carrots/yams and sauté for another 2 to 3 minutes. Add all the remaining ingredients except for the last three and sauté another 2 minutes. Break up the bouillon cubes, if used, in the stir-fry and mix them well with everything else. Stir regularly.

Remove the mixture from the heat when done. Mix the remaining three ingredients together well and add the vegetable mixture to them, mixing thoroughly. Form the mixture into balls, using ⅛ to ¼ cup for each ball. Bake the balls on an oiled flat pan for 18 to 22 minutes, until firm, browned, and hot.

Serve these delicious balls with a gravy, tomato sauce, Mock Tomato Sauce, or any special sauce along with other vegetables and whole grains or legumes. The balls keep for 5 to 7 days refrigerated or may be frozen, although they are best eaten within several days of preparation. One-half cup Jerusalem artichokes may be substituted for ½ cup of water chestnuts if desired.

Mock Meat Loaf

Serves 4

1 recipe for Mock Meatballs II
Natural oil (for oiling pan)

Optional: 1 to 2 tablespoons sesame or
sunflower seeds, raw, hulled

Optional: paprika

Preheat the oven to 375°F. Generously oil a large loaf pan or small square casserole dish. Line the bottom of the pan with wax paper and oil it again. (Omit wax paper for corn allergies.) Gently press the mixture into the pan and shape it with a smooth, slightly rounded top. Press sesame or sunflower seeds into the top of the loaf and sprinkle with paprika for added color if desired. Bake for 40 to 50 minutes, uncovered, until nicely browned and firm. Cool for 5 to 10 minutes before slicing. Serve with a favorite sauce or gravy and vegetable side dishes. Keeps for up to 7 days refrigerated or may be frozen.

Black Bean Vegetable Goulash

Serves 6 to 8

1½ cups dry black beans,* soaked 6 to 8 hours

4 medium carrots, sliced in ⅓- to ½-inch chunks

3 to 4 small white and purple turnips, chopped in 1-inch chunks, or 1 small head cauliflower

1 stalk broccoli (1½ to 2 cups), chopped

Optional: 4 to 6 Jerusalem artichokes, chopped small

5 to 6 stalks celery, sliced in 1-inch chunks

1 to 2 red bell peppers, chopped in 1-inch chunks

1 small zucchini or yellow summer squash, quartered and cut in 1-inch chunks

1 extra large or 2 medium onions, chopped

2 tablespoons simmered tamari soy sauce or substitute

4 teaspoons Homemade Vegetable Broth Powder, or 2 Homemade Vegetable Bouillon Cubes

⅓ cup fresh chopped parsley or 2 tablespoons dried

1 teaspoon *each* sea salt, basil, and dill weed

½ teaspoon paprika or cumin powder

¼ teaspoon *each* sea kelp and thyme

Several dashes cayenne to taste

Optional: 8 to 12 water chestnuts, chopped or sliced, or ½ to 1 cup mung bean sprouts

Cook the beans until tender. Steam the carrots, turnips, broccoli, and artichokes (if any) for 9 to 12 minutes until slightly tender. When the beans are done, drain off all except 2 cups of the cooking water. Then add the precooked and other vegetables along with the herbs and all remaining ingredients except for mung bean sprouts, if any. Simmer everything together on low to medium heat for 25 to 30 minutes until the flavors mingle and the vegetables are all tender but not mushy. (Add the mung bean sprouts 12 to 15 minutes before the goulash is finished cooking.) Serve hot and enjoy. A complete meal by itself, this is especially high in protein and calcium. Keeps for up to 7 days refrigerated and freezes well.

---

*Pinto or kidney beans can be substituted for black beans for a different flavor and a brown color, as well as a few less nutrients.

Rainbow Lentil Stew

Serves 6

1½ cups brown/green lentils, dry

3 to 4 medium carrots, sliced in ¼- to ⅓-inch pieces, or 1 large yam, chopped and rinsed 2 to 3 times to remove excess starch

2 cups chopped cauliflower

1 stalk broccoli (1½ to 2 cups), chopped, or 1½ cups kohlrabi, peeled and chopped small

1½ to 2 cups chopped asparagus, or 4 to 5 stalks celery, sliced in ¾-inch chunks

1 to 2 red bell peppers, chopped in 1-inch chunks

1 small zucchini or yellow summer squash, quartered and cut in 1-inch chunks

1 extra large or 2 medium onions, chopped

Optional: ½ to 1 cup fresh or frozen green peas

Optional: 2 to 3 Jerusalem artichokes, chopped

2 tablespoons simmered tamari soy sauce or substitute

1 tablespoon Homemade Vegetable Broth Powder, or 2 Homemade Vegetable Bouillon Cubes

⅓ cup fresh chopped parsley or 2 tablespoons dried

1½ teaspoons basil

1 teaspoon *each* sea salt and dill weed

½ teaspoon paprika or cumin powder

¼ teaspoon *each* sea kelp and thyme

Several dashes cayenne to taste

Cook the lentils for 50 to 60 minutes, until tender but not too soft. Use only enough water to cook them properly and end up with about 2 cups of extra liquid when cooked.

Steam the carrots or yam, cauliflower, broccoli or kohlrabi, asparagus, and artichokes (if any) for 9 to 12 minutes, until slightly tender. When the lentils are done, drain off all except 2 cups of the cooking water. Then add the precooked and other vegetables along with the herbs and all remaining ingredients. Simmer everything together on low to medium heat for 20 to 25 minutes, until the flavors mingle and the vegetables are all tender but not mushy. Serve hot and enjoy. This is a complete meal by itself. Keeps for up to 7 days refrigerated or may be frozen.

Festival Vegetable Rice Pie

Serves 4

2½ to 3 cups cooked brown rice (1¼ to 1½ cups short grain dry rice)

1 cup finely chopped onion

1½ to 2 tablespoons natural oil

1 cup chopped broccoli, ½-inch chunks

1 cup chopped carrot, ½-inch chunks

1 cup chopped zucchini or yellow summer squash, quartered, ¼-inch chunks

1 red bell pepper, chopped small

3 to 4 teaspoons dried parsley or ⅓ cup finely chopped fresh parsley

1½ teaspoons basil

1 teaspoon *each* sea salt, paprika, thyme, and dill weed

¼ teaspoon sea kelp and cumin powder

Several dashes cayenne

10 to 12 ounces regular tofu, or 2 extra large eggs or 3 medium or large eggs, whites and yolks separated

½ cup Brown Bean Juice

2 tablespoons simmered tamari soy sauce or substitute

Preheat the oven to 350°F. Precook 1¼ to 1½ cups dry brown rice with extra water (3½ to 4¼ cups), until completely tender and soft. Let it cool. Oil a standard 9-inch glass pie plate and gently press the brown rice into it to form a ½-inch-thick bottom and side crust. Do not line the top edge with rice.

In a large skillet, sauté the onion in hot oil on high heat for 1 minute, stirring regularly. Add the broccoli and carrot and sauté another 2 to 3 minutes, until semi-tender. Add the remaining vegetables and all the herbs and dry seasonings and sauté for another 2 minutes. Stir regularly.

In a food processor or food mill, blend the tofu with the bean juice and tamari soy sauce until smooth, or use a hand mixer to beat the eggs whites until stiff peaks form and gently stir in beaten yolks, bean juice, and tamari soy sauce. Fold the tofu or egg mixture into all except 1 cup of the vegetable mixture and mix well. Smooth it into the rice piecrust. Spread the remaining

(continues)

vegetable mixture over the top of the pie and press it into the top for a colorful surface topping. Bake with tofu for 40 to 45 minutes, until firm, browned, and hot throughout. Bake with eggs for only about 30 minutes, more or less. This pie is a full meal and can be served alone or with a gravy, sauce, or Acidophilus Yogurt. Keeps for 3 to 5 days refrigerated. Do not freeze.

Mediterranean Vegetable Rice Pie

Serves 4

2½ to 3 cups cooked brown rice (1¼ to 1½ cups short grain dry rice)

1 cup finely chopped onion

1½ to 2 tablespoons natural oil

2 cloves garlic, chopped

1 cup chopped broccoli, ½-inch chunks

1 cup chopped zucchini, quartered, ¼-inch chunks

1 red bell pepper, chopped small

½ cup chopped artichoke hearts (packed in water and drained)

½ cup chopped black olives

⅓ cup finely chopped fresh parsley

1½ teaspoons basil

1 teaspoon *each* sea salt, paprika, thyme, and dill weed

¼ teaspoon *each* sea kelp and cumin powder

Several dashes cayenne

10 ounces regular tofu, or 2 extra large eggs or 3 medium or large eggs, whites and yolks separated

3 to 4 tablespoons (2 ounces) crumbled goat feta cheese, or 2 ounces extra tofu

½ cup Brown Bean Juice

2 tablespoons simmered tamari soy sauce or substitute

Optional: 2 to 3 cups tomato sauce or Mock Tomato Sauce

Preheat the oven to 350°F. Precook 1¼ to 1½ cups dry brown rice with extra water (3½ to 4¼ cups), until completely tender and soft. Let it cool. Oil a standard 9-inch glass pie plate and gently press the brown rice into it to form a ½-inch-thick bottom and side crust. Do not line the top edge with rice.

In a large skillet, sauté the onion in hot oil on high heat for 1 minute, stirring regularly. Add the garlic and broccoli and sauté another 2 to 3 minutes, until semi-tender. Add the remaining vegetables and all the herbs and dry seasonings and sauté for another 2 minutes. Stir regularly.

In a food processor or food mill, blend the tofu and feta cheese (if any) with the bean juice and tamari soy sauce until smooth, or use a hand mixer to beat the egg whites until stiff peaks form and gently stir in beaten yolks, bean juice, and tamari soy sauce. Fold the tofu or egg mixture into all of the vegetable mixture (except for 1 cup) and mix well. Smooth it into the rice piecrust. Spread the remaining vegetable mixture over the top of the pie and press it into the top for a colorful surface topping. Bake with tofu for 40 to 45 minutes, until firm, browned, and hot throughout. Bake with eggs for only about 30 minutes, more or less. Use a pie server to slice and serve. This pie is a full meal and can be served alone or with Homemade Tomato Sauce or Mock Tomato Sauce as a topping. Keeps for 3 to 5 days refrigerated. Do not freeze.

Taco Bean Rice Pie

Serves 4

2½ to 3 cups cooked brown rice (short grain is best)

½ recipe for Mexi-Taco Beans (follows)

1 tablespoon arrowroot or kudzu powder

1½ cups chopped, seeded tomatoes or red bell peppers, or 1 cup Homemade Salsa

2 cups zucchini, quartered and chopped

1 to 2 cups yellow summer squash, quartered and chopped, or yellow bell peppers, chopped

Optional: 1 to 1½ cups chopped bell peppers (green, orange, purple, or red if not already used)

Optional: ½ cup chopped or sliced black olives

Optional extras: Guacamole and/or plain Acidophilus Yogurt

Preheat the oven to 350°F. Pre-cook 1¼ to 1½ cups dry brown rice with extra water (3½ to 4¼ cups), until completely tender and soft. Let it cool. Oil a standard 9-inch glass pie plate and gently press the brown rice into it to form a ½-inch-thick bottom and side crust. Do not line the top edge with rice.

(continues)

Place a ¾- to 1-inch layer of the taco beans mixed with the arrowroot inside the crust and top with the vegetables in the order given. Save the Guacamole and/or yogurt to serve over the pie after baking. Bake for 30 to 40 minutes, or until the vegetables are brown on the top edges and the beans are hot throughout. Scoop the taco/rice pie onto plates, top with extras, and enjoy. For this meal in itself, salad is optional. Leftovers keep for a few days refrigerated and cannot be frozen.

Quick-and-Easy Broiled Taco Beans
Serves 4

½ recipe for Mexi-Taco Beans (follows)

1½ cups chopped, seeded tomatoes or red bell peppers, or 1 cup Homemade Salsa

2 cups zucchini, quartered and chopped

Optional: 1 to 1½ cups chopped bell peppers (green, orange, yellow, purple, or red if not already used)

Optional: ½ cup chopped or sliced black olives

Optional extras: 1 sliced avocado and/or plain Acidophilus Yogurt

Preheat the broiler. Position the oven rack 3 to 4 inches from the heat source. Place the beans in an oiled, small casserole dish, cover with toppings, and broil for 12 to 18 minutes, until hot throughout and the vegetables are tender. Serve with extras and enjoy. Leftovers keep for 1 to 2 days refrigerated. Do not freeze.

Mexi-Taco Beans

Serves 6 to 8

2 cups dry black beans, pinto, or kidney beans, or mixture of two

1 large onion, finely chopped

2 cloves garlic, chopped small

2 tablespoons simmered tamari soy sauce or substitute, or 2 Homemade Vegetable Bouillon Cubes

1 tablespoon chili powder, or 1 tablespoon Your Own Chili Powder

1 teaspoon sea salt

¼ teaspoon sea kelp

⅛ teaspoon or less cayenne to taste

Optional: 1 teaspoon crushed red chili peppers, cooked with the onions

Cook the beans until tender and add the onion and garlic to cook with them for the last half hour of cooking. Onions and garlic can also be sautéed separately in 2 to 3 teaspoons oil for added flavor. Drain the cooked beans, retaining 1 to 2 cups of liquid to mash with the beans. (Extra bean cooking liquid can be saved for Brown Bean Juice to use in other recipes.) Mash the beans easily with a small-holed hand masher or in a food processor. Add all the remaining ingredients while mashing and serve hot with raw or steamed vegetable dippers, as a side dish with or over whole grains, or in another recipe calling for taco beans. Beans keep for 6 to 8 days refrigerated or may be frozen.

Mexican Layered Salad

Serves 4 to 6

Layer 1: ½ recipe for Mexi-Taco Beans (see previous recipe)

Layer 2: Homemade Salsa and/or Guacamole, about 1 cup or more

Layer 3: Chopped leaf lettuce or spinach, about 2 cups

Layer 4: Chopped tomatoes or red bell peppers, about 2 cups

Layer 5: Acidophilus Yogurt or Tamari Tofu Sauté, 1½ to 2 cups

Layer 6: Quartered and chopped zucchini or English cucumber

Layer 7: Guacamole (if not used earlier), about 1 cup

Layer 8: *Optional:* Steamed black olives, ½ cup or more

Use freshly made Mexi-Taco Beans that are still hot or have been reheated for optimum nutrient absorption and good digestion, as well as to deter parasites that may develop on stored food. Do not use cold beans. Find a clear glass bowl with a flat bottom that is evenly deep so the salad can be viewed in layers through the sides of the bowl if desired. Begin with the warm bean layer and add layers as listed. Can be a full meal alone or served with Chickpea Chapatis. Serve immediately and enjoy. Prepare enough for one meal and no leftovers.

Orange Yam Pie with Crunchy Crust

Serves 4

Crust:

½ cup ground raw sunflower seeds

½ cup ground raw almonds, filberts, or pecans

½ cup amaranth or teff flour

½ cup arrowroot powder

¾ teaspoons cinnamon

⅛ teaspoon sea salt, or a bit more

3 tablespoons natural oil

1½ tablespoons apple juice (or pear, peach, or apricot juice, or 1 teaspoon honey or maple syrup mixed well with 4 teaspoons water)*

*Because this is cooked over 20 minutes, Candida is not affected by this. See Controversial Foods in Chapter 4.

Filling:

5½ to 6 cups (about 3 large) chopped orange yams, peeled or unpeeled, ½-inch chunks

2 to 3 teaspoons natural oil

1 large onion, finely chopped (1¼ to 1½ cups)

2 cloves garlic, minced

1 tablespoon butter and ¼ teaspoon sea salt, or 1 Homemade Vegetable Bouillon Cube (or other substitute), mashed with hot yams

1 tablespoon milk powder or soy milk powder or tapioca flour, or use 1 of the optionals

1 tablespoon arrowroot powder

½ teaspoon cinnamon

Few dashes *each* allspice, nutmeg, and ground cloves

Optional: 1 tablespoon powdered egg replacer, or 1 well-beaten large egg (for firmer pie)

For the crust: Preheat the oven to 350°F. Mix all the dry ingredients together thoroughly. Mix the oil and juice together and slowly add them to the dry ingredients with a fork until a moist, crumbly mixture is formed. Press the mixture into an oiled 9-inch glass pie plate to get about a ¼-inch layer on the sides and bottom of the pan. Reserve 1 to 2 tablespoons of the crust mixture for the top of the pie. Do not cover the top flat edge of the pie plate with crust. Bake the crust for 4 to 5 minutes and remove immediately to cool.

For the filling: Preheat the oven to 350°F. Steam the yams until very tender. One-half cup of Jerusalem artichokes may be substituted for ½ cup of the orange yams if desired. In a skillet, heat the oil on high heat and sauté the onion and garlic until tender. Mash the yams until smooth and mix them with the onion mixture and all the remaining ingredients. Place the yam mixture in the cooled piecrust and smooth the top with a knife or rubber spatula. Sprinkle with reserved crust mixture. Bake for 50 to 60 minutes, until firm and browned. Cool for at least 5 minutes before slicing and serving with a pie server. Serve with a green vegetable or salad and optional legume dish. Keeps for 4 to 5 days refrigerated. Do not freeze.

Confetti Carrot Pie with Crunchy Crust

Serves 4

Crust:

½ cup ground raw sunflower seeds

½ cup ground raw almonds, filberts, or pecans

½ cup amaranth or teff flour

¼ cup arrowroot powder

¾ teaspoon cinnamon

⅛ teaspoon sea salt, or a bit more

3 tablespoons natural oil

1½ tablespoons apple juice (or pear, peach, or apricot juice, or 1 teaspoon honey or maple syrup mixed well with 4 teaspoons water)*

Filling:

4 to 4½ cups 7 to 8 medium) chopped carrots, ½-inch chunks

2 to 3 teaspoons natural oil

1 large onion, finely chopped (1¼ to 1½ cups)

½ cup asparagus or broccoli, ⅓- to ½-inch chunks, presteamed 5 minutes, or ½ cup fresh or frozen green peas

½ cup red or purple bell pepper or black olives, ⅓- to ½-inch chunks

½ cup zucchini or celery, ⅓- to ½-inch chunks

½ cup yellow summer squash or yellow bell pepper, ⅓- to ½-inch chunks; or ½ cup cauliflower or parsnips, ⅓- to ½-inch chunks, presteamed 5 minutes

2 cloves garlic, minced

1 tablespoon butter and ¼ teaspoon sea salt, or 1 Homemade Vegetable Bouillon Cube (or other substitute), mashed with hot yams

1 tablespoon milk powder or soy milk powder or tapioca flour, or use 1 of the optionals

1 tablespoon arrowroot powder

1 tablespoon fresh chopped parsley, or 1 teaspoon dried

½ teaspoon *each* dill weed, basil, and thyme

Several dashes cayenne

Optional: 1 tablespoon powdered egg replacer, or 1 well-beaten large egg (for firmer pie)

---

*Because this is cooked over 20 minutes, Candida is not affected by this. See Controversial Foods in Chapter 4.

For the crust: Preheat the oven to 350°F. Mix all the dry ingredients together thoroughly. Mix the oil and juice together and slowly add them to the dry ingredients with a fork until a moist, crumbly mixture is formed. Press the mixture into an oiled 9-inch glass pie plate to get about a ¼-inch layer on the sides and bottom of the pan. Reserve 1 to 2 tablespoons of the crust mixture for the top of the pie. Do not cover the top flat edge of the pie plate with crust. Bake the crust for 4 to 5 minutes and remove immediately to cool.

For the filling: Preheat the oven to 350°F. Steam the carrots until very tender. One-half cup Jerusalem artichokes may be substituted for ½ cup of the carrots if desired. In a skillet, heat the oil on high heat and sauté the onion and garlic until tender. When the carrots are steamed, remove them from the steamer and steam any other vegetables that require it, together. Mash the carrots until smooth and mix them with the onion mixture and all the remaining ingredients and extra steamed vegetables (if any). Place the carrot mixture in the cooled piecrust and smooth the top with a knife or rubber spatula. Sprinkle with reserved crust mixture. Bake for 50 to 60 minutes, until firm and browned. Cool for at least 5 minutes before slicing and serving with a pie server. Serve with green vegetable or salad and optional legume dish. Keeps for 4 to 5 days refrigerated. Do not freeze.

Planter's Pie
(Vegetarian Version of Shepherd's Pie)

Serves 4

1 batch Mock Meat Gravy, or 2½ to 3 cups Homemade Tomato Sauce or Mock Tomato Sauce

2 medium heads of cauliflower, or 4 to 6 large orange yams, or 1 large butternut or buttercup squash

3 to 4 teaspoons natural oil (canola, sunflower, or sesame are best)

1 to 1¼ cups diced onions (1 medium)

1 cup diced carrots, ⅓-inch chunks

1 cup diced celery, broccoli, or asparagus, ⅓-inch chunks

1 cup diced zucchini, or 1 cup fresh or frozen green peas

8 to 10 ounces regular tofu, mashed

2 to 3 teaspoons butter or natural oil

Several dashes sea salt

Prepare the sauce or heat up a premade sauce. Steam the cauliflower, yams, or squash (squash may be baked if desired) until very tender. Heat the 3 to 4 teaspoons oil in a large skillet, preferably cast-iron. Sauté the onion for 1 minute, add the vegetables except for the peas, and sauté for 2 to 3 minutes until somewhat tender. Add the tofu and sauté 1 to 2 minutes more. Preheat the oven to 350°F.

Mash the hot cauliflower, yams, or squash with the 2 or 3 teaspoons butter or oil and salt until smooth and all lumps are gone; set aside. The mashed vegetables should equal 3½ to 4 cups. Mix the hot sauce with the sautéed mixture (and peas if any) and spread it in a 2½-quart, low baking dish 2 to 3 inches high. (A 9 × 13-inch pan works well.) Spread an even layer of mashed vegetables over this and smooth the top. Bake for 40 to 45 minutes, until hot throughout, very tender, and the mashed vegetables on top have set and become a bit firm. This is a complete meal in itself but may be served with salad if desired. Bake to reheat. Keeps for 4 to 6 days refrigerated and is best if not frozen.

Chickpea and Carrot Casserole

Serves 8 to 10

1 cup dry chickpeas, soaked 12 to 24 hours

2 cups carrots, finely grated, or 1½ cups carrots and ½ cup beets, finely grated

1½ to 2 cups milk or milk substitute, or Brown Bean Juice

1 cup celery or zucchini, chopped small

1 large onion, finely chopped

2 cloves garlic, minced or pressed

2 large beaten eggs, or 2 tablespoons dry egg replacer with ½ cup extra milk or milk substitute

⅓ cup amaranth or teff flour, or ⅓ cup ground sunflower or sesame seeds

1 to 2 tablespoons natural oil or melted butter

1 tablespoon simmered tamari soy sauce or substitute, or 1 Homemade Vegetable Bouillon Cube, mashed with hot beans

¼ cup finely chopped fresh parsley or 2 tablespoons dried

2 teaspoons *each* basil, paprika, and dill weed

½ teaspoon sea salt

Several dashes *each* sea kelp and cayenne

Topping: sesame seeds or coarsely ground sunflower or pumpkin seeds

Optional: paprika

Preheat the oven to 375°F. Cook the chickpeas until tender and use a small-holed hand masher, meat grinder, or food processor to mash them until smooth. Mix all the ingredients together well, except for the topping. Spread the mixture evenly into a large oiled casserole dish and press the topping into the surface. Sprinkle on paprika for color if desired and topping. Bake for 40 to 50 minutes, or until browned, firm, and cooked throughout. Serve hot along with green vegetables and/or salad with optional whole grains. Keeps for 4 to 6 days refrigerated or may be frozen.

Winter Squash with Wild Rice Stuffing

Serves 2 to 4

½ cup dry wild rice

1 medium or large butternut or buttercup squash

Optional: 2 tablespoons butter, or 1 tablespoon natural oil

¾ to 1 teaspoon cinnamon

½ teaspoon sea salt

Several dashes nutmeg

1 cup asparagus, chopped in ½-inch pieces, or broccoli, artichoke hearts packed in water, or chopped kohlrabi

⅔ cup water chestnuts, pine nuts, almonds, filberts, or pecans, chopped small (use raw or Home-Roasted Nuts for added flavor)

2 to 4 green onions, chopped small

2 tablespoons fresh chopped parsley

Preheat the oven to 400°F. Cook the dry wild rice in 1¼ to 1½ cups water for 1 hour or more, until tender. Cut the squash in half from top to bottom; scoop out and discard the seeds and pulp. Place the squash pieces, open side down, on a flat, unoiled, metal baking sheet and bake for 20 to 30 minutes, until the squash is tender but not mushy. Scoop out an extra ¾ cup (or a bit less) of squash from the inside of each half (about 1½ cups in all). Mash and mix the scooped-out hot squash with the butter or oil (if used), cinnamon, sea salt, and nutmeg; set aside.

Cook the asparagus or other green vegetable with the rice during the last 15 to 20 minutes of cooking time. Mix the cooked rice and vegetable with the nuts, onions, and parsley, then mix them with the mashed squash mixture and heap them equally into the partially hollowed-out squash shells. Place the upright stuffed squash back in the oven and lower the temperature to 350°F. Bake for 20 to 25 minutes more, until hot throughout and the flavors mingle. Serve at once with extra butter, sea salt, or an added topping or sauce if desired. Great served with a salad or green vegetable and optional bean dish. Keeps refrigerated for 2 to 3 days. Do not freeze.

Spaghetti Squash with Special Sauce

Serves 2

1 medium spaghetti squash

1 batch of Special Sauce: Homemade Tomato Sauce, Mock Tomato Sauce, Sesame Tahini and Ginger Sauce, Toasted Sesame Sauce, Toasted Almond and Filbert Sauce, Toasted Nut and Vegetable Sauce, Green Garlic Sauce, Nutty Garlic Sauce, or Savory Sweet Onion Sauce (see recipes)

Boil a whole spaghetti squash in a pot full of water for 55 to 75 minutes, or until tender enough for a knife to slide in and out easily. While the squash is cooking, prepare and/or heat the sauce in a saucepan until hot throughout. When the squash is ready, cut it in half, lengthwise, and use a spoon to scrape out and discard the seeds and pulp. Use a fork to scrape the edible squash from its skin and place it on a plate.

If preferred, cut the squash in half lengthwise, remove the seeds and pulp, and bake in a preheated 350°F oven, upside down on a flat baking sheet, for 35 to 45 minutes, or until tender.

Cover the hot squash with the heated sauce and enjoy. Serve with a green vegetable or salad and optional legume dish. The squash can be steamed or baked to reheat and keeps for 4 to 6 days refrigerated.

Spinach Tofu-Stuffed Zucchini

Serves 4

6 small zucchinis, cut in half lengthwise, ends removed

3 large bunches (or 4 small) fresh spinach, lightly chopped

3 to 4 teaspoons natural oil (sunflower, sesame, canola, or olive are best)

6 to 8 green onions, chopped small

1 medium red or orange bell pepper, chopped small

¼ cup pine nuts, sunflower seeds, chopped raw almonds, or other chopped raw nuts (Home-Roasted Nuts may be used)

8 to 10 ounces regular tofu, crumbled

2 cloves garlic, minced

3 tablespoons fresh chopped parsley, or 1 tablespoon dried

1 teaspoon *each* sea salt, curry powder,* and basil

¼ teaspoon *each* marjoram, dill weed, and thyme

Several dashes cayenne

1½ tablespoons simmered tamari soy sauce or substitute, or 2 Homemade Vegetable Bouillon Cubes (mashed into tofu while sautéeing), or 2 teaspoons Vegetable Broth Powder

Preheat the oven to 350°F. Steam the zucchini pieces for 5 to 7 minutes, until slightly tender. Steam the spinach separately until tender. In a large skillet, heat the oil on high heat. When the oil is hot, sauté the onions, bell pepper, and nuts for 2 minutes, stirring constantly. Add the tofu and all the remaining ingredients and sauté for another 2 to 3 minutes while stirring. Remove from heat and mix with the steamed spinach.

Place the strips of zucchini, cut side up and touching each other, in a low baking dish, with ¼ inch or more of water on the bottom. Cover the zucchini with the spinach-tofu mixture. Bake for 12 to 16 minutes, until hot and tender throughout. Serve immediately all by itself or covered in a gravy, Homemade Tomato Sauce, or Mock Tomato Sauce. Serve with whole grains and optional salad. Keeps for 2 to 4 days refrigerated. Do not freeze.

---

*Try Your Own Curry or Your Own Chili Powder if not able to tolerate regular curry powder. See recipes.

Whole Grain-Stuffed Red Bell Peppers

Serves 4

1 cup dry brown rice or kasha, or ¾ cup millet or quinoa

1½ tablespoons natural oil

1 large onion, finely chopped

1 cup finely grated carrot

2 tablespoons finely chopped fresh parsley or 1 tablespoon dried

1 teaspoon *each* sea salt and basil

½ teaspoon *each* oregano, paprika and thyme

⅛ teaspoon *each* marjoram and sea kelp

1 to 2 tablespoons raw hulled sesame seeds or sunflower seeds, ground

Several dashes cayenne

Optional: 2 to 4 small artichoke hearts packed in water, drained, and chopped small

4 large red bell peppers, cut in half lengthwise and seeded

Preheat the oven to 350°F. Cook the brown rice or other grain until tender and fairly dry. In a large skillet, heat the oil on medium-high heat and sauté the onion and carrot for 1 to 2 minutes, stirring regularly. Add the herbs, spices, seeds, and artichoke hearts (if any), and continue to sauté another 2 minutes, until the vegetables are slightly tender. Add the cooked grain to the skillet and sauté for 3 to 4 minutes more, stirring constantly, so the flavors can mingle. Place the raw red bell peppers in a large, uncovered baking dish (about 9 × 13 × 1½ inches), and fill them with heaping amounts of the grain-vegetable mixture. Fill the bottom of the baking dish with about ½ inch of water. Bake the peppers for 18 to 25 minutes, until the grain is lightly browned and the peppers tender but still a little crisp. Serve with a hot gravy, Homemade Tomato Sauce, or Mock Tomato Sauce. Serve with salad or green vegetable and optional legume dish. Keeps for 1 to 2 days refrigerated. Do not freeze.

Parsley and Whole Grain Casserole

Serves 4 to 6

7 cups cooked whole grains (2¼ to 3⅓ cups dry), brown rice, basmati brown rice, millet, or quinoa (no other grains)

4 teaspoons natural oil

1 medium onion, chopped small

3 to 4 cloves garlic, minced

½ cup pine nuts, chopped water chestnuts, chopped raw nuts, or mung bean sprouts

2 cups broccoli, chopped tiny, ¼- to ⅓-inch pieces

2 Homemade Vegetable Bouillon Cubes, or 2 teaspoons Homemade Vegetable Broth Powder

1 cup milk substitute, milk, bouillon, broth, or Brown Bean Juice

¼ cup ground raw nuts, seeds, or chopped water chestnuts

2 tablespoons amaranth or teff flour

¾ to 1 cup dried parsley flakes or 1½ cups finely chopped fresh parsley

1 teaspoon *each* sea salt, dill weed, and paprika

Several dashes cayenne

Optional: 2 teaspoons simmered tamari soy sauce or substitute

Optional: 1 to 2 well-beaten eggs (for texture and extra protein)

Extra paprika and/or sesame seeds

Preheat oven to 375°F. While the whole grain is cooking, heat the oil in a large skillet and sauté the onion for 2 minutes. Add the garlic, nuts, and broccoli and continue to sauté for 2 to 3 minutes more, until the broccoli is tender but still firm. The bouillon cubes can be broken up in the hot sautéed mixture or in the hot whole grain when it is just finished cooking. If millet or quinoa are used, do not cook them too tender with too much water.

Add the sautéed mixture to the hot whole grains and remaining ingredients, except paprika, and combine thoroughly but gently so as not to mash the grain. Place the mixture in a lightly oiled, deep, 9- or 10-inch large casserole dish and smooth the top. Sprinkle on extra paprika and/or spread on sesame seeds and press them into the top of the casserole for added eye appeal. Bake for 30 to 35 minutes, until hot and somewhat firm throughout. Serve immediately. Because this is a meal in itself, salad is optional. Keeps refrigerated for 5 to 7 days. Best if not frozen.

Quinoa with Zucchini or Broccoli

Serves 2

1 cup dry quinoa (white or
brown, see below)

3 cups water

1 cup zucchini, quartered,
chopped in ¼-inch pieces, or 1
cup broccoli florets, chopped
tiny, ¼-inch pieces

2 to 3 tablespoons tamari soy sauce or
substitute

1 to 2 teaspoons dried parsley

⅛ teaspoon *each* crushed basil, dill
weed, and paprika or cumin

Several dashes *each* sea salt, sea kelp,
and cayenne

Optional: 1 to 2 teaspoons butter or
natural oil (can be olive or
flax oil)

Sort the quinoa grains and discard any that are not uniform. Quinoa always needs sorting; remove the black or darker ones as these tend to be gritty and crunch distastefully with a mouthful of tender quinoa. Rinse the quinoa by rubbing it together in cool water. Discard the water and add 2½ to 3 cups fresh water. Bring the grain and water to a boil on high heat, scoop off the foamy part, and discard. Turn the heat to low and add the zucchini or broccoli. Continue to cook for 10 to 25 minutes. The brown quinoa takes 10 to 15 minutes to cook and has a more robust, grainy texture and is an acquired taste. The white quinoa takes about 18 to 25 minutes to cook and has a pleasant, delectable flavor that is enjoyed by almost everyone. The brown may be a bit more nutritious and requires several rubbings and washings to remove an outer "saponin" coating that can aggravate digestion if not removed. White quinoa needs only one rubbing and rinsing. Despite the saponin, quinoa is a well-tolerated, nutritious, mild, delicious, quick-cooking, and desirable grain, especially good for sensitive stomachs and allergies.

While the food is cooking, heat the tamari soy sauce and all the remaining ingredients to a boil in a tiny saucepan, and simmer on low heat for 5 minutes until flavors mingle. These must be heated to destroy possible bacteria.

Unlike other grains, quinoa should be totally tender, not crunchy or chewy, when ready, for optimum nutrition and digestion. Serve the quinoa hot with vegetables and sauce, and enjoy. Serve alone or with a legume dish and optional orange vegetable. Leftovers can be reheated with a tiny bit of water on low heat; keeps for 3 to 5 days refrigerated. Do not freeze.

One-Pot Vegetables and Brown Rice

Serves 2

3 to 4 cups precooked brown rice (short grain is best; basmati brown rice may be used occasionally)

2 cups broccoli spears

2 cups carrots, chopped in ¼-inch rounds

1 red, purple, or yellow bell pepper, cut in strips, or ½ yellow summer squash or zucchini, quartered and chopped

½ cup sliced water chestnuts or mung bean sprouts

2 to 4 tablespoons simmered tamari soy sauce or substitute

1 to 2 teaspoons dried parsley

⅛ teaspoon *each* crushed basil, dill weed, and paprika or cumin

Several dashes *each* sea salt, sea kelp, and cayenne

Optional: 1 to 2 teaspoons butter or natural oil (can be olive or flax oil)

Optional: 2 to 3 tablespoons pine nuts or lightly chopped raw almonds or filberts

Optional: 1 to 2 green onions, chopped in ½- to 1-inch pieces

Heat some water to boiling in a steaming pot and turn down to a low bubbling boil. Put the rice on one side of the pot and the broccoli and carrots (covered with nuts and onions, if any) on the other side, cover, and steam for 10 minutes. Be sure that there is enough air circulation so the steam can properly cook the vegetables in the allotted time or extra cooking time may be required. After 10 minutes, add the remaining vegetables and water chestnuts (if any) and continue to steam for another 4 to 8 minutes, until hot throughout, tender but not mushy. Avoid crunchy vegetables; they are harder to digest and oil-soluble vitamins are less easy to assimilate.

While the food is cooking, heat the tamari soy sauce and all the remaining ingredients in a tiny saucepan to a boil and simmer on low heat for 5 minutes until flavors mingle. These must be heated to destroy possible bacteria. Serve the rice hot, covered with vegetables and the sauce, and enjoy. Serve alone or with optional legume dish and/or salad.

Create dozens of variations of this meal by using other precooked steamable whole grains like kasha and brown pot barley and an array of other vegetables. Millet and quinoa do not always steam well. This is a complete, simple, quick, hearty, and nourishing meal. Best not to save leftovers. Prepare only enough for one meal.

Spanish Rice Paella

Serves 2 to 4

1 cup dry brown rice (short grain is best), or basmati brown rice

8 ounces Tamari Tofu Sauté, or Broiled Tofu Slices, in chunks

2 to 3 tablespoons olive oil or natural oil

1 large onion, chopped small

3 cloves garlic, minced

1 cup asparagus, kohlrabi, or broccoli, chopped small

1 red or orange bell pepper, chopped small

½ small zucchini or yellow summer squash, quartered and chopped small

½ cup artichoke hearts packed in water, drained and chopped

12 to 16 pitted black olives, sliced in rings or cut in half

2 medium tomatoes, chopped small

2 Homemade Vegetable Bouillon Cubes, or 3 teaspoons Homemade Vegetable Broth Powder

¼ cup Brown Bean Juice, broth, bouillon, or tomato juice

½ teaspoon powdered saffron, or 1 gram saffron strands

2 to 3 tablespoons chopped fresh parsley

Sea salt and cayenne to taste

Optional: 2 tablespoons lemon juice

Garnish: Parsley sprigs

Cook the rice. Prepare the tofu fresh. (See recipes.) In a large skillet or wok, heat the oil and sauté the onion and garlic until slightly tender, about 2 minutes. Add all the vegetables except the tomatoes and sauté until tender but still a bit crispy and firm, 3 to 5 minutes. Add the tomatoes, bouillon cubes (break them up) or powder, liquid, spices, and lemon juice (if any) and sauté for another 2 to 3 minutes. Add the hot, cooked rice to the skillet and mix gently; cook for another minute. Remove from heat and keep covered for 3 to 4 minutes. Serve garnished with parsley sprigs. A complete meal in itself. Keeps for 3 to 5 days refrigerated and can be baked to reheat. Do not freeze.

Asian Vegetable Stir-Fry with Tofu

Serves 2

1 to 2 cups precooked whole grain, brown rice, basmati brown rice, kasha, millet, quinoa, or brown pot barley; or 3 to 4 cups steamed turnips, cauliflower, or baked spaghetti squash

2 to 3 tablespoons natural oil (toasted sesame oil is best for stir-frys, but olive, sunflower, or canola may be used)

1 medium onion, chopped or sliced in rings*

6 to 10 slices peeled fresh ginger

1 small stalk broccoli, small spears or chopped, or chopped zucchini

2 small carrots, sliced in a long diagonal, then sliced in half lengthwise, ⅛ inch thick

2 stalks celery, chopped in ¼-inch moons

2 to 4 cloves garlic, minced*

1 to 2 teaspoons finely grated, peeled ginger, or ⅛ to ¼ teaspoon powdered ginger

1 to 2 cups kale, chard, or bok choy (green, leafy part only), chopped in thin strips

1 small red, yellow, or purple bell pepper, cut in strips

½ to 1 cup tofu chunks, ½- to ¾-inch pieces, presteamed

10 to 14 snow peas (edible pea pods), ends removed and deveined

Optional: ½ cup sliced water chestnuts, chopped lotus root, or mung bean sprouts

Optional: 1 to 2 Jerusalem artichokes, sliced

2 to 4 tablespoons simmered tamari soy sauce or substitute

Optional: Several dashes cayenne, cumin, or coriander

Most of the vegetables can be substituted or eliminated if required. Heat the oil on high heat in a wok or large iron skillet (or fry pan) and add the onion and ginger when the oil is hot. Test for hotness by putting a tiny piece of onion in cool oil and adding the rest when it sizzles noisily. Stir the onion/ginger regularly for 1 to 2 minutes, then add the broccoli and carrots;

---

*Instead of onions and garlic, ½ to 1 teaspoon prepared horseradish can be added with the green leafy vegetables and ginger.

sauté and stir for another 2 to 3 minutes. Add the celery, garlic, extra ginger, green leafy vegetables, bell pepper, and sauté for another 1 to 2 minutes until the greens shrink a bit. Keep the heat on high so the pan is always sizzling. Stir regularly, but not necessarily constantly, for even cooking and no scorching. Add the tofu next and sauté for another 1 to 2 minutes. Add all the remaining ingredients, sauté for another 1 to 2 minutes, and serve immediately over a bed of hot whole grains or starchy vegetables. A meal in itself. Make only enough of the stir-fry for one meal so there will be no leftovers. Does not store well.

Tamari Tofu Sauté

Serves 1

4 ounces regular tofu, cut in ½-inch chunks

1 to 2 tablespoons tamari soy sauce or Mock Tamari Soy Sauce

Optional (1 or more of the following): ½ teaspoon dried, crushed parsley flakes, crushed basil, cayenne, and/or few pinches cumin

Rinse the tofu and presteam it for 5 to 7 minutes before using in this recipe. Heat the tamari soy sauce and seasonings to a low boil and simmer for 5 minutes. Heat a small fry pan on fairly high heat with the preheated tamari soy sauce and add the tofu when it is hot. Stir the tofu constantly for 1 minute. Sauté until most or all of the tamari soy sauce is absorbed and the tofu has a rich, brown seared coating and is hot throughout.

Serve as a side dish, main dish, or snack. This little treat can keep you going for hours when time is limited. Serve with or over cooked whole grains or starchy vegetables, with green vegetables and/or a salad for a complete meal. A gravy or sauce can be put over the tofu. This tofu tastes terrific all by itself; the sauté process adds exceptional flavor. The pan will look hard to clean but wipes clean easily if soaked in water for a few minutes. Double the recipe for two. Make only enough for one meal or snack.

Leftovers can be reheated but are lacking in moisture and flavor. Can also be used in a variety of recipes.

Broiled Tofu Slices

Serves 2

8 ounces regular tofu, cut in ¼-inch slices

⅓ cup water, stock, or broth and 2 to 3 tablespoons simmered tamari soy sauce or substitute; or ½ cup Brown Bean Juice and 1 teaspoon Vegetable Broth Powder

½ to 1 teaspoon dried, crushed parsley

⅛ teaspoon *each* dried, crushed basil and dill weed

Sea salt or vegetized sea salt

Cayenne or cumin

Optional: several dashes paprika, onion powder, and/or garlic powder

Heat the broiler and place a rack about 4 inches below it. Place the tofu slices about ¼ inch apart in a lightly oiled low baking pan or dish. Beat all the remaining ingredients together well and pour over the tofu pieces. Broil the tofu for 8 to 14 minutes on the first side until well browned and 6 to 10 minutes on the other side. Add a bit of extra water, stock, or broth only if the liquid runs out, to keep the tofu moist. Broiling time varies widely as broilers vary; watch the tofu carefully and turn or remove it from the oven when browned and still moist.

Enjoy this snack like the Tamari Tofu Sauté or cut it into chunks and use it in other recipes like One-Pot Vegetables and Brown Rice, Spanish Rice Paella, or Broiled Vegetable and Tofu Kebabs.

Broiled Vegetable and Tofu Kebabs

Serves 2

Zucchini, cut in ¼-inch rounds

Yellow summer squash, cut in ¼-inch rounds

Broccoli florets, presteamed 5 minutes

Cauliflower florets, presteamed 5 minutes

Red, orange, yellow, purple, and/or green bell pepper, 1-inch chunks

Onion wedges

Tomato wedges

White grapefruit sections

Edible pea pods

Broiled Tofu Slices, cut in chunks

Use ½- to ¾-inch pieces, 1 to 1½ inches long, for the preceding vegetables and foods (2 to 3 cups per person):

Use one or more of the following sauces:
Simmered tamari soy sauce or Mock Tamari Soy Sauce
Homemade Tomato Sauce or Mock Tomato Sauce
Homemade Tomato Sauce or Mock Tomato Sauce mixed half and
    half with simmered tamari soy sauce or Mock Tamari Soy Sauce
Garlic French Dressing
Nutty Garlic Sauce

Heat a broiler and prepare the kebabs. Use two or more skewers about 1 foot long per person. Bamboo or stainless steel skewers (spears) may be used.* Use a variety of ingredients. Begin and end each spear with zucchini or yellow squash wheels and include one or two of them in the middle to hold up the kebab and help it to heat evenly. Cut the vegetables in the sizes indicated or they will not finish cooking at the same time. Alternate ingredients on each skewer and place them on a low baking pan 4 inches or so below the broiler. No need to turn them. Broil for 6 to 12 minutes, depending on the broiler, or until well browned on the edges and tender. Serve over cooked whole grains or starchy vegetables for a complete meal. Salad is optional. Prepare only enough for one meal. These do not reheat or store well and they do not taste good cold. (Fish or precooked chicken can be used.)

MAIN DISHES THAT REQUIRE DAIRY PRODUCTS

Check with your doctor before using any of the following recipes.

All phases of the Candida diet—I, II, III, and IV—can use recipes for well-cooked, soft cheeses if your doctor permits and you do not have dairy allergies. These cheeses have no difficult-to-digest rennet enzymes (enzymes from a calf's stomach), high mold content like hard cheeses, or excessive additives like other cheeses. The "good" cheeses for cooking are feta cheese (preferably goat's milk feta), ricotta cheese, farmer's cheese, and quark. These may be added to other recipes as well and used 1 time per week or so as your doctor allows. See chapter 14 for breakfast recipes with cheese and/or eggs.

---

*If barbecuing outdoors, bamboo skewers must be soaked in water for 30 minutes or more before using.

Mediterranean Vegetable Briam (with Dairy)*

Serves 6 to 8

1 large cauliflower, chopped in chunks or 1-inch florets (3 to 4 cups)

4 to 5 teaspoons olive oil (or other oil if desired)

1 large onion, finely chopped (1½ to 2 cups)

2 medium zucchini, sliced in ¼-inch rounds or chopped

4 to 5 large tomatoes, chopped, or 1 (28-ounce) can tomatoes, drained, cored, and chopped

4 to 8 artichoke hearts packed in water, drained, and quartered (if large, cut in eighths), or 1 cup chopped asparagus

3 to 4 tablespoons finely chopped fresh parsley or 2 tablespoons dried

1½ teaspoons basil

1 teaspoon oregano

½ teaspoon *each* dill weed and thyme

½ teaspoon sea salt

1 pound feta cheese, crumbled or chopped into small bits

½ to ¾ cup tomato juice or juice from canned tomatoes

Optional: several dashes cayenne

Optional: ½ to ¾ cup black olives, cut in half lengthwise

Optional: ½ cup chopped water chestnuts or pine nuts

Preheat the oven to 375°F. Presteam the cauliflower until tender. Heat the oil in a large skillet and sauté the onion for a minute or two. Add the zucchini and sauté for a few minutes more, until semi-tender.

Last, add the tomatoes, artichokes or asparagus, and herbs (and cayenne, if any) and continue to sauté for another 2 to 3 minutes. Remove from heat and add the tomato juice (and olives or nuts, if any) to the vegetables.

Place the vegetable mixture in a lightly oiled 9 × 13-inch baking dish or into small individual baking dishes and cover with the feta cheese. Bake for 20 minutes or more, until fully tender and the cheese is melted and browned on the edges. Can be enjoyed as a side dish or as a main dish all by itself. Best served with other protein dishes like egg or meat dishes. A salad is optional with this. Keeps for 3 to 5 days refrigerated. Do not freeze.

---

*If doctor allows.

NOTE: The Mediterranean Vegetable Briam is originally a Greek recipe, usually prepared with potatoes and sautéed eggplant instead of cauliflower, artichokes or asparagus, and black olives.

Spinach and Cheese-Stuffed Zucchini (with Dairy)*

Serves 4

6 small zucchinis, cut in half lengthwise, ends removed

3 large bunches (or 4 small) fresh spinach, lightly chopped

3 to 4 teaspoons natural oil (sunflower, sesame, canola, or olive are best)

6 to 8 green onions, chopped small

1 medium red or orange bell pepper, chopped small

¼ cup pine nuts, sunflower seeds, chopped raw almonds, or other chopped raw nuts (Home-Roasted Nuts may be used)

2 cloves garlic, minced

3 tablespoons fresh chopped parsley or 1 tablespoon dried

1 teaspoon *each* sea salt, curry powder,** and basil

¼ teaspoon *each* marjoram, dill weed, and thyme

Several dashes cayenne

1½ tablespoons simmered tamari soy sauce or substitute, or 2 Homemade Vegetable Bouillon Cubes (mashed into tofu while sautéeing), or 3 teaspoons Homemade Vegetable Broth Powder

10 to 12 ounces feta or farmer's cheese, crumbled

Preheat the oven to 350°F. Steam the zucchini pieces for 5 to 7 minutes, until slightly tender. Steam the spinach separately until tender. In a large skillet, heat the oil on high heat. When the oil is hot, sauté the onions, pepper, and nuts for 2 minutes, stirring constantly. Add all the remaining ingredients except for the cheese and sauté for another 2 to 3 minutes, stirring.

(continues)

---

*If doctor allows.

**Try Your Own Curry or Your Own Chili Powder if not able to tolerate regular curry powder. See recipes.

Remove from heat and mix with the steamed spinach and cheese. Place the strips of zucchini, cut side up and touching each other, in a low baking dish with ¼ inch or more of water on the bottom. Cover the zucchini with the spinach-cheese mixture. Bake for 10 to 15 minutes, until everything is hot and tender throughout. Serve immediately all by itself or covered in a gravy, Homemade Tomato Sauce, or Mock Tomato Sauce. Serve alone or with egg or meat dishes and optional salad. Keeps for 2 to 4 days refrigerated. Do not freeze.

Cheese-Stuffed Red Bell Peppers (with Dairy)*
Serves 4

3 to 4 teaspoons natural oil

1 large onion, finely chopped

1 cup finely grated carrot

2 tablespoons finely chopped fresh parsley, or 1 tablespoon dried

1 teaspoon *each* sea salt and basil

½ teaspoon *each* oregano, paprika, and thyme

⅛ teaspoon *each* marjoram and sea kelp

Several dashes cayenne

4 large red bell peppers, cut in half lengthwise and seeded

2 cups ricotta, quark, or feta cheese

1 to 2 tablespoons raw hulled sesame seeds or sunflower seeds, ground

Optional: 2 to 4 small artichoke hearts packed in water, drained, and chopped small; or ½ cup chopped asparagus, ½-inch chunks

Optional: 2 well-beaten eggs (mixed with the cheese)

Preheat the oven to 350°F. In a large skillet, heat the oil on medium-high heat and sauté the onion and carrots for 1 to 2 minutes, stirring regularly. Add the seasonings and artichoke hearts or asparagus (if any), and continue to sauté for another 2 minutes until the vegetables are slightly tender. Place the bell peppers in a large, low, uncovered baking dish (9 × 13-inch). Mix the cheese with seeds and vegetable sauté and fill the peppers with heaping amounts of the mixture.

---

*If doctor allows.

Fill the bottom of the baking dish with about ½ inch of water. Bake the peppers for 15 to 20 minutes, or until the peppers are tender but still a little crisp and everything is hot throughout. Serve with a hot gravy, Homemade Tomato Sauce, or Mock Tomato Sauce. Serve with salad or green vegetable and optional egg or meat dish. Keeps for 1 to 2 days refrigerated. Do not freeze.

Herb and Cheese-Stuffed Tomatoes (with Dairy)*

Serves 2

2 large ripe tomatoes

½ cup feta, farmer's, ricotta, or quark cheese

4 to 5 teaspoons simmered tamari soy sauce or substitute

2 tablespoons finely chopped fresh parsley

2 to 3 teaspoons chopped fresh basil or mint leaves

2 teaspoons finely chopped chives or green onion tops (green part only)

½ teaspoon fresh or dried dill weed

Couple dashes cayenne

Preheat the broiler. Position the oven rack 3 to 4 inches from the heat source. Wash and core the tomatoes: Remove at least a 2-inch circle from the top of each tomato and 4 tablespoons of the inner pulp so they can be stuffed with the cheese and herbs. Create a wide opening that is not too deep so the cheese is fully cooked in the broiling process and does not contribute to yeast growth. Mix all the remaining ingredients together in a bowl and stuff them into the tomatoes. Broil the tomatoes for 15 minutes or more, until well browned, very tender (soft), and bubbly. Enjoy as a side dish or main dish. Serve with another protein dish like eggs, fish, or chicken, or with whole grains. Include a green vegetable and/or salad for a complete meal. Serve immediately. Do not store.

---

*If doctor allows.

Fish is light and can be served with other protein dishes or with whole grains, but not with legumes. Here are a few wholesome fish recipes for those days when you want a little easy-to-digest meat protein. Shellfish of all types should be avoided during any of the phases of Candida diet. (See Foods to Eliminate list in chapter 10.) For fish safety and selection tips and more fish recipes, see my book *Jeanne Marie Martin's Light Cuisine: Seafood, Poultry, and Egg Recipes for Healthy Living.*

Baked Salmon Fillets

Serves 2

12 to 16 ounces salmon fillet(s)

3 to 4 tablespoons simmered tamari soy sauce or substitute, or Mock Tamari Soy Sauce

2 to 3 teaspoons fresh lemon or lime juice

1 to 2 teaspoons parsley leaves, crushed

¼ to ½ teaspoon paprika

¼ teaspoon basil leaves, crushed

Several dashes sea salt

Few dashes cayenne

Optional: ⅛ teaspoon tarragon or dill weed

Optional: 1 to 2 teaspoons butter

Garnishes: lemon or lime wedges and/or parsley sprigs

Preheat the oven to 375°F. Wash the fish and place skin side down in a lightly oiled glass baking dish with ¼ to ⅓ inch water around the fish. Pour the tamari soy sauce or substitute over the fillets, followed by the citrus juice. Sprinkle the parsley and other seasonings evenly over the fish. Pat with butter if desired. Bake the fillet(s) for 9 to 14 minutes, until it flakes, changes color, and is cooked evenly throughout. Baste once or twice so that it stays moist and tender.

Add a bit of extra hot water around the fish if it all evaporates before cooking is complete. (Cool water could crack the dish.) Serve the salmon with lemon or lime wedges, parsley sprigs, and/or fresh chopped parsley, chives, or green onion tops (green part only). Serve with whole grains or other protein dishes with eggs or cheese. Serve with green vegetables and/or a salad. Keeps for 1 to 2 days and may be frozen, but is best if not frozen.

Herb-Baked Sole or Cod

Serves 2

1 pound fresh or thawed sole or cod fillets

2 tablespoons butter or clarified butter, or 1 tablespoon natural oil plus 1 tablespoon broth or stock

1 tablespoon amaranth or teff flour, or 1 tablespoon ground almonds or filberts

2 green onions, finely chopped, or 3 tablespoons finely chopped chives

1 small clove garlic, pressed

2 tablespoons finely chopped fresh parsley

1 teaspoon finely chopped fresh dill weed, or ½ teaspoon dried

½ teaspoon basil and/or chervil

¼ teaspoon *each* thyme and marjoram

⅛ teaspoon sea salt

Couple dashes tarragon

Several dashes cayenne

Garnishes: lemon or lime wedges and/or parsley sprigs

Preheat the oven to 450°F. Wash the fish and place in an oiled low baking dish with a cover. Heat the butter or oil mixture and all the remaining ingredients in a small saucepan for 2 minutes, stirring to remove any lumps. Pour the sauce over the fish and bake, covered, for 25 minutes, or until the fish flakes easily with a fork and has a uniform texture throughout. Garnish and enjoy. Can be served with whole grains or protein dishes like cheese or eggs. Serve with green vegetables and/or a salad. Keeps for 1 to 2 days refrigerated and may be frozen, but is best not frozen.

Stuffed Trout or Salmon with Sun-Dried Tomatoes

Serves 4 to 6

1 large, whole rainbow trout or salmon, fresh or thawed (2 to 3 pounds, 1 to 1.35 kg)

1 to 2 tablespoons butter or natural oil (olive, canola, sunflower, or sesame)

1 medium onion, chopped (1 to 1¼ cups)

2 cloves garlic, minced

3 tablespoons chopped sun-dried tomatoes (dry, not packed in oil)

2 tablespoons lightly chopped fresh parsley

2 to 3 teaspoons chopped fresh basil or ¼ teaspoon dried

¼ teaspoon *each* oregano, dill weed, and thyme

⅛ teaspoon sea salt, or less

Several dashes cayenne

3 to 4 green onions, chopped

2 to 3 lemons (or limes if allergic), cut in ¼-inch rounds

Wash the fish and clean it if required. Remove the fins but leave the head and tail intact. Slice the fish along the belly lengthwise from the head to the tail. Remove large bones if desired.

Preheat the oven to 450°F.

In a large frying pan or skillet, heat the butter or oil and when hot, sauté the onion and garlic for 2 minutes, until fairly tender. Add the sun-dried tomatoes and all the seasonings and sauté for another 1 to 2 minutes. Remove from heat and mix the raw green onion into the mixture.

Stuff the sautéed mixture evenly into the fish and top with a layer or two of lemon slices. Brush the outside of the fish all over with oil to seal in the juices and place it in a lightly oiled baking dish. Bake for 20 to 25 minutes, until the flesh is opaque and flakes easily. Serve immediately with green vegetables and/or a salad. Cheese, egg, or other vegetable side dishes are optional. Keeps refrigerated for 1 to 2 days and may be baked or steamed to reheat. May be frozen but is best if not.

POULTRY AND MEAT MAIN DISHES

There are no red meat (pork, beef, veal, lamb, or game) recipes in this book, mainly because I never cook or eat these but also because they are heavy, hard-to-digest foods for a Candida or healing diet of any kind.

You may use your own red meat recipes if desired, without sweeteners, mushrooms, or other foods that agitate Candida. Pork and all game meats must be completely avoided on a Candida diet, as well as any processed, ground, deli, cold, or luncheon meats. This means no bacon, hamburgers, hot dogs, or sausages. (See Foods to Avoid List in chapter 10.) Quality cuts of beef, veal, or lamb may be eaten occasionally but should be limited to one to three times per week total, unless your doctor says otherwise. Choose steaks, roasts, chops, or stew meats only.

Poultry, including chicken, turkey, quail, and Cornish hens, may be eaten one to three times per week and are best if free-range, organic, or grown without hormones and fed wholesome foods. Goose or duck are best avoided as they are fatty meats. Avoid ground, deli, cold, and luncheon poultry meats. See my book, *Jeanne Marie Martin's Light Cuisine: Seafood, Poultry, and Egg Recipes for Healthy Living,* for safe handling and selection tips and additional recipes.

Turkey Vegetable Soup

Serves 10 to 14

12 to 14 cups light broth, stock, or water

Bones of 1 turkey

3 to 4 cups turkey pieces, cut or torn into small bits

2 large onions, chopped small

3 to 4 cloves garlic, minced

4 cups celery, chopped

3 medium carrots, quartered and chopped small

2 small zucchinis, quartered and chopped

1 to 2 tablespoons butter or natural oil

1 tablespoon Homemade Vegetable Broth Powder

3 Homemade Vegetable Bouillon Cubes

¼ cup simmered tamari soy sauce or substitute

½ cup chopped fresh parsley, or 3 tablespoons dried

1 to 2 teaspoons sea salt to taste

2 teaspoons dried, crushed basil leaves

½ teaspoon *each* thyme and dill weed

⅛ teaspoon sea kelp or dulse

Several dashes cayenne to taste

Bring the broth or water and turkey bones on high heat to a boil, then turn down to medium-low until the water is barely bubbling; simmer, covered, for 2 to 4 hours to make flavorful, nutritious turkey stock and draw the calcium from the bones into the water. Strain and save the stock and discard the bones, retaining any leftover, wholesome bits of meat.

Sauté the onion, garlic, and vegetables in the oil or butter until somewhat tender, in a large skillet on high heat, stirring constantly. Add the sautéed mixture to the turkey stock along with the remaining ingredients. Simmer everything together for 1 to 2 hours on low heat. Add a bit of extra water if needed. Serve hot or save until the next day for fuller flavor. This soup is better the second to fifth day as the flavors have developed more; 1 to 2 cups of the soup can be blended thoroughly and added back to the soup for a quick flavor enhancer. Serve with salad and other optional protein dishes. Keeps for 4 to 5 days refrigerated or may be frozen.

Warm Chicken Salad

Serves 2

2 cups or more spinach or exotic mixed greens (without endive, escarole, or radicchio)

1 small red (yellow, orange, or purple) bell pepper, cut in thin strips; or 1 tomato cut in thin wedges; or 1 cup steamed asparagus

3 to 4 teaspoons natural oil (olive, canola, sunflower, or sesame best)

1 small or medium whole, boneless chicken breast, cut into thin (½ inch or less) strips*

1 tablespoon finely chopped fresh parsley, or 2 teaspoons dried

½ teaspoon *each* paprika, dill weed, and basil

Several dashes sea salt and cayenne to taste

Spread the vegetables decoratively on a medium-size plate. Heat the natural oil in a large skillet, preferably cast-iron. Add the chicken pieces and seasonings when the oil is hot and stir almost constantly, over medium-high heat, until the chicken is cooked throughout, browned, and no longer pink inside, 6 to 10 minutes depending on heat level and size of chicken strips. Serve immediately over the salad greens and vegetables. A meal in itself, or serve with vegetable side dishes or protein dishes. Acidophilus Yogurt is a nice accompaniment and helpful digestive aid. Chicken may be steamed to reheat. Keeps for 1 to 3 days refrigerated or may be frozen.

---

*Turkey may be used instead of chicken.

Yogurt and Spice Chicken (with Dairy)*

Serves 4

4 large, boneless, skinless chicken breasts

1 cup plain yogurt (lowfat)

⅓ cup fresh lemon juice

3 to 4 cloves garlic, pressed

2 teaspoons curry powder or Your Own Curry Powder

1 teaspoon cinnamon

½ teaspoon cumin powder

¼ teaspoon sea salt

A dash or two nutmeg and allspice or cloves

Several dashes cayenne

Cut the breasts in half, wash the chicken, and pat it dry. Make small cuts in the chicken so it can absorb the marinade. Mix the remaining ingredients together in a glass bowl and add the chicken. Turn the chicken to coat well and let marinate, covered, in the refrigerator for 4 hours. Turn the chicken 2 to 3 times while it marinates. After marinating, preheat the broiler. Set rack about 2 inches from heat source. Place the chicken on an oiled, low broiling pan and baste the chicken with extra marinade. Broil for 7 to 9 minutes on each side, basting once or twice for each side. Garnish with lemon wedges and parsley sprigs. Serve immediately with green vegetables and/or salad. Other vegetables or protein side dishes are optional for a complete meal. Keeps for 1 to 3 days refrigerated or may be frozen.

TIP: Never marinate in a metal bowl if lemon or citrus juice is used.

---

*If doctor allows.

Herb Garlic Chicken

Serves 2

4 large pieces chicken (breasts or legs with thighs), with or without skins

¼ cup tamari soy sauce or substitute, simmered

6 very large or 10 to 12 small gloves garlic, crushed

Lots of dried parsley and paprika

½ teaspoon *each* basil and thyme

Sea salt to taste

Several dashes cayenne

Preheat oven to 350°F. Place the washed chicken in a 9- or 10-inch glass baking dish with about ¼ to ⅓ inch water in the bottom. The chicken skin does hold in natural juices and flavors and is best left on the chicken. The herbs can be scraped off the skin and the skin discarded later, if desired. Pour the tamari soy sauce over the chicken pieces. Sprinkle each piece very generously with dried, crushed parsley leaves, covering the entire surface of each piece of chicken. Next, sprinkle on just as much paprika. Sprinkle the basil and thyme over each piece of chicken and add sea salt. Place the garlic cloves in the water surrounding the chicken. Bake for 35 to 45 minutes. After the first 10 minutes, baste every 10 to 14 minutes with the garlic and juices from the bottom of the dish until crispy, and cooked throughout. Serve with green vegetables and/or salad. Other vegetables and protein dishes are optional. Herb and Cheese–Stuffed Tomatoes are good with this chicken. Keeps for 3 to 4 days refrigerated or may be frozen.

Herb-Baked Chicken Kiev

Serves 2

Herb Butter:

¼ cup (½ stick) butter, softened

2 tablespoons finely chopped parsley

1 tablespoon chopped chives or green onions

1 teaspoon chopped basil or chervil

½ teaspoon fresh lemon or lime juice, or ⅛ teaspoon corn-free, unbuffered vitamin C crystals

⅛ teaspoon dried, crushed tarragon leaves, or dill weed

1 to 2 cloves garlic, pressed

Chicken recipe:

2 large, whole, boneless, skinless chicken breasts

Sea salt

Cayenne

¼ cup milk or milk substitute

½ teaspoon paprika

⅓ cup amaranth or teff flour, or ground almonds, filberts, or sunflower seeds

Mix all the Herb Butter ingredients together and form them into two rectangular sticks, about 2½ inches long, in an oiled, low, flat bowl or pan. Cover them and freeze solid for 30 minutes or more. Preheat the oven to 425°F. Flatten each chicken breast on an oiled surface, by using the flat side of a meat mallet or rolling pin to pound each chicken piece into a rectangular piece about ¼ inch thick. Turn the chicken several times while flattening. Be careful not to tear or mash the chicken. Sprinkle the chicken lightly with sea salt and a bit of cayenne pepper. Place one stick of the herb butter in the center of each flattened chicken breast. Roll it up, jelly-roll style, tucking the ends in and sealing well. Use toothpicks if necessary to seal each piece properly. Dip the chicken in the milk and paprika and coat it with the flour or ground nuts or seeds. Place the chicken pieces, seam side down, in an oiled glass pie plate or low Corningware dish. Bake uncovered for about 30 minutes or a bit more until browned and tender. Remove toothpicks, if any, and serve garnished with lemon wedges and fresh parsley sprigs. An elegant dinner for two. Serve with green vegetable and/or salad. Other vegetable or protein dishes optional. Keeps for 2 to 4 days refrigerated or may be frozen.

Mediterranean Chicken or Turkey Stew

Serves 4

4 cups Homemade Tomato Sauce or Mock Tomato Sauce

1 medium or large chicken, skinned and cut into pieces, or 2 to 3 large pieces of turkey

8 to 10 artichoke hearts packed in water, drained and sliced

1 cup black olives, sliced in half lengthwise

½ cup or more chopped water chestnuts or substitute

5 to 6 green onions, chopped

1 to 2 cloves garlic, pressed

Water, broth, or stock

Sea salt and cayenne to taste

½ cup lightly chopped fresh parsley

Optional: 4 to 6 cups cooked spaghetti squash or steamed cauliflower

Heat the sauce in a large saucepan until hot throughout. Wash the chicken pieces and remove any fatty parts or gristle. Add the chicken to the sauce along with the vegetables, onions, and garlic.

Cover the pot and simmer on low heat for 60 to 75 minutes, or until the chicken falls off the bone and is very tender. Add ½ cup or a bit more of liquid as needed while cooking, if mixture is too thick. Add sea salt and cayenne for added flavor if desired. Wonderful served over cooked spaghetti squash or cauliflower. Top each serving with fresh, chopped parsley. Serve with green vegetables and/or a salad. Keeps for 2 to 4 days refrigerated or may be frozen.

Roasted Chicken with Berry Berry Sauce

Serves 2 to 4

1 large, fresh chicken

Water

Butter or natural oil (sunflower, sesame, or canola are best)

Sea salt

Amaranth or teff flour

1 to 2 batches Berry Berry Sauce

Preheat oven to 350°F. Wash the chicken briefly and pat it dry. Place the bird on a rack in a roasting pan, breast side up, and rub it completely with oil or preferably butter to seal in the juices and flavors. Salt the entire bird lightly if desired. Pour about 1 inch or a bit more water in the bottom of the roasting pan and set in oven.

Baste the bird with pan drippings every 10 to 12 minutes. After the first 30 to 40 minutes, when the chicken is nearly done, baste it again and sprinkle it all over with the flour until it is lightly coated. Bake for another 10 to 15 minutes, until the bird is completely browned and tender, juicy but not dry. Baste one last time and let cook another 5 to 8 minutes before removing from the oven and serving. Carve it like a turkey and serve with the Berry Berry Sauce or another (grain-free) gravy if preferred. The floured coating creates a delicious, crispy skin. Serve with green vegetables and/or a salad. Great with one of the cheese recipes and/or other cooked vegetables. Keeps for 2 to 4 days refrigerated or may be frozen.

Chapter 19

SIDE DISHES AND SPECIAL RECIPES

Versatile vegetable dishes, seasoning blends, condiments, a few flour-free breads, and information on crackers and breads compose this innovative chapter of specialties and substitutes. Enjoy these wholesome versions of altered favorites as well-rounded additions to the Candida diet.

VEGETABLE SIDE DISHES

Globe Artichokes

1 to 2 artichokes (1 per person)   Butter and/or fresh lemon juice

Choose firm, uniformly green, unwrinkled artichokes (no purple or "fuzz") with preferably pointy rather than rounded leaves. With each artichoke, wash and cut off all the stem or stalk. Pull off and discard the first row or two of leaves around the stalk. With a sharp, serrated knife, trim ¾ to 1 inch off the tip of each artichoke and discard. Snip ¼ to ½ inch off the tip of each remaining leaf with scissors or knife. Place the vegetables upside down (top down, stalk up) in a vegetable steamer over medium boiling water and steam for 45 to 55 minutes or until very tender. When a knife slides in and out easily, it is done.

Starting with the bottom row of leaves nearest the stalk end, pull off one leaf at a time and dip the part that was attached to the artichoke in melted

(continues)

butter and/or fresh lemon juice. With the inner part of the leaf facing upwards, pull the base of the leaf between your teeth, pulling off all tender, easy-to-chew parts. (These are the edible parts.) Discard the rest of each leaf. As you get closer to the center, you can eat more of each leaf as they get progressively more tender. When you reach the "choke," scrape off the stringy, prickly part and discard. What's left is entirely edible! Dip it in the sauce and enjoy the best part—the heart, a delectable treat. Savor the delicious, stimulating after-taste of the artichoke in your mouth. Artichokes are very healing for the liver.

Homefries

Serves 2

3 to 4 small white and purple turnips, peeled or unpeeled

Natural oil

Optional: sea salt

Preheat the oven to 350°F. Chop the turnip into french fry–size strips and use a brush to coat each one lightly with oil. Lightly salt each one if desired. Place the fries on an oiled, flat baking sheet and bake for 20 to 25 minutes, or until the fries are browned and tender. Serve hot and enjoy. Do not store.

Hot and Spicy Homefries

Serves 2

3 to 4 tablespoons natural oil

Strip of jalapeño or other hot pepper

Several dashes cayenne

3 to 4 small white and purple turnips, peeled or unpeeled

Optional: sea salt

Optional: ¼ teaspoon paprika

Preheat the oven to 350°F. Measure the oil into a small dish and add the hot pepper, cayenne, and paprika (if any), stirring for a minute or two to blend the flavors. (If you really want the fries hot, blend the oil, spices, and hot pepper together.) While the oil and spices mingle, chop the turnip into french fry–size strips. Remove the pepper strip and use a brush to coat each fry lightly with seasoned oil. Lightly salt each one if desired. Place the fries on an oiled, flat baking sheet and bake for 20 to 25 minutes, or until the fries are browned and tender. Serve hot and enjoy. Do not store.

Herb Homefries

Serves 2

3 to 4 tablespoons natural oil

1 teaspoon dried, crushed parsley

½ teaspoon dried, crushed basil

¼ teaspoon thyme or dill weed

Few dashes each sea kelp and cayenne

3 to 4 small white and purple turnips, peeled or unpeeled

Sea salt

Preheat the oven to 350°F. Measure the oil into a small dish and add all the herbs except for the sea salt. Beat the herbs into the oil to blend the flavors. While the oil and herbs mingle, chop the turnip into french fry–size strips. Use a brush to coat each fry lightly with seasoned oil. Lightly salt each one if desired. Place the fries on an oiled, flat baking sheet and bake for 20 to 25 minutes, or until the fries are browned and tender. Serve hot and enjoy. Do not store.

Carrot Cauliflower Medley

Serves 1 to 2

1 cup cauliflower, chopped in 1-inch florets, steamed 5 to 7 minutes

1 medium or large carrot, finely grated

Optional: several dashes sea salt

Optional: ¼ teaspoon cinnamon

Optional: 2 to 4 teaspoons ground nuts or seeds (almonds, filberts, pumpkin, or sunflower seeds)

Preheat the oven to 350°F. Mix the cauliflower with the carrot and sprinkle with one or more of the optionals, if desired. Place the mixture in an oiled, small baking dish and bake for 18 to 22 minutes, or until the carrots are tender and the mixture is hot throughout. Serve and enjoy. Can be refrigerated for 1 to 2 days then reheated, but is best if not stored.

Citrus Beet Treat

Serves 1 to 2

1 medium or large fresh beet, finely grated

3 to 4 teaspoons fresh lemon or lime juice

Choose fresh, bright red beets, preferably ones purchased with beet green tops rather that old, slightly moldy storage beets.

Mix the beet and citrus juice together and enjoy. The citrus makes the beet taste very sweet. This is a nutritious and healthful treat for the tastebuds and the liver. Serve as a snack, side dish, or instead of a salad. Do not store.

Broiled Stuffed Tomatoes

Serves 2

2 large, ripe tomatoes

1 cup Fat-Reduced Falafel Spread, or
1 cup Herb-Scrambled Tofu

Preheat the broiler and place a rack 6 to 8 inches from the heat. Wash and core the tomatoes. Scoop out a third to half of the insides of each tomato and save for other recipes. Stuff the tomatoes with one of the fillings and broil until browned, hot and bubbly. Serve all by itself or topped with Guacamole or one of the gravies. Make only enough for one meal's side dish or for a snack. Do not store.

Asparagus with Parsley-Lemon Butter

Serves 2

1 small or medium bunch
asparagus

2 to 3 teaspoons softened butter or
natural oil

1 teaspoon finely chopped fresh
parsley

1 to 2 teaspoons fresh lemon juice (or
lime juice if preferred)

Several dashes sea salt

Optional: dash or two cayenne

Optional: 1 to 2 fresh mint leaves or
fresh basil leaves, finely
chopped

Break off the bottom quarter to third of each asparagus stalk; if green, they can be peeled and cooked with the rest of the asparagus (or saved for later and peeled and eaten raw or cooked in other recipes). If the bottoms are white or tough, discard them. Steam the asparagus until tender, 8 to 12 minutes. Mix the soft butter or oil with the remaining ingredients and spread or pour them over the asparagus when ready. Eat hot and enjoy. Best to eat when prepared; however, may be stored in the refrigerator for 1 to 2 days and reheated if desired.

Mashed Orange Yams or Squash

Serves 2

2 medium orange yams, or ½ butternut or buttercup squash

Several dashes sea salt or cinnamon

Optional: ⅛ to ¼ cup milk substitute,
simmered

Optional: 1 to 3 teaspoons butter, or 1
to 2 teaspoons natural oil

Bake the squash the quick and easy method (follows) or steam the peeled squash or yams sprinkled with the cinnamon (if any) until very tender. Mash the very tender vegetables with a small-holed hand masher or use a food mill or food processor. Add simmered milk substitute and/or butter or oil to the mashed vegetables for a lighter consistency if desired. Keeps refrigerated for up to 4 to 5 days and can be baked to reheat. Do not freeze.

Quick and Easy Winter Squash

Serves 2 to 4

1 medium or large acorn, turban,
spaghetti, butternut, buttercup, or
other medium winter squash, or 2
large pieces cut hubbard or other
large winter squash

Optional: sea salt

Optional: butter or natural oil

Preheat the oven to 400°F. Cut the squash in half lengthwise or from top to bottom and scoop out the seeds and pulp. Place the pieces cut-side down on a lightly oiled, flat metal sheet and bake for 25 to 40 minutes, until tender and a knife passes through easily. The skin should be only slightly browned or wrinkled. This is one of the fastest ways to prepare large pieces of winter squash. Serve with sea salt and butter or natural oil as desired. Refrigerate for up to 4 to 5 days and steam to reheat. Do not freeze.

Cinnamon-Baked Squash

Serves 2 to 4

1 medium butternut or buttercup
squash

Water

Cinnamon

Preheat the oven to 400°F. Use a sharp knife to cut the squash in half from top to bottom. Scoop out the seeds and pulp and discard. Fill the hollowed-out section of each half with water and sprinkle the entire cut section generously with cinnamon. Place the squash halves in a low (about 2-inch deep) baking dish with ¾ to 1 inch water around the bottom of each squash in the pan. Bake for 50 to 65 minutes, or until a knife moves in and out of the squash easily and it is very tender. Cut and serve hot. Keeps refrigerated for 3 to 4 days and may be reheated by baking, steaming, or placing the scooped-out squash in a little water in a covered saucepan and simmering.

CONDIMENTS AND SPECIAL SEASONINGS

Homemade Ketchup

Makes ¼ cup

2 tablespoons tomato paste

2 to 4 tablespoons water

½ teaspoon simmered tamari soy
sauce or substitute, or salted
bouillon, or 1 teaspoon Brown
Bean Juice (black bean is especially nice) and ⅛ teaspoon sea
salt

Optional: small squirt fresh lemon or
lime juice, or ¹⁄₁₆ teaspoon
corn-free, unbuffered vitamin C crystals

Simmer everything on low to medium heat for 5 minutes or more in a covered saucepan. Stir regularly. Serve immediately on burgers or other dishes or use in recipes calling for ketchup. Eat fresh or refrigerate for up to 2 to 3 days or freeze for use in recipes.

Clarified Butter

1 pound butter

Heat the butter in a heavy saucepan on very low heat for 1 hour, until the butter is melted and has separated. Skim off the foamy white milk solids from the top of the liquid. Save the yellow liquid below it, but be careful not to include the whey and milk solids on the bottom of the pan. Store in a jar in the refrigerator. It will re-solidify. Keeps for 2 to 3 weeks if kept bacteria-free. (Keep fingers, other foods, and licked utensils out of it!) Most people who are allergic to butter can tolerate it in this form.

Gomashio/Sesame Salt (No Oil Added)
Makes about ¾ cup

1 cup hulled, white sesame seeds*   2 to 3 tablespoons sea salt

Preheat oven to 300°F. Spread the seeds on a low, dry baking pan and let them bake for 4 to 5 minutes or so. Stir them well and bake for another 2 to 4 minutes. Stir again and bake for another 2 to 3 minutes, until a bit browned and toasty smelling. Remove them from the oven and cool for 5 minutes or more.

A second way the sesame seeds can be heated is in a dry iron skillet on medium-high heat, stirring almost constantly until browned. When the seeds have cooled, grind them ¼ cup at a time in a blender or all at once in a food processor or coffee mill. Traditional gomashio leaves half the seeds whole and grinds the rest. For easier digestion during a Candida diet, grind all the seeds until as finely ground as possible. Mix in the sea salt and keep the gomashio in the freezer, in a jar, so you will not have to reheat it before you use it each time. Freezing will prevent bacteria growth. Sesame seeds are high in calcium, and Gomashio adds flavor and nutrients to simple dishes as well as improving fancy dishes.

---

*Sunflower seeds may be substituted if desired.

Your Own Chili Powder

Makes 1 tablespoon

Chili Powder #1

1 teaspoon dried red chili peppers, ground

½ teaspoon cumin powder

½ teaspoon dried oregano leaves, ground

¼ teaspoon each onion and garlic powder

⅛ teaspoon ground celery seed or ground caraway

⅛ teaspoon ground coriander or ground cardamom

⅛ teaspoon ground cloves

1/16 to ⅛ teaspoon cayenne (if allergic, use ⅛ teaspoon black or white pepper)

Optional: 1/16 teaspoon extra oregano if less cayenne is used

Chili Powder #2

1½ teaspoon dried red chili peppers, ground

½ teaspoon cumin powder

½ teaspoon dried oregano leaves, ground

¼ teaspoon ground celery seed or ground caraway

⅛ teaspoon ground allspice

⅛ teaspoon powdered horseradish, or ⅛ teaspoon extra oregano

1/16 to ⅛ teaspoon cayenne (if allergic, use ⅛ teaspoon black or white pepper)

Mix one group of ingredients together or create your own similar version, omitting any items to which you are sensitive. Grind all ingredients to a powder before mixing thoroughly.

Use an herb grinder, coffee mill, or blender to grind. The recipe amount should equal about 1 tablespoon all together. Each recipe makes 1 tablespoon chili powder. Use in recipes instead of regular chili powder if you prefer or if you have trouble digesting store-bought chili powder. See the Substitution Chart in chapter 11 for more help with alternative spices.

Your Own Curry Powder

Makes 1 tablespoon

Curry Powder #1

1 teaspoon turmeric

¾ teaspoon ground coriander

½ teaspoon ground ginger

¼ teaspoon *each* ground cardamom and cumin powder

⅛ teaspoon ground fenugreek seed

¹⁄₁₆ to ⅛ teaspoon cayenne (if allergic, use ⅛ teaspoon black or white pepper)

Curry Powder #2

1¼ teaspoons dried red chili peppers, ground

1 teaspoon ground coriander

¼ teaspoon ground fenugreek seed

⅛ teaspoon each dry mustard and ground ginger

Cayenne to taste (if allergic, use ⅛ teaspoon black or white pepper) or ¹⁄₁₆ to ⅛ teaspoon cayenne

⅛ teaspoon turmeric or extra dry mustard

Mix one group of ingredients together or create your own version, omitting any items to which you are sensitive. Make sure they are all ground to a powder before mixing thoroughly. Flavor will alter with substitutions.

Use an herb grinder, coffee mill, or blender to grind. The recipe amount should equal about 1 tablespoon curry powder all together. Use in recipes instead of regular curry powder if you prefer or if you have trouble digesting store-bought curry powder. See the Substitution Chart in chapter 11 for more help with alternative spices.

Oven-Dehydrated Vegetables

Makes about ⅔ cup

1½ cups chopped carrots, orange yams (rinsed thoroughly), or small, peeled turnips, cut into ¼-inch chunks

1 cup chopped red bell pepper, seeded tomato, zucchini or yellow summer squash, cut into ⅓-inch chunks

2 cups chopped celery, peeled broccoli stalks, or green pepper, cut into ⅓-inch chunks

1½ cups white or yellow onion, cut into ⅓-inch chunks*

Preheat the oven to 200°F. Wash and dry the vegetables to be cut. Chop the vegetables into uniform pieces so they cook for the same length of time (except for the first group of carrots, yams, or turnips: these are cut smaller as they usually contain more moisture and dry more slowly).

Spread the cut vegetables on a flat, dry baking pan and place them in the oven. After 1 hour, stir the vegetables in the pan so they heat evenly, and put them back in the oven. After 30 minutes, stir the vegetables again. Repeat this 30-minute process two more times; bake vegetables 2½ hours, stirring four times, including when removing them from the oven.

Let the vegetables cool for 1 to 2 hours at room temperature, then use a blender, herb grinder, or coffee mill to grind, or freeze for later grinding. If using a blender, it takes several minutes to grind; stop the blender often so it does not overheat and make sure it does not vibrate off the countertop. May be frozen for up to 1 month or more. It takes three to four batches of oven-dehydrated vegetables to make one batch of Homemade Vegetable Broth Powder or Homemade Vegetable Bouillon Cubes.

---

*If onions are not used in the dried vegetables, ½ to 1 teaspoon horseradish powder or "wasabi" can be used for added flavor.

Homemade Vegetable Broth Powder

Makes 1¼ cups

½ cup finely ground, dried (dehy-drated) vegetables (vegetable pow-der): onion, green onion, leek, carrot, celery, green and/or red bell pepper, parsley, and sometimes tomato and cabbage

2 tablespoons chickpea or amaranth flour (soy or teff flour may be used but are not as good)

2 tablespoons arrowroot powder

1 tablespoon dried parsley flakes

1 teaspoon sea salt

1 teaspoon dried basil leaves

1 teaspoon dried oregano leaves

½ teaspoon ground sea kelp or ground dulse

½ teaspoon dill weed

½ teaspoon dried alfalfa leaves, or ½ teaspoon extra parsley

¼ teaspoon cumin powder or paprika

⅛ teaspoon dried mint leaves, or extra basil or oregano

⅛ teaspoon cayenne

2 tablespoons natural oil (canola, sunflower, or sesame are best)

Vegetable powder or dried vegetables can be purchased at many health food stores and specialty markets. Vegetables can also be dehydrated at home in the oven or a food dehydrator. If not already ground, a coffee grinder works the best and is the fastest way to grind the dehydrated vegetables. A blender or food mill may be used, but they take longer to grind vegetables. (See Oven-Dehydrated Vegetables.) Sift or strain powder if needed before measuring for this recipe. The flour needs to be heated on medium-high heat in a small, dry skillet and stirred constantly until it is toasty smelling and lightly browned. Then mix it with the vegetable powder and arrowroot and set aside.

All the seasonings must be ground in the coffee or herb mill or blender until they are a fine powder. Then mix them with the other dry ingredients thoroughly. Lastly mix in the natural oil; use a fork or your fingers to mix completely. Store the vegetable broth powder in a jar in the freezer (or a dou-ble plastic bag if preferred). Keep in the freezer for up to 3 to 6 months if kept airtight. Pull out as needed for use in soups, main dishes, and other recipes. The powder should cook for at least 20 minutes in recipes, for optimum flavor, digestibility, and to avoid any possible bacteria.

Store-bought vegetable broth powders may contain corn, soya, hydro-genated soya or vegetable protein, MSG, potato starch, peanut oil, lactose, and other ingredients that agitate Candida yeast and allergies.

Homemade Vegetable Bouillon Cubes

Makes about 24 cubes

1 batch Homemade Vegetable Broth
Powder

6 tablespoons cooked, hot, mashed
beans (pinto, kidney, adzuki,
romano, or red beans are best), with
no liquid

3 tablespoons arrowroot powder

3 to 4 teaspoons natural oil (canola,
sunflower, or sesame are best)

Mix all the ingredients together and use a fork or your fingers to mash
and mix everything thoroughly. Use 1 tablespoon of the mixture to make each
cube. Shape them into traditional squares or roll them into balls if preferred.
Store in jars, aluminum foil (shiny side in), or double plastic bags in the
freezer for up to 3 to 6 months if kept airtight. These should cook for at least
20 minutes in recipes, for optimum flavor, digestibility, and to avoid any possible bacteria. Store-bought vegetable bouillon cubes contain most of the same
agitating ingredients as the store-bought vegetable broth powders.

Mock Tamari Soy Sauce

Makes 1 to 1¼ cups

2¼ cups Brown Bean Juice, from
black beans (allow juice to settle; use clear, dark juice on top,
not the cloudy part)

¾ to 1 teaspoon sea salt

⅛ to ¼ teaspoon sea kelp

⅛ teaspoon vegetable powder (or
ground, dried vegetables)

Mix everything together well and bring to a boil on medium-high heat in
a covered saucepan. Reduce the heat immediately to low and simmer for 90
minutes, covered. Stir every 15 minutes or so.

Use a knife to scrape any spices off the side of the pan while stirring and
mix them back into the liquid. Keeps for 5 to 7 days refrigerated and must be

(continues)

re-simmered before each use. It is best to freeze 2-tablespoon servings of the Mock Tamari in individual ice cube tray sections for later use. Once frozen, place the cubes in a freezer bag or freezer jar in the freezer so they will stay fresh. Take them out and use in each recipe calling for tamari soy sauce, as desired.

GRAIN-FREE BREADS

No grain flours are recommended for regular Candida treatment or the Phase II Diet in this book. There are a few bean/legume and seed flours that may be used occasionally as a bread substitute. However, these should not be overused or heavily relied upon. Bean and seed flours can be hard to digest when eaten alone or on a regular basis. Save these for an occasional treat, one to three times per week at most. When Phase II is over, or for Phase I, III, and IV, occasional yeast-free (usually wheat-free) whole grain breads can be used, as well as whole grain rye crackers, rice cakes, and plain pancakes if recommended by your doctor or health specialist. For more yeast-free, whole grain breads and other recipes, see my *All Natural Allergy Cookbook*. Wheat-free, yeast-free breads are a bit tricky to make and require many guidelines, so read the baking chapters in the allergy cookbook carefully before attempting to make breads from it.

Amaranth or Teff Flatbreads

Makes 8

1 cup amaranth or teff flour*

2 tablespoons arrowroot powder

Optional: 2 to 4 teaspoons whole flaxseeds

1 tablespoon natural oil

½ cup water

¼ to ½ cup extra amaranth or teff flour for kneading

Preheat the oven to 400°F. Sift the flour with the arrowroot powder to lighten it by adding air to it. Add the flaxseeds if desired. Beat the oil and water together with a fork in a separate bowl and add the flour slowly to it, stirring as it is added.

---

*Chickpea or soy flour can also be used to make these breads.

Work the dough with the fork and then your hands. Knead briefly and roll it into a ball. Divide the ball into 8 parts. Roll each part into a ball and pat flat. Sprinkle each ball with extra flour and roll it between two sheets of wax paper with a rolling pin or strong glass tumbler. (If wax paper cannot be used because of corn content, keep turning bread while rolling and use extra flour so it will not stick.) Turn over frequently while rolling, and lift the wax paper occasionally to add flour so the dough does not stick. The bread should be somewhat rounded and ⅛ inch thick.

Lightly oil a frying pan or griddle and heat to medium-high heat. Put one flatbread in the pan and heat for 15 to 20 seconds on each side. Immediately put the bread in the oven and bake it for 3 minutes. Turn the flatbread over and bake for another 1½ to 2 minutes. The bread should puff up a bit in the oven, but not as much as a traditional pita because it has no yeast. Re-oil the pan with a paper towel dipped in oil, and repeat procedure for each flatbread. Cool the breads but refrigerate them within 4 hours of baking. Keep refrigerated for 3 to 6 days. Lightly toast or heat leftovers in foil in the oven to discourage bacteria.

This is a protein, seed-flour bread—not a grain-flour bread. Enjoy 1 to 2 flatbreads (and/or chapatis or other seed or legume breads) every second or third day on the Candida diet. Limit flatbread intake to this amount as pure seed bread takes extra work to digest and the bowels should not be overburdened during treatment, or at any time. Eat slowly, chew well, and enjoy.

Chickpea Chapatis

Makes 8 to 10

1 cup chickpea flour (also called garbanzo, chana, or besan flour)

2 tablespoons arrowroot powder

⅛ to ¼ teaspoon sea salt

⅓ cup water

1 tablespoon natural oil

Sift the first 3 ingredients together and add them to the water and oil. Mix well and roll into 1-inch balls and pat flat. With a rolling pin, roll out

(continues)

pastry-like rounds about ⅛ inch thick or a bit thicker. (Can roll like flatbreads between wax paper although it is not needed.) Heat a lightly oiled frying pan or griddle until very hot. Reduce heat to medium-high and heat each round for 1 to 2 minutes on each side, until warmed and slightly browned. Serve hot or cool and refrigerate within 4 hours.

Keep refrigerated for 3 to 6 days. Lightly toast or heat leftovers in foil in the oven to discourage bacteria.

This is a protein, legume-(bean) flour bread—not a grain-flour bread. Enjoy one to two chapatis (and/or flatbreads or other seed or legume breads) every second or third day on the Candida diet. Limit chapatis intake to this amount as pure bean bread takes extra work to digest and the bowels should not be overburdened during treatment or at any time. Eat slowly, chew well, and enjoy.

Popcorn

Popcorn can be hard to digest, but it is a whole grain and a helpful treat that can be enjoyed once a week or less. Use digestive aids if necessary (HCL, plant enzymes, Beano, bile salts, or other non-prescription aids can be helpful. Consult a health specialist if needed.) Melted butter and sea salt may be added to the popcorn if desired. Use organic, yellow popcorn cooked in natural oil or hot air-popped only. Do not use microwave popcorns, colored corn, or corn with any additives whatsoever. Maximum 2 to 4 cups popped popcorn per serving. Those who have serious problems digesting popcorn should avoid it.

Chapter 20

TREATS THAT ARE NOT TOO SWEET

```
┌─────────────────────────────────────────────┐
│                                               │
│        Anything Sweet Feeds the Yeast!        │
│                                               │
└─────────────────────────────────────────────┘
```

FRUIT

Studying other Candida books, I was surprised and dismayed to see that many of them count carbohydrate points for fruits and say that fruits like bananas are okay, while grapefruit is not good for a Candida diet because of higher carbohydrate points. Anything sweet feeds the yeast! If a fruit is especially sweet, like many southern, tropical, and exotic fruits such as bananas, mangoes, grapes, melons, oranges, pineapple, star fruit, lychee nuts, and others, yeast will love it and thrive on it!

These same books say to eat fruit after a meal, as you are less likely to be upset by fruit eaten after a meal than by fruit eaten before. The reason an empty stomach is upset by fruit before a meal is that the fruit is too sweet and feeds the yeast. When yeast are fed, they get strong and you get weak. An upset or queasy stomach after eating fruit denotes that the yeast have had a treat and are strong, or sometimes it means that you are allergic or sensitive to the food just consumed, or you have trouble digesting raw foods.

To suggest fresh, raw fruit after a meal is terrible food combining and causes the prior eaten food and the fruit to be improperly digested. It may lead to fermentation of foods in the digestive tract and these fermented foods then become even better food for the yeast. If the proper nonsweet, tart, subacid fruit is eaten 15 to 30 minutes or more before a meal and eaten in proper sequence—fruit first then other foods—foods are properly digested and do not spoil in the body and provide food for the yeast or make one's stomach upset. During severe Candida problems, it is better to eat no fruit except the lemons, limes, white grapefruit, avocados, or cooked berries mentioned in the Phase II diet plan. One can easily survive without fruit. The body can take care of its need for carbohydrates with whole grains and vegetables and get its enzymes from tart fruits, tomatoes, yogurt, and acidophilus (or lactic acid–fermented vegetables, if allowed), or from supplements.

Instead of counting carbohydrates in sweet and starchy foods, this book counts the attributes and abilities of certain fruits and foods to be tolerated, digestible, and nutritious and to have the tendency to discourage yeast growth. One should only eat fruits that the yeast do not like to eat!

WAYS TO MAKE FRUIT MORE DIGESTIBLE

Fruits are easy to digest, except for some individuals with digestive troubles. The skins and seeds of certain fruits do not break down well in some digestive tracts. If this is the case, peel apples, pears, and other subacid fruits before eating them during Phase I or IV Diets, for children on Phase III Diets, and adults on Phase III diets—if allowed by the doctor!

Eat one type of fruit—alone—at a time, unless citrus (except oranges) is included. Lemon, lime, or white grapefruit juice can be used to soak cut fruit in to help it break down easier for better digestion; this serves the dual purpose of counteracting any bacteria or hidden mold that might delight the yeast.

Use food-combining methods (see chapter 9) as another yeast deterrent. Chew a fruit to water in your mouth. Crunchy fruits are better for discouraging Candida, but they need to be chewed very well. Always buy and eat organic fruits if good quality is available.

One way to assist in fruit digestion is to eat subacid fruits with Acidophilus Yogurt. The acidophilus helps to counteract yeast looking for "good time fruit." Dairy products are not usually good with fruits; since real, plain yogurt is a high-enzyme food, it is okay to eat yogurt with tart or subacid fruits occasionally. Wait at least 30 to 60 minutes after eating fruit and yogurt before eating other foods!

Fruits allowed on Phase I diet:

Apples, avocados, nonsweet pears, Japanese pear apples, kiwi (tender-firm, not too soft or ripe), papayas (if not too sweet), grapefruit, fresh lemon juice, fresh lime juice, strawberries, blackberries, blueberries, raspberries, other berries, watermelon.

PHASE I FRUIT AND YOGURT

Fruit is limited on this diet, after freely eating any fruit you choose in the average diet, but this is temporary. Wait 30 to 60 minutes after eating these fruits (except with avocados) before eating other foods. Try the following singular fruits or combinations of fruit and/or yogurt as pre-breakfast fruit or a separate daytime snack, up to five to six times weekly:

1. Peel apples, pears, papayas, or kiwis and eat them alone, or cut and soaked in fresh lemon or lime juice, or cut them and serve with Acidophilus Yogurt.
2. Eat plain, firm berries, one type, alone or with Acidophilus Yogurt (cut off and discard any soft spots on berries).
3. Eat ½ avocado stuffed with fresh berries, alone or topped with Acidophilus Yogurt. See above.
4. Always eat watermelon totally alone.
5. Eat ½ grapefruit, pink or white, alone or with plain, natural yogurt or Acidophilus Yogurt.
6. Eat ½ avocado stuffed with chopped grapefruit sections, alone or topped with Acidophilus Yogurt. See above.

7. Eat any of the Phase II fruit combinations.

Fruits allowed on Phase II diet:
Avocados, white grapefruit, fresh lemon juice, fresh lime juice, cooked berries (if doctor approves).

PHASE II FRUIT AND YOGURT

Fruit is quite limited on this diet, but this is temporary. Remember to wait 30 to 60 minutes after eating these (except with avocados) before eating other foods. Try the following singular fruits or combinations of fruit and/or yogurt as pre-breakfast fruit up to 3 to 4 times weekly:

1. Drink the juice of one small lemon or lime straight and drunk with nothing else (or ½ large lemon or lime).
2. Eat ½ white grapefruit alone, or cut it and serve with Acidophilus Yogurt.
3. Eat ½ avocado filled with chopped white grapefruit sections.
4. Try chopped avocado with lemon or lime juice.
5. Eat ½ to 1 small or medium avocado eaten alone.
6. Have Acidophilus Yogurt with cut avocado and/or grapefruit sections.
7. Eat plain, natural yogurt with fresh lemon or lime juice alone.
8. Make cooked berries or Berry Berry Sauce (if allowed) mixed with Acidophilus Yogurt.
9. Try ½ avocado or ½ white grapefruit topped with cooked berries or Berry Berry Sauce (if allowed).

Fruits allowed on Phase III diet:
(for children and some adults if allowed by doctor)
Apples, avocados, nonsweet pears, Japanese pear apples, kiwi (tender-firm, not too soft or ripe), papayas, grapefruit (white only), fresh lemon juice, fresh lime juice, strawberries, blackberries, blueberries, raspberries, other berries.

PHASE III FRUIT AND YOGURT

These fruits may be eaten by children and by adults only if the doctor permits during a Phase III diet with treatment. Raw fruit must be limited to one serving daily for children and three to six servings per week for adults as pre-breakfast fruit. These limitations are temporary. Remember to wait 30 to 60 minutes after these (except with avocados alone) before eating other foods. Try the following singular fruits or combinations of fruit and/or yogurt as pre-breakfast fruit up to three to six times weekly.

1. Peel apples, pears, papayas, or kiwis and eat them alone, or cut and soak in fresh lemon or lime juice or cut them and serve with Acidophilus Yogurt. (You can eat the skins of organic apples and pears if they are chewed well.)
2. Eat fresh, plain berries, one type, alone or with Acidophilus Yogurt.
3. Eat ½ white grapefruit alone or with plain, natural yogurt or Acidophilus Yogurt.
4. Eat any of the Phase II fruit combinations.

Frozen Berry Sorbet

Phases I and IV; if allowed, Adults II and III

Frozen treats can be eaten 1 to 2 times per week if allowed (3 to 4 times per week for children). The fruit is not cooked; it is frozen, which destroys live fruit enzymes that can slow or hurt digestion when eaten after a meal. Freezing also helps kill Candida on fruit.

3 cups frozen berries (strawberries, raspberries, blueberries, or black-berries)

1 to 2 teaspoons fresh lemon or lime juice

Take one type of berries out of the freezer and let sit at room temperature for 1 hour or more until soft. Use a food processor or blender to purée these until smooth. Place in a clean plastic container or freezer jar about ¾ full and freeze solid. Remove from freezer 10 minutes before you wish to eat this. Enjoy ½ cup of this alone, 30 minutes before meals or 1 to 1½ hours after a meal. For a smoother, less-icy sorbet, soften frozen sorbet slightly at room temperature and process or blend a second time and re-freeze before enjoying.

Frozen Fruit Sorbet

Phases I, IV, and Children; if allowed, Adults III (not II)

Frozen treats can be eaten 1 to 2 times per week if allowed (3 to 4 times per week for children). The fruit is not cooked, it is frozen, which destroys live fruit enzymes that can slow or hurt digestion when eaten after a meal.

3 cups frozen cut papayas, kiwis, sometimes pears

1 to 2 teaspoons fresh lemon or lime juice

Take one type of fruit out of the freezer and let sit at room temperature for 1 hour or more until soft. Use a food processor or blender to purée until smooth. Place in a clean plastic container or freezer jar about ¾ full and freeze solid. Remove from freezer 10 minutes before you wish to eat. Enjoy ½ cup alone, 30 minutes before meals or 1 to 1½ hours after a meal. Process twice, as with Frozen Berry Sorbet, for smoother sorbet.

Berry Berry Sauce

Phases I, IV, and Children; if allowed, Adults II and III

Adults may enjoy this once or twice a week, children two to four times per week. Keeps for 1 to 3 days refrigerated; must be reheated before each serving.

3 to 4 cups fresh or frozen berries (strawberries, raspberries, blueberries, or blackberries)

2 to 3 teaspoons fresh white grapefruit juice, or 1 to 2 teaspoons fresh lemon or lime juice, or ⅛ teaspoon corn-free unbuffered vitamin C crystals

Chop the fresh or frozen berries or purée them in a food processor or blender until smooth. Heat them in a covered saucepan on medium-high heat. Once they come up to a boil, turn the heat to low and simmer for 4 to 6 minutes, until cooked and hot throughout. Remove from heat and serve hot over pancakes, cereals, or meat dishes. They can also be quick-chilled in the freezer for 15 minutes or so and served with Acidophilus Yogurt.

Baked Apples or Pears

Phases I, IV, and Children; if allowed, Adults III

1 nonsweet pear or baking apple, per person (Macintosh, Spartan, golden delicious, Rome, or other)

Optional: cinnamon

Optional: dash of sea salt

Optional: bit of butter

Preheat oven to 375°F. Peel and chop the fruit and place in a lightly oiled, low, glass or Corningware baking dish. Sprinkle with cinnamon and extras if desired. Bake for 20 to 35 minutes or until tender throughout. Serve as a side dish or dessert 1 to 2 times per week (more for children, about 2 to 5 times per week). Keeps refrigerated for 1 to 3 days; must be reheated to serve.

Homemade Applesauce

Phases I and IV and Children only

5 pounds baking apples (Macintosh or Spartan are good)

3 to 4 tablespoons water

Peel, core, and chop the apples into 1-inch pieces and place them with water in a pot with a tight-fitting lid. Put them on an electric burner already pre-set at high or on a high gas flame and stand with the pot for 1 to 2 minutes or so until you hear (or peek and see) the water sizzling. Turn the heat immediately to low and stir.

Simmer, covered, for 55 to 75 minutes, until the apples are so tender they either fall apart by themselves or can easily be hand-mashed with a square- or round-holed hand masher. (A potato masher will not work.) Check them and stir every 20 minutes or so. Mash thoroughly, especially for children who do not like lumps. The sauce is naturally sweet.

Serve the sauce warm with meals, over meat, or 1 to 1½ hours after meals. Do not eat on a totally empty stomach! Serve 1 to 2 times per week, 1 to 3 times per week for children. Keeps refrigerated for 3 to 6 days; must be

(continues)

reheated to serve. Can be quick-chilled in the freezer for 15 to 25 minutes before serving if desired. If apples taste too naturally sweet, add a teaspoon or two of fresh lemon or lime juice when serving or serve occasionally with Acidophilus Yogurt.

Jicama and Lime

For All Phases

½ to ¾ cup chopped, raw jicama per person, peeled

3 to 5 teaspoons fresh lime juice per serving

Peel and cut the crunchy jicama (hee-ca-ma) vegetable and rinse it thoroughly. Mix it with the lime juice. Enjoy this crunchy sweet-tart delight as a separate snack 30 minutes or more before a meal, or 1½ hours or more after a meal. Jicama is too starchy a vegetable to eat alone; however, it may be eaten this way once every 5 to 6 days or more. Eat fresh. Do not store.

Roasted Carob Pod Treats

Phases I, II, and III

These are best if eaten 30 to 60 minutes after a meal. These tasty treats are not familiar to many people. Carob tastes a bit like cocoa and has ten times less fat than chocolate and contains no caffeine or oxalic acid. The pods grow on a tree and are common in the Middle East. They are also called St. John's bread, as it is claimed that St. John the Baptist ate these in the desert to sustain himself. These are in the legume family.

Purchase pre-roasted carob pods from a specialty food market or have them specially ordered from a natural foods store; most do not stock whole carob pods. Wash them, shake or pat dry, and place them in a preheated 325° to 350°F oven for 5 minutes until warmed throughout. The baking kills any bacteria and softens them. Cool a few minutes until just a bit warm and enjoy chewing this tasty, malt-like treat as a dessert. Eat everything but the seeds. Spit out the seeds and chew well. Enjoy this treat about once a week if allowed.

SPECIAL ADDITIONS FOR RECIPES

Phases I, IV, and sometimes III. Have once to three times per month unless otherwise stated.

1. Bake or broil papaya slices with meats; they are good for helping to digest meat better.
2. Roast quartered apples or pears with a roasted chicken.
3. Kiwi and white grapefruit chunks mix well together as a little fruit salad for special occasions or have with Acidophilus Yogurt.
4. Use cut chunks of white grapefruit on a leafy green salad instead of tomatoes. (Can be enjoyed once a week in all phases.)
5. Bake avocados inside or on top of casseroles and vegetable pies. (These can be enjoyed one to three times weekly during all diet phases.)

Part III

PROTECTING YOUR FUTURE, PREVENTING CANDIDA RECURRENCE, AND BEYOND

BY DR. ZOLTAN P. RONA AND
JEANNE MARIE MARTIN

Chapter 21

WHAT TO DO IF CANDIDA IS NOT HEALING

POSSIBLE CONTRIBUTING FACTORS

BY ZOLTAN P. RONA

I often see patients in my practice who have been treating conditions like chronic fatigue syndrome, allergies, irritable bowel syndrome, and many other fungal connection illnesses for several years. Many have made the rounds of internal medical specialists, naturopaths, chiropractors, and other health-care practitioners. For some of these people, the battle against fungi has become a 24-hour preoccupation. Each case is unique, and several areas of diagnosis and treatment need to be investigated to fully heal more stubborn cases. For this, the help of an open-minded doctor or holistic medical practitioner is usually necessary.

Following are diagnoses and treatment options that may have been overlooked or unaddressed in the course of battling the fungal connection.

- Clinical depression is a real factor and the number one reason for the failure of months or years of antifungal therapy to clear symptoms such as chronic fatigue, spaciness, eating disorders, incurable food allergies, insomnia, memory loss, and multiple somatic complaints. This diagnosis is often resisted by chronically ill patients. A significantly high percentage of these victims have been sexually or otherwise abused in childhood. Long-term psychotherapy and low-side-effect antidepressants may be warranted.

- Subclinical hypothyroidism or Wilson's disease (see chapter 3), especially in cases where body temperatures are consistently below 98.6°F or 37°C.
- Toxic heavy metal excess or hypersensitivity, especially to mercury in dental amalgams, but also to lead, cadmium, aluminum, copper, arsenic, and nickel (see chapter 3).
- Vitamin deficiencies, especially of B-complex vitamins, notably folic acid and vitamin B_{12}, which may be poorly absorbed by the intestines of chronically ill individuals. Injections may be necessary until gut healing can take place.
- Mineral deficiencies or imbalances involving zinc, copper, selenium, calcium, magnesium, chromium, manganese, silicon, boron, iodine, and lithium.
- Essential fatty acid and amino acid deficiencies can mimic the symptoms of chronic fungal illness and come about due to malabsorption caused by digestive enzyme deficiencies. Amino acids are precursors to all the neurotransmitters responsible for optimal brain and nervous system function.
- Masked or delayed food allergies or chemical hypersensitivities, which can only be determined by elimination provocation testing or blood tests like RAST or ELISA/ACT.
- Hypoglycemia or hyperglycemia due to endocrine gland dysfunction other than the thyroid (pancreas, adrenal, gonadal disease).
- Alcohol, tobacco, or other drug; substance abuse victims require long-term addiction therapy, in a hospital or detox clinic setting. As an initial act, look into 12-Step support groups for guidance.
- Chronic parasitic infestations due to poor or inappropriate medical testing procedures.
- Low stomach acidity or low pancreatic enzyme production in response to food intake.
- Other undiagnosed viral or bacterial infections (HIV, *Helicobacter pylori*, or others).

COMPLETING CANDIDA TREATMENT

BY JEANNE MARIE MARTIN

If Candida treatment was not successful and there are no other underlying causes, look at your choice of drug or herbal treatment(s)or at your diet. See Regulation of Treatment in chapter 5 and Types of Treatment in chapter 3 and discuss an alternative treatment with your doctor.

Perhaps diet is the problem. More than half of my nutrition counseling clients cheat on their Candida diets one or more times per week. It is difficult to starve the yeast if you keep feeding them foods they like. If you took a not-too-serious approach to your diet and cheated weekly or often, you need to get serious for six to eight weeks or more about diet, while repeating treatment, or choose alternative treatment(s). Follow the Phase II Diet religiously, with any important changes suggested by your doctor or dictated by food allergies. Read over the sections on cleaning and preparing raw foods and stick with this book's other food guidelines as carefully as possible. If you have specific problems with the diet, get experienced advice from a qualified nutrition counselor.

In addition to proper diet, be careful to use flushing agents or digestive aids while doing the diet with treatment to assure that toxins do not build up, flood the body, and interfere with the treatment and your healing. Use flushing foods like yogurt, citrus and tomato juices, miso or lactic acid–fermented vegetables (if allowed), raw veggies or vegetable juice, or flushing agents like acidophilus, oxygen capsules, flaxseed, psyllium, or laxative teas. Continue proper treatments and diet with proper flushing for a longer period of time than previous treatment. Use regulated treatment that is not too heavy or light and is consistent or about the same intensity every day.

When you finish another round of treatment and the Phase II diet, go into the Phase III diet for three to six weeks more, without treatment, until your energy levels pick up. (Use flushing foods and agents here, too, if needed.) Once this is completed, stay on a Phase IV diet for an indefinite length of time and avoid any foods that agitate you in any way! Follow the extra tips in chapter 22 for preventing Candida reoccurrence. Sometimes a complete body-cleansing program done several weeks after treatment can take care of removing extra body toxins left over after yeast treatment. Toxins that may have piled up during treatment need to be thoroughly moved through the body. It is not enough to kill the yeast; their poisons are sometimes left behind and need to be purged from the body or they can contribute to future health problems and renewed yeast growth. The Phase II diet (or sometimes Phase III diet) is usually best to follow during most cleansing programs unless the product(s) states another specific diet. A 10- to 21-day detox cleanse will often do the trick.

If your body refuses to get better even though you did everything right during a second (or additional) treatment, you have done a good cleanse, and your body remains in a weakened state because of other health problems, stay on the Phase II or III Diet (including any doctor-recommended changes and treatments) until the other health problems are healed or under control.

Chapter 22

STAYING HEALTHY ONCE CANDIDA TREATMENT IS OVER

POST-CANDIDA TREATMENT

BY ZOLTAN P. RONA

People who recover from the effects of the Candida syndrome are usually empowered to get on with their lives. Sometimes they forget what made them ill and how they got better, and return to old, unhealthy habits.

To prevent a recurrence, healed Candida victims must remain vigilant about their diet and lifestyle. The fact that you experienced this illness is a sign that your body, mind, and spirit are more susceptible than those of your friends or neighbors who did not. Recurrence is indeed possible if you let down your guard.

My advice is to follow, as closely as possible, the basic general principles of boosting the immune system discussed in chapter 7 for the rest of your life. Since each case is unique, lifestyle, diet, and supplement recommendations will be different from person to person. Work with a natural health-care practitioner to design a long-term maintenance program. Visit your naturopath, holistic medical doctor, or therapist on a regular basis (at least twice a year) when you are well, not only when symptoms occur.

Health is intimately connected to knowledge. You need not take a course in naturopathic medicine, but do read what you can get your hands on about health issues on a regular basis. Spread the good word about natural and alternative medicine. Millions of people are suffering needlessly, treating chronic illnesses with toxic drugs. One way you can help others is to pass this book on to your family, friends, and concerned health-care practitioners.

HEALTH MAINTENANCE AFTER CANDIDA

BY JEANNE MARIE MARTIN

Healing Candida can be a temporary victory for many people because once you have had a problem with Candida overgrowth, there is always a potential for a recurrence if you fall into old ways of abusing your body again. Sometimes people quickly return to old habits and sometimes they gradually go downhill until they are back where they were with Candida symptoms and side effects.

If you follow the Phase IV diet for the rest of your life, you have a better chance of avoiding recurrences than by abandoning all diet guidelines and eating everything in sight. The Phase IV diet allows you to eat many "normal foods" while giving special guidelines for preparation, food combining, food types, and amounts.

Special supplements can be continued to help prevent new yeast from getting a firm foothold in the body. The tips here have helped many of my clients stay healthy and avoid recurrence.

Use these tips especially around the holidays! That is the time when many people "fall off the wagon" and return to their worst old diet patterns. These tips can make living easier, more enjoyable, and definitely more "yeast-free." This is a good list to make a copy of, after treatment is over, and tape inside a kitchen cupboard door or the medicine cabinet door so you can refer to it often.

Now that Candida is healed, keep the critters (yeast) under control and enjoy life a little. You worked hard during treatment, now savor your victory and make sure it is a lasting one! May you enjoy a healthy, happy life!

HEALTH AND DIET GUIDELINES FOR LIFETIME CANDIDA CONTROL

1. Do not eat any sweets on an empty stomach. Have a meal first or a complex carbohydrate or protein snack before desserts or sweets.
2. Do not eat sweets first during a meal. If having eggs and pancakes, eat the eggs first, then the pancakes if they include syrup. If the pancakes are plain or covered in unsweetened, cooked fruit sauce, they are not a sweet and can be eaten first in a meal. If having sweet applesauce with a meal, eat a quarter of the meal, or several bites, before the applesauce is eaten.
3. Whenever possible, eat desserts 1 to 1½ hours after a full meal of foods. If possible, limit desserts to one serving daily or less.
4. Every time you eat a real sweet food or dessert, take a Biotin tablet (300 to 500 micrograms). This helps inhibit the yeast and keeps new yeast from growing. Up to two or three tablets can be taken daily (900 to 1,500 micrograms). Take at least one, preferably two (or sometimes three or four if many sweets are eaten that day), and B50-complex daily as well when using biotin.
5. Take a vitamin B50-complex once or twice daily for life and at least 500 milligrams of vitamin C daily—1,000 to 2,000 milligrams daily is the ideal (more if desired or required). Allergy C, Sago palm–derived C, Ester C, or buffered C are the best types of vitamin C to take.
6. If drinking alcohol, limit yourself to two to three drinks maximum. Never drink on an empty stomach! Always have a meal first or at least a large complex carbohydrate or protein snack. Take an extra one to two vitamin B50-complex before drinking (with food if possible), along with 1,000 milligrams vitamin C, 300 micrograms biotin, and an extra 100 milligrams of B_6. (Always have B_6 with a B50-complex.)
7. It is best not to drink alcohol until an hour after a full meal. The day after drinking, take two to four capsules of B50-complex, 1,000 to 2,000 milligrams vitamin C, two to three biotin tablets (at separate meals), and 50 milligrams more of B_6. Take the B_6 in the morning, especially if you have a hangover. (If so, you're treading dangerous waters and a Candida reoccurrence is likely!) Be sure to eat especially good meals the day before and the day after drinking. Avoid drinking alcohol more than two to eight days monthly, depending on your body's ability to handle it, and drink lightly. Avoid highly sweetened red wines and mixed drinks. Avoid alcohol altogether if possible!

8. Do not eat raw eggs, raw mushrooms, overripe fruits or veggies, or any undercooked protein foods, especially red meats, shellfish, or poultry. Avoid raw sushi and sashimi. Choose cooked sushi varieties.

9. If you have just eaten a huge meal that is weighing you down, take an acidophilus capsule or other flushing agent or digestive aid and do some slow exercise like walking or doing the dishes. Take acidophilus daily or several times weekly if your stomach acid is low or digestion is sluggish.

10. If feeling low and susceptible to colds, flu, or sickness, or if you have been close to or intimate with someone sick, take garlic capsules and/or citrus seed concentrate (Citricidal) one to two times daily until symptoms or weakness passes. Take 2,000 milligrams of vitamin C daily (can be taken all at once or preferably 500 milligrams four times during the day at least four to five hours away from bedtime). Lemon or lime juice can be taken straight one to two times daily, during the daytime, away from foods. Take these items along when you travel.

11. During holidays (and every day) eat two to three wholesome meals daily. Do not just snack or munch on goodies all day long.

12. Follow food-combining principles (chapter 9) three to six days per week to assist digestion. Follow them every day when you have low energy, feel sick, or are under excessive stress.

13. Continue to use the healthful lifestyle suggestions in chapter 7 as needed: chiropractic, massage, deep breathing, meditation, strengthening techniques, Epsom salt baths, hot/cold showers, and other methods of your choosing.

14. If you need to take antibiotics in the future, take acidophilus daily (and eat yogurt if possible) throughout treatment, and for 10 to 14 days after the antibiotics are completed to keep a healthy balance of friendly bacteria in your system and protect from yeast overgrowth recurrence.

15. Do not smoke cigarettes, cigars, or marijuana; chew tobacco; or take pleasure drugs or unnecessary prescription drugs. These weaken the body immensely and invite Candida to multiply rapidly.

16. Do a nonsweet, herbal, or natural cleansing program two to four times per year for optimum health. (No sweet fruit juices or maple syrup should be used.) If you feel you need something more after Candida treatment, rest a month or two and then do a cleansing program.

17. Take digestive aids or laxative teas occasionally if required. Do not overuse these products. If digestive problems persist, see your doctor.

18. Drink tested spring water whenever possible. This will add years to your life and life to your liver, kidneys, colon, and other organs. Use distilled/demineralized and ozonated water only when cleansing, NOT when fasting.

19. Follow the Phase IV diet as much as possible—for life—for optimum health and well-being.

20. Keep a balanced lifestyle. Do not overwork excessively. Get enough exercise, rest, sunshine, fresh air, play, and other elements of a healthful lifestyle. Keep a positive attitude and employ healing aids when needed from chapter 7.

21. Educate yourself about healthful living. Read health books, newsletters, and magazines and attend talks or seminars if possible to learn everything you can about how to stay healthy, prevent disease, and utilize what you learn. Then: Enjoy life! Be practical and realistic and let loose a little once in a while, too.

Ask your holistic doctor or holistic nutrition consultant for more information on the right program(s) for you.

Remember: Buzzards do not fly in circles around an oasis! Keep healthy and strong and not even the yeast will be able to get you down!

Chapter 23

BEYOND CANDIDA

How to Use This Book's Recipes and Diets for Other Diseases

BY JEANNE MARIE MARTIN

ABOUT THE DIETS

Candida, as discussed throughout this book, is sometimes a forerunner or complication of another disease or diseases. Sometimes Candida treatment alone is not enough. If your Candida is severe, does not respond successfully to treatment, and is not cured within two to six months, you need to look for an underlying cause or possible contributing factors. (See Possible Contributing Factors in chapter 21)

Tests including allergy testing (ELISA/ACT test), Vega testing, B.E.V. (BioEnergetics of Vincent), blood tests, urine tests, stool analysis, hair analysis, kinesiology testing and/or others may be required to determine health problems or diseases that may be weakening the body and therefore not allowing Candida to heal.

When and if another health problem is discovered, concentration must shift to focus diet and medical treatment on the underlying cause of the Candida. Only when the cause or contributing factor (disease) is healed can one hope to alleviate the symptoms and side effects of Candida successfully.

Even if there is no Candida problem, the diets and some of the treatments recommended in this book can be beneficial for treating other health problems and diseases listed further on. In chapter 2, Dr. Rona gives a good account of fungal/Candidiasis connections to other diseases. Here in this chapter, diets that support the healing of various diseases are outlined, using the four phases of diet in this book and the recipes.

Health problems/diseases have a better chance of being cured if proper diet is used along with various medical treatments and some of the health aids found in chapter 7. I tell my students and clients: "A person only has a fifty-fifty chance of healing a disease if treatments, medicines, and/or herbal remedies alone are given. There is as much as a 90 percent chance of healing if *proper diet* also is used to assist the healing process."

This book can be a powerful aid to assist healing diseases. Use the guidelines further on and check the books *Prescription for Nutritional Healing, Healthy Healing,* and Dr. Rona's *Return to the Joy of Health* (See References—Nutrition Guidebooks) for additional information, as well as consulting holistic doctors and medical specialists. Vitamins, supplements, remedies, and treatments are not given here for diseases and should be recommended by your physician(s).

Cleansing is also beneficial to all diseases. First stabilize the body with proper diet. Consult your holistic doctor or health expert before beginning a cleanse and have him or her assist you in choosing a cleansing program that is right for your needs. Some cleanses and fasts are given here.

Of course, your personal physician(s) advice supersedes all information given here. Be sure to get more than one doctor's opinion regarding cancer and all major diseases.

ALLERGIES OR FOOD SENSITIVITIES

See your doctor for food and environmental allergy testing and for information on elimination and rotation diets. (See Rotation Diets in chapter 15 also.) If major changes need to be made in your diet (and lifestyle), do a Phase I diet first along with any doctor-recommended changes. Next move to a Phase II diet, also with doctor-recommended changes. Nearly all the recipes in this book can be used except for those containing foods you have tested positive to for allergies. Use the substitution chart in chapter 11 to help eliminate unwanted foods in the recipes.

Food combining is very important for allergies. Do not eat sweet fruit on an empty stomach; avoid them or eat them one hour after breakfast or lunch, never after supper.

Have your doctor do parasite, thyroid, digestive, and vitamin/mineral deficiency (or overabundance) testing as well, to rule these out as problems, as they are possible contributing factors for allergies. Digestive aids (chapter 3) and/or energizing supplements and healing aids (chapter 7) may also be required.

Once the diet is regulated and possible treatments underway or completed, a total body-cleansing program of 10 to 21 days can be very beneficial to expel toxins that may be contributing to allergy reactions. Two or more yearly cleanses may also be helpful.

ADDITIONAL ALLERGY DIET TIPS

1. Drink tested spring water.
2. Eat lots of stabilizing warm cooked whole grains, legumes, orange yams, winter squash, and carrots (unless allergic).
3. Avoid common allergenic foods like most dairy products (real yogurt and kefir are the most tolerated), wheat, gluten, eggs, strawberries, caffeine, potatoes, shellfish, red meats, soy, corn, peanuts, mushrooms, yeast, sweet fruits, sugar, excessive sweets, aspartame, MSG, sulfites, artificial colors and flavors, and junk foods of all kinds.
4. Enjoy healthful vegetable juices several times a week, as well as four to six servings of vegetables daily.
5. Use Rotation Diets. (See Rotation Diets in this book and my *All Natural Allergy Cookbook*—see Recommended Reading.) Yeast- and gluten-free breads and desserts can also be found in my allergy cookbook. Consult your doctor for more information.
6. Do a vegetable fast occasionally, as needed, one to four times monthly if your doctor permits. This helps rest the digestive tract and purge some body toxins. (See Cleansing further on.)
7. Keep a food diary and watch for reactions to specific foods or combinations of foods. Also notice which foods agitate an empty stomach. Inform your doctor of the results.
8. For more information about allergies, see my book *Your Natural Medicine Chest*.

ASTHMA AND ECZEMA

Follow the basic guidelines for chronic fatigue syndrome with a few changes. Eat largely raw foods and include green food products like alfalfa and spirulina in the diet. Get allergy testing (for dairy and gluten in particular, as well as for other foods and environmental factors) and for children especially, heavy metal testing. Avoid almost all dairy products (and sometimes eggs, too), except possibly some butter or clarified butter and a little goat milk yogurt and cooked feta cheese if tolerated. Meats and preservatives must be avoided. Take digestive aids as needed and/or avoid gassy foods. Enjoy unsweetened cranberry and citrus juices (except orange). Avoid high-mucus refined foods and excessive whole grain breads and crackers. Gluten (mainly wheat, oats, barley, and rye) may also be a problem, so include it in the allergy testing. (Pasta is best left alone.) Avoid living in, or visiting for long periods of time, homes with gas stoves in them; avoid as well any toxic fumes. Helpful teas include pau d'arco, ginger, and fenugreek. Use lobelia during asthma attacks. The Phase II or III diets with some doctor-recommended changes are best. Get more specific details from your doctor and nutritionist.

BOWEL PROBLEMS

The Phase II diet is excellent for most severe bowel problems including: irritable bowel syndrome (IBS), colitis, ulcerative colitis, diverticulitus, spastic colon, ileitis, and chronic constipation. Study chapter 9 in particular for food combining and severe digestion information essential to healing bowel problems.

Bowel problems are often related to food allergies, heavy metal overdose, parasites, and/or Candida. Getting medical testing for these problems as well is essential.

Raw vegetables sometimes have to be eliminated from the diet for severe problems because they scratch the colon and are very hard to digest. If this is the case, daily fresh vegetable juices are essential to the diet. See chapter 15 for acceptable vegetables to eat raw (if tolerated) and for the cooked vegetables that are recommended for bowel problems. Vegetable selection and storage guides are also in this chapter.

Additional Bowel Problem Diet Tips

1. Drink tested spring water and occasionally (steam) distilled when cleansing.
2. Avoid drinking mineral waters, especially sparkling mineral waters.
3. Especially no corn chips, popcorn, or other corn products; nuts or seeds (except ground nuts and seeds or butters cooked into some recipes may be tolerated); red meat; poultry; or any scratchy, hard-to-digest foods. Soft, natural, whole foods are best.
4. The Vegetable Fast is excellent one or more days per week, excluding all raw veggies except for juices.
5. An occasional one day (nonsweet—see recommended fruits under Fasting) fruit fast, two to six times per month can be healing.
6. Bowel cleansing can be very helpful. Ask your holistic doctor to recommend correct programs for you.
7. Make sure that whole grains and legumes are very well cooked with extra water and eaten while warm and very tender, or better yet, blended or mashed in most recipes.

CANCER

When cancer has been diagnosed, the severity of the condition and the type of cancer affect what diet particulars are required.

Begin with a Phase I diet if major diet changes need to be made and caffeine, alcohol, and/or smoking need to be eliminated. As quickly as possible, move to the Phase II diet. This diet contains all the most important elements of a macrobiotic diet, blended with other holistic, healing foods. Vegetables, brown rice, and brown legumes should make up 80 to 95 percent of the diet. Also read over the Chronic Fatigue Syndrome diet for additional understanding of simple, easy-to-digest diets.

Additional Cancer Diet Tips

1. Drink tested spring water (and occasionally distilled if doctor recommends).
2. Fruits and fruit juices are best limited to one to two servings daily in the morning. Phase I fruits may usually be eaten throughout (plus some

peaches and apricots), as well as fresh-squeezed apple juice and black cherry or currant juices if doctor permits.

3. Do a Vegetable Fast one to three days weekly as doctor permits. (Better every other day than three days in a row.)

4. The enzymes found in raw vegetables and juices, miso, seaweed, raw onions and garlic, and sometimes yogurt, are helpful on a regular basis.

5. Avoid all dairy products except a little yogurt and kefir about one to three times weekly. (Unless allergic) A little butter or clarified butter may be had occasionally.

6. Enjoy cruciferous vegetables steamed until tender (not mushy or crunchy) or juiced: broccoli, brussels sprouts, cabbage, and cauliflower daily. (Rotate so none are eaten every day.)

7. Enjoy orange vegetables: carrots, yams, or winter squash one to two times daily. (Rotate.)

8. Enjoy leafy green vegetables two to three times daily (raw and tender cooked): chard, beet greens, mustard greens, kale, collards, spinach (if allowed), Boston lettuce, bibb lettuce, leaf lettuce, red lettuce, exotic greens (without radicchio, endive, or escarole), and others. (No iceberg [head], romaine, or white, stalky parts of other lettuces.)

9. Enjoy one or more high-germanium (high-oxygen) foods daily: aloe vera, shiitake mushrooms, onions, garlic, ginseng, or comfrey or suma teas.

10. All foods, especially *raw foods,* must be *chewed to water* before swallowing! Gandhi said: "Chew your liquids, drink your foods." Whole grains must be cooked overtime with 3 to 4 cups water per 1 cup grain. Legumes must be blended, mashed, or mashable with the tongue. *Both* must be eaten warm! Cooked veggies must be tender throughout, never crunchy! Raw vegetables must be eaten first in a vegetarian meal (second after red meats or poultry). Only the veggies in chapter 15 may be had raw and must be chewed to water before consuming. If raw veggies are too much work to chew, raw vegetable juices can be had instead, one to three glasses daily as doctor permits. Each glass must be slowly drunk for 20 minutes each, swished in the mouth, and mixed with lots of saliva.

11. Consume no soy products except well-cooked, warm soybeans (consume no cold beans!), miso, and wheat-free soy sauce only every other day! One to three servings can be had every other day, as doctor permits. Cooked, warm tofu may be had once or twice weekly maximum if permitted, on days when soy is eaten.

12. Do not use stir-frys! Mainly steam and occasionally, two to three times weekly, bake or broil (without oil) vegetables. Avoid using oil to cook with or added to foods.

13. Fish and flaxseeds (ground) or flax oil may be beneficial. Consult your physician for your particular needs. Usually 1 to 3 servings every other day.

14. Seven to 10 organic apricot kernels or almonds may be enjoyed four to five days per week, eaten alone, and chewed to water for healing natural B15 (laetrile) they contain.

15. Definitely no microwaving!

16. Besides teas in the beverage chapter (chapter 12), ask your doctor about which of the following herbal teas may be beneficial for you: dandelion, organic green tea, red clover, ginseng, pau d'arco, or suma. Also ask about taking singular green foods/products like: barley green, green kamut, spirulina, wheat grass, chlorella or blue green algae, or others.

FOR EARLY STAGES OF CANCER AND LESS CHRONIC CASES:

- a little butter is okay
- do a Vegetable Fast one day weekly
- eat 40 percent or more vegetables daily
- most or all food should be organic
- no junk foods
- some salmon, white fish, veal, and lamb may be allowed
- some wheat- and yeast-free whole grain breads and pancakes may be consumed, if allowed

FOR ADVANCED STAGES OF CANCER, CHRONIC CASES, AND ESPECIALLY THOSE AFFECTING DIGESTIVE ORGANS

- avoid butter
- do a Vegetable Fast two to three days weekly
- eat 60 percent or more vegetables daily
- all-organic foods are essential
- no non-healing foods
- eat fish only if doctor permits
- no breads or pancakes except those mentioned in this book

CHRONIC FATIGUE SYNDROME

The cause or causes of chronic fatigue syndrome (CFS) are still debated among health professionals. CFS has been connected to Epstein-Barr virus and sometimes to low blood sugar, Candida, anemia, or thyroid problems. What *is* known is that the immune system is impaired, often severely. The diets in this book are designed to boost the immune system with high-nutrient, digestible, quality foods while avoiding agitating, nutrient-depleted foods that demand excessive energy to digest.

Meats, hard cheeses, pale or whitish lettuces, dry cereals, corn, potatoes, wheat, and other foods not included in this book all require tremendous body energy to digest. With CFS, a person's body is too weak to process these and other agitating foods. Junk foods also provide little energy and actually deplete the body further.

The key to CFS diets is simplicity. Each individual food consumed processes differently. The more foods eaten at one time, the more body energy goes to digestion.

As soon as possible, begin the Phase II diet. The overall diet can include all the variety of Phase II, but each meal or snack needs to be very simple with limited types of food in each. Digest-Aid-Meal-in-a-Soup is perfect for CFS. Also, hearty soup recipes like Lentil Vegetable Soup, Blended Black Turtle Bean Soup, Broccoli Wild Rice Soup, Taco Bean Soup, and Brown Bean and Broccoli Soup digest well.

Since digestion is almost always impaired with CFS, it is best to enjoy blended soups, very tender steamed vegetables, raw vegetable juices, yogurt, and nonsweet fruits (without seeds) as mainstays of the diet. Tips from the Low Blood Sugar diet should also be employed.

If those with CFS can handle it, well-cooked *whole* grains and *whole* legumes can be eaten if cooked with extra water and prepared tender enough to mash easily in the mouth. These grains and beans can be prepared in big batches, plain, and kept refrigerated up to eight days (beans can be frozen up to three months or more). To flavor these, make batches of nutritious yam or nut butter sauce or one of the others in the sauce chapter (chapter 17). Stick with these basic options for all the nutrients required for healing.

Digestive aids and/or laxative teas can be very helpful here as well. (See chapter 3.) Make sure to have at least one bowel movement per day.

It is helpful if someone else can prepare foods for those with CFS as they have little energy to cook and the energy they do have should be spent on special exercise and healing. However, cooking at least some of their own foods can be good exercise for those with CFS, provided they are willing.

ADDITIONAL CHRONIC FATIGUE SYNDROME DIET TIPS

1. Drink tested spring water.
2. Drink five to six glasses of carrot/beet/green food (like barley green powder—about ¼ teaspoon) juice per week. Mainly carrot with ½ small or medium beet. Drink slowly and swish in the mouth for 20 minutes minimum to absorb all the nutrients. Between meals is best.
3. Do a Vegetable Fast occasionally to rest the digestive tract and assist healing. (About one to four times monthly as desired.)
4. Enjoy antiviral foods (and remedies) like garlic, onions, lemons, limes, grapefruits, and individual green foods. (Take the green foods, in small amounts, one at a time for 30 to 45 days or so or every other day.)
5. Enjoy digestive helps such as flax meal, yogurt, kefir, acidophilus, miso, and seaweed.
6. Enjoy globe artichokes one to two times per week if possible, eaten last in the meal or alone (with butter and lemon is okay). Also, include Jerusalem artichokes whenever possible in meals to aid the blood sugar and help with Candida as well. (Three or more times per week is great, when available.)
7. Stick with only the raw vegetables in the Phase II diet. See chapter 15 and #10 under Cancer Diet.
8. No junk foods, refined foods, pastas, dry cereals, rice wraps, rice crackers, or rice cakes. Avoid bread, crackers, or pancakes except those in this book. Although these items are not included in the Phase II diet, it is important to state these items plainly here as they greatly interfere with healing CFS.

CLEANSING

Cleansing is a rather complex issue and it requires a huge book to cover all the possible types and methods of cleansing. Some titles are listed in the back of this book, although none of them is truly complete. Look for a future book from me entitled *Complete Cleansing and Fasting Guidebook*.

Cleansing means that specific healing foods are consumed along with flushing or purging natural remedies or herbs to remove built-up toxins in the body that interfere with good health. There are full body cleanses and cleanses for the liver, colon, and other specific organs. One can do a food cleanse, toxin-purging cleanse, parasite cleanse, an antiviral cleanse, a cleanse for a specific disease, and many more types, including those with dual or multiple purposes.

Some cleanses require enemas or colonics and many do not. Sometimes digestive teas and/or laxatives are required and sometimes these come with the cleanse and need to be reduced for some individuals. If you do a package cleanse or specific cleansing program: *Do what it recommends!* If you don't, digestive problems or illness could follow for even six months or a year later! Do not do more than one cleanse at a time unless your holistic doctor recommends a particular combination for your specific needs and monitors your progress. Multiple cleanses can be very dangerous, even life threatening in some instances!

It is possible and all right to eat three meals per day plus snacks and still do a very beneficial cleansing. The Phase II and Phase III diets in this book are excellent for cleansing, and unless you are doing a special package cleanse with definite diet instructions, use this book's Phase II and III diets for most cleanses. If you are purging too deeply during a cleanse, increase your food intake to lessen the intensity of the cleanse. If you feel you are not cleansing enough, eat less food for deeper purging of toxins.

A cleanse can last 24 hours or up to 90 days, on rare occasions (for a very mild cleanse) longer. Most average cleanses last 10 to 21 (or 30) days. Generally, it is best to limit cleansing to a maximum of 90 days total per year except in special circumstances, such as for cancer or specific chronic diseases.

One cannot consume drugs (pleasure or medicinal), drink alcohol, or smoke *anything,* during *most* cleanses as these items are counterproductive. One drink (or cigarette) can have the effect of 10 in the body while cleansing.

Some food cleanses are given in this book under Healing Foods in chapter 4. For other types of cleansing, refer to the cleansing books listed under the references *and* get advice from your holistic physician. Health food stores are full of cleansing products and kits; however, it is best to get authoritative advice from your holistic doctor or a cleansing expert rather than most salespersons. Some are quite knowledgeable while many are not and just try to sell products.

DIABETES AND LOW BLOOD SUGAR (HYPOGLYCEMIA)

Those with blood sugar problems do well on Phase II or Phase III diets, including lots of vegetables, legumes, and complex carbohydrates such as whole grains, orange yams, and winter squash. Chromium-rich millet and blood sugar–balancing legumes are particularly beneficial. See chapter 6, Nutrition Consultations # 5 and # 3, for important information.

ADDITIONAL DIABETES AND LOW BLOOD SUGAR DIET TIPS

1. Drink mainly tested spring water as a beverage.
2. Yogurt is better than milk, digestion-wise and blood sugar-wise.
3. All sweet fruits must be avoided, including bananas, grapes, oranges, kiwis, tropical fruits, and dried fruits.
4. Avoid fatty foods and hard-to-digest foods, as well as sweets and refined starches.
5. If sweets *are* eaten, never eat them on an empty stomach but preferably one hour or so after a full, well-balanced meal. (Take with B-complex, biotin, and, if not at night, vitamin C to help handle the sugars—hopefully natural sugars.)
6. Exclude rice wraps, rice cakes, most corn products, dry cereals, all pastas, and most crackers and breads from the diet. Some whole grain breads and pancakes may be enjoyed occasionally, preferably if wheat-free.
7. Vegetable juices with a bit of singular green food are excellent four to six times weekly.
8. A Vegetable Fast can be very beneficial two to four times a month as desired.
9. Foods that help balance the blood sugar are: legumes, Jerusalem artichokes, garlic, and blueberry leaf tea.

FASTING

Fasting gives the body and especially the digestive organs a rest from the constant work of processing foods. It increases energy and longevity and helps the body to heal.

To some, fasting means only drinking water for one 24-hour day (or more) from sun up one day to sun up the following day. Actually, one can fast on vegetable juices, fruit juices, vegetables, and/or fruits. For beginners, it is best not to fast completely on liquids. (Cleansing is easier for novices because food can be eaten.) It is best to choose fruits OR vegetables for a one-day (or more) fast.

The fruit fast is easiest. One can fast on many fruits or choose just one for special healing purposes. Do not make fruit salads! Chew all veggies and fruits slowly and thoroughly. Choose organic produce whenever possible. Follow the Phase II diet the day before a cleanse and the day after and avoid all meats. Eat less the day before rather than more and the fast will be easier.

One cannot fast at all while smoking nor drink alcohol within three days before or after a one-day fast. Avoid alcohol for longer (seven days or more) for a longer fast. For more complete fasting information, see my book *For the Love of Food: The Complete Natural Foods Cookbook*.

THE MONO FRUIT FAST

1. Drink lots of tested spring water—a minimum of eight glasses each day of fasting, preferably more.
2. Choose one type of fruit to fast on: (A) watermelon, (B) bananas (not too ripe with a dash of green on one end), (C) apple juice and peeled and cored apples, (D) peach juice and fresh peaches (in season), OR (E) pear juice and fresh, tender pears (in season). These are the best fasting fruits.
3. Choose organic fruit and fruit juices whenever possible.
4. Have juices separately from whole fruits, at least one hour apart. Chew thoroughly or sip slowly!
5. You can eat as much fruit as you like, within reason, but limit juices to two to four glasses per day.
6. Avoid fruit juices closer to bedtime. Whole fruits should be eaten last, an hour or two (or more if desired) before bed if possible.

THE MIXED FRUIT FAST

1. Follow the main guidelines for the mono fruit fast.
2. Eat only one type of fruit (one or more pieces) at a time, at least one hour apart from different fruits.
3. Only choose one type of juice, if drinking juice, per day.

THE VEGETABLE FAST
(Can be done while taking cancer drugs or other medication)

1. Drink at least four to eight glasses of tested spring water during the day away from meals. Drink more in hot weather. Sip and drink slowly.
2. For breakfast, eat a plate of steamed carrots (no butter or seasonings), orange yams, or baked winter squash. (Squash can also be boiled whole.) Or if preferred, drink one glass of mixed vegetable juice, including mainly carrots, ½ small or medium fresh beet, and ¼ teaspoon singular green food powder (or add a sprig of parsley, celery stalk, cabbage wedge, handful of spinach, or other green veggie instead of green food powder). If you have bowel problems, have the cooked vegetables, not the juice.
3. For snack, if desired, chew on ½ red bell pepper, a carrot stick, half an avocado, or grated beet with lemon juice OR if you didn't have juice for breakfast or if you have bowel problems: have the veggie juice suggested previously (or the avocado).*
4. For lunch, eat a plate of steamed vegetables (from accepted veggies in chapter 15)—one to three different types maximum. Include first a green veggie (like asparagus, broccoli, cooked greens, etc.), then if having two or three: an orange veggie, like one from breakfast and either another green veggie or cauliflower, turnips, or parsnips. Eat a satisfying amount. For those who do not have bowel problems, a salad of grated zucchini/carrot/beet and optional peeled kohlrabi may be had *instead*—only if chewed to water before swallowing! The salad may be sprinkled with fresh lemon, lime, or grapefruit juice for better digestion, nothing else!
5. For snack, same as # 3.*
6. For supper, same as # 4, only no raw vegetables allowed.
7. For snack if desired, half an avocado, one cup or less steamed orange vegetable, OR if you have not had two glasses of juice already today, one could be had now.*
8. Chew all foods to water. Swish juices in the mouth, and take 20 minutes to drink one glass. Drink and eat s-l-o-w-l-y.

---

*In one of the places where the three asterisk are, a steamed artichoke may also be had as a snack option once daily, dipped in fresh lemon, lime, or grapefruit juice only or eaten alone. Do not eat with lemon, lime, or grapefruit juice if having at night.

9. Eat all the foods suggested for meals here (and hopefully snacks, too), especially if taking medication.

NOTE: For bowel problems, eat no raw vegetables except in juices! Raw avocado is okay.

FIBROMYALGIA

The guidelines for this diet are basically the same as for chronic fatigue syndrome. The few differences are that raw foods and juice should be increased unless there are significant digestive or bowel problems, then only increase raw vegetable juices. Enjoy high magnesium foods like whole grains and black-eyed peas. Eat smaller meals and eat more often.

MULTIPLE SCLEROSIS

Follow the basic guidelines for chronic fatigue syndrome with a few changes.

Make sure all foods are organic if possible. Eat plenty of green vegetables, three or more servings daily, including a green food (rotate green foods). Eat lots of raw veggies and more juices. Drink lots of tested spring water, preferably at least eight glasses daily. Enjoy natural, lactic acid–fermented vegetables like sauerkraut. Get tested for food allergies, especially a gluten allergy. Eat high potassium foods like: avocados, kiwi, dried fruit, winter squash, yams, well-cooked brown rice, dulse, and garlic.

ALL OTHER HEALING DIETS

Adapt diets from this book with doctor's changes and also see the source books mentioned at the beginning of this chapter for additional information.

Glossary of Special Foods

This section gives more information on special foods and products for Candida Diets and discusses why some products are not good for Candida. Items already discussed within the book are not included here.

Amaranth (seed, flour, or puffed)   Made from a tiny grain-like seed, smaller than the head of a pin, from a tall plant native to Mexico but now grown in the United States and a little bit in Eastern Canada. The ancient Aztecs were nourished on this high-energy food, considered a complete protein, high in calcium and other nutrients. This is not a grain. Use it in grain-free recipes. It has a robust, pleasant, nut-like flavor. Do not eat the puffed amaranth on Candida Diets but seeds and flour may be enjoyed often in cooking.

Arrowroot   A white powdered thickening agent high in minerals. Use this as a healthy alternative to cornstarch or baking soda, in equal proportions, in soups, stews, and gravies or casseroles. May be used in small amounts, often, when mixed with other foods.

Besan   Same as chickpea flour. A legume flour, grain-free.

Calcium carbonate   An alkaline ingredient sometimes used in baking powder recipes instead of baking soda.

Calcium phosphate   An acidic ingredient sometimes used in baking powder recipes instead of cream of tartar.

Cashews   A nut that is not a true nut and is higher in mold content than most other nuts. Do not use on Candida diets.

Cayenne (Same as red pepper):   Tastes stronger than black pepper but is actually milder on the stomach and very beneficial and healing to the body. Good for heart problems, circulation, and ulcers. Red pepper is a vegetable, not a stomach-irritating spice like black pepper. Use instead of black whenever possible. If allergic to red pepper, then black, white, or pink pepper may be used in small amounts, or use ground horseradish, onion, or garlic powder for a healthier choice.

Chana flour   Same as besan or chickpea flour.

Chickpea flour (chana, besan)   A high-protein legume flour that can be used to add protein to recipes and may be used occasionally instead of grain flours. Used commonly in East Indian foods like chapatis, an unleavened flat bread.

Cilantro   Also known as coriander, or Mexican or Chinese parsley.

Cornstarch   May contribute to constipation, diarrhea, or digestive troubles and may rob the body of vitamin C and other nutrients. Arrowroot may be used as a more wholesome substitute in equal proportions in recipes.

Couscous   A partial wheat grain not good for any Candida diet.

Cream of tartar   An acidic ingredient used in making baking powder.

Eggs   Buy free-range or organic eggs when possible. Quail, duck, or other eggs can be substituted for those allergic to hen's eggs. One hen's egg is about ¼ cup liquid, so measure other eggs accordingly. Eggs must be well cooked for Candida diets.

Egg substitutes   Packaged, natural egg substitutes may be purchased. Follow the package directions or use the substitutes suggested in many of this book's recipes or see the Substitution Chart (chapter 9).

Feta cheese   See goat cheese.

Flaxseed   Highly nutritious with high essential fatty acids omega-3 and -6. The oil can be taken by the spoon but may be hard for some to digest if other oils are. Use digestive aids (or bile salts) or grind seeds in food processor or blender and sprinkle on cereals or whole grain dishes for added nutrients. These are not generally high in mold content and so may be eaten raw and are more beneficial raw.

Gluten grains and flours   Technically, all true grains contain at least a small amount of gluten. However, most people allergic to gluten grains can tolerate everything except the four high-gluten grains: wheat, rye, barley, and oats. Spelt and kamut also contain more gluten as they are a form of wheat. No gluten grains or flours or any grains flours at all are recommended for most Candida diets. See diet Phases for the few exceptions (chapter 10).

Gluten-free grains and flours   Grains containing only minute amounts of gluten. These include buckwheat (kasha), rice, millet, corn, and some say quinoa. (Quinoa's status is debated: Is it a grain or seed?)

Goat cheese and milk   Fifty percent or more of people allergic to cow's milk products can tolerate goat dairy products. Goat milk is closer to human milk in quality, is easier to digest, and is generally lower in fats and cholesterol. Goat products are mild tasting if male goats are kept separate from the female goats. On a Candida diet, cooked goat's milk and occasional cooked goat feta cheese are allowed in some Phases.

Grain-free flours   Those who are allergic or intolerant of grains cannot eat any grains and may use these flours: amaranth, arrowroot, carob, cassava, potato, tapioca, and teff. Also, seed, nut, and legume flours, including soy, lentil, chickpea, sunflower seed, sesame seed, almond, cashew, filbert/hazelnut, and other flours and meals. Celiacs cannot tolerate any whole grains or grain flours. For Candida diets avoid carob flour/powder, potato, and minimize the use of cassava, arrowroot, and tapioca. No cashew flour or meal can be used.

Guar gum powder   A thickener and binder used to help gluten-free, yeast-free baked goods keep their rise. Can be mixed into cold or hot foods to thicken salad dressings and casseroles. Derived from an East Indian seed, guar gum can be used instead of eggs, liquid lecithin, or arrowroot in some recipes. Good as a mild laxative, for ulcers, and as a mild appetite suppressant in very small amounts.

Gums   See Guar gum and Xanthan gum.

Hato mugi   See Job's tears.

Herbs   Herbs are generally the green, leafy parts of plants or mild seeds, as opposed to spices, which are strong seeds, roots, and barks. On a Candida diet, herbs can be eaten plentifully if cooked. Spices should be eaten sparingly as they may agitate the digestive tract. All herbs used in the recipes in this book are dried unless fresh is specified.

Job's tears (hato mugi)   Sometimes called pearl barley, this unique grain is nothing like the small, white, round, refined pearl barley available in many stores. It is really not barley at all. It looks somewhat like puffed brown rice and is the seed of an annual wild grass. This biblically named seed has been used for thousands of years. One macrobiotic sourcebook claims Job's tears will counteract the effect of eating animal proteins and fats and that it is a cooling-off food, good for cancers and other growths like warts and moles. Use the seeds in soups and stews, or instead of barley or brown rice. It is a robust seed with a pungent flavor and not easy to find. Available or orderable from some health food stores or allergy shops. A good substitute whole grain for Candida diets if one is allergic to other whole grains. Cook like brown rice until tender. Gluten and grain-free.

Kamut (pronounced "ka-moot")   A Mediterranean variety of wheat more digestible and nutritious than regular wheat but not allowed on most Candida diets.

Kelp   See Sea kelp.

Kudzu (kuzu)   A starch-like extract of a Japanese root that often comes in crumbly white chunks. Used like arrowroot as a thickener and prized for its medicinal properties, it is also a plentiful weed in the southern United States.

Legume flours   Non-grain, high-protein bean flours that include soy, chickpea, pinto, black bean, and lentil flours. These contain no gluten and may be used often but must be well cooked to be digestible. Avoid green split pea or white bean flours.

Margarine Dr. Rona calls it "plastic butter." Dr. Rudolph Ballantine, M.D., author of *Diet and Nutrition*, says the rise in heart disease directly parallels the rise in the use of margarine. He states: "It seems increasingly likely that eating margarine, instead of preventing heart attacks, actually accelerates the process that causes them." It is not recommended for Candida or any diet!

Natural foods Foods that are in as whole a state as possible, with nothing important added or taken away. No artificial additives, preservatives, chemicals, hormones, colorings, flavorings, or anything unnatural added.

Natural oils Oil-pressed without solvents like most supermarket or commercial oils. These are cold-pressed or expeller-pressed oils made without chemicals or additives. Use only natural oils on Candida diets! See Shopping Guide (chapter 11) for good brand names and the References and Recommended Reading section for books on the subject. Important: Keep all natural oils refrigerated after opening! Discard after date on label or after three to six months stored in the refrigerator. Shelf storage length is usually printed on the bottle. Do not let perspiration, saliva, or bacteria get into the oil bottle and do not let it sit out of the fridge too long, especially on a hot day. Once oil is poured out of its bottle, never pour it back into the bottle, as it may easily collect bacteria or dust once poured. Oil poisoning is very painful and dangerous! See recipes for recommended varieties. Safflower oil may also be used on a Candida diet if doctor allows.

Nuts and seeds Purchased roasted nuts and seeds must be avoided as they are often rancid and may be loaded with preservatives, additives, and even sweeteners. They are also hard to digest, high in fats and calories, and many are high in mold content and can contribute to feeding yeast. However, some nuts and seeds can be enjoyed on a Candida diet if they are purchased raw and are high quality, preferably organic. Cook all nuts by the Home-Roasting method (see recipe) or use them in cooked recipes. Nuts are more digestible when eaten in small amounts and cooked into other foods. Rotate them in the diet and only eat every second or third day. Nuts should be ground for recipes or used in nut butter form and should be eaten warm. Seeds are usually a little easier to digest than nuts.

Whole Home-Roasted Nuts may occasionally be eaten alone as a snack if your digestion is good or you use helpful digestive aids like HCL, Beano, Plant Enzymes (sometimes bile salts if one has trouble digesting fats), or another doctor-recommended aid. Nuts (and seeds) eaten this way should be chewed completely to powder before swallowing. The best types of nuts to use on a Candida diet include almonds, filberts, pecans, and sometimes Brazil nuts. Avoid all others! (Use pecans only in recipes!) Pine nuts, though not true nuts, are included. Healthful seeds include flax, sesame, sunflower and especially pumpkin.

Oils See natural oils.

Potassium bicarbonate Low-sodium baking soda.

Puffed cereals These are too starchy for Candida Diets.

Quinoa (pronounced "keen-wah") A quick-cooking, essentially gluten-free, high-protein grain, excellent for Candida or allergy diets. The "mother grain of the Incas" is grown in South and North America. It is not a true grain, but is excellent used in place of rice or millet as a cereal or main-dish grain. It is naturally protected by an agitating substance called saponin, which is often removed by a dry process and home washing. Once the saponin is removed, the quinoa is quite digestible. Delicious quinoa is high in amino acids/protein and many nutrients.

Sea kelp A seaweed or ground seaweed powder high in minerals, used to flavor foods. It enhances natural flavors and adds body and depth to recipes. See Healing Foods (chapter 4) for more information.

Sea salt Derived from vacuum-dried sea water. Contains all the natural minerals found in salt that are usually refined out of earth salt or regular table salt. Earth salt is harder to digest and contains corn sugar in the form of dextrose, so it must be avoided for all Candida diets. Regular table salt may contain chemicals to help preserve it, keep its color, and retard moisture, as well as other additives. Sea salt has none of these extras and does not cause the body to retain as much water. Sea salt is sometimes finer than earth salt; if so, use ¼ teaspoon sea salt per one teaspoon table salt. Recipes in this book call for sea salt only. See Shortcuts (chapter 11) for salt tips for doubling recipes. Salt spreads further when used in cooking rather than at the table, and people who eat more carbohydrate vegetables, whole grains, and legumes in their diet can tolerate higher amounts of salt than the average frequent meat-eater!

Seeds   See Nuts and seeds

Sesame tahini   A peanut butter–like ground seed butter, only stickier. High in calcium, protein, and other nutrients. Made from hulled, white sesame seeds, sometimes roasted for better flavor, usually mixed with oil. Oil can be drained off for less calories and fat. Cook this into nut sauces or use in recipes. Do not eat tahini raw, cold, or by itself! Must be heated and cooked to kill any mold or bacteria content before it is eaten.

Spelt   A European grain closely related to wheat. A high-gluten grain like kamut, more digestible than regular wheat, though not recommended for most Candida Diets.

Tahini   See Sesame tahini.

Tapioca flour   A gluten-free, grain-free flour usually derived from cassava root. Tapioca is a somewhat starchy, slightly sweet, white, powder-like flour that mixes especially well with amaranth. It can be used instead of milk powder in some recipes. May be used occasionally if cooked with other foods.

Tartaric acid   An acidic ingredient sometimes used in baking powder.

Teff (seeds or flour)   An Ethiopian seed whose name translates as "lost," a consequence of dropping this smallest of "grains." One grain of wheat weighs about the same as 150 grains of teff. This seed ranges in color from ivory or tan to brown and reddish varieties. It contains five times the iron, calcium, and potassium of any grain, is high in protein and fiber, and is gluten- and grain-free. Teff has been used for thousands of years to bake Injera, a starchy Ethiopian flat bread. Use whole teff cooked with another cereal grain or as a flour in recipes often. Half a cup can also be used instead of one cup sesame seeds in many cooked or baked recipes. The flour can be used in place of other grain flours and is especially good for allergy cooking.

Tempeh   A fermented soy product usually avoided during Candida treatment.

Tofu   A processed soy product that looks like white feta cheese but tastes bland alone. The beauty of tofu is that it absorbs and complements flavors used with it in cooking. It actually enhances other flavors. A good meat or dairy substitute that is high in protein, calcium, phosphorus, potassium, and iron, tofu is more digestible than some types of legumes. Must be well cooked for Candida diets to avoid bacteria that can easily grow on most processed foods. Store completely covered in pure water in a jar. Keeps for up to two to three weeks refrigerated, if water is changed every few days or so. Plain tofu is fresh as long as it retains its milky white color and has no scent or taste. If the tofu smells a bit, rinse it thoroughly. If no smell remains, it can be used if cooked well. Needs pre-steaming for 4 to 9 minutes for some recipes (4 minutes if being cooked again). Soft (silken), medium, firm/regular, extra firm, or pressed tofu varieties are available. Do not use the sweetened dessert tofu available.

Tofu cheese   A basically non-dairy cheese substitute available in cheddar (amber), mozzarella (Italian-style), Monterey jack, jalapeño, and other flavors. Useful for most dairy-free diets, except these usually contain casein, a protein dairy derivative used to harden the cheese. There are non-casein varieties but they are sorely lacking in flavor and quality. The casein varieties taste similar to cheese and can be used occasionally on Candida diets if fully cooked into recipes, about one to four times a month if allowed. This soy cheese grates and melts like cheese and is a good substitute for most recipes that contain cheese.

Walnuts   A nut that is often high in mold content and almost always impossible to get fresh unless cracked out of the shell. Avoid for all Candida diets.

Wehani rice   A tasty, nutritious, natural red rice sold separately and in mixed rice blends. It may be used one to three times monthly.

Xanthan gum   A corn-derived thickener and emulsifier. It is a good binder and thickening agent in dressings and other recipes. Also used commercially in the packaging of meat and poultry. Those with corn allergies should use guar gum instead, in equal amounts.

References and Recommended Reading

BY JEANNE MARIE MARTIN

CANDIDA COOKBOOKS

The Yeast Connection Cookbook, William G. Crook, M.D., and Marjorie Hurt Jones, R.N., Professional Books, ISBN 0-93347816-X

The Candida Albicans Yeast-Free Cookbook, Pat Connolly and Assoc. of Price-Pottenger Nutrition Foundation, Keats Publishing, Inc., ISBN 0-87983-409-9

The Candida Directory & Cookbook, Helen Gustafson and Maureen O'Shea, Celestial Arts, ISBN 0-89087-714-9

CANDIDA INFORMATION BOOKS WITH RECIPES

Back to Health, Dennis W. Remington, M.D., and Barbara W. Higa, R.D.,Vitality House International, Inc., ISBN 0-912547-03-0

Who Killed Candida, Vicki Glassburn, TEACH Services, Inc., ISBN 0-945383-12-6

CANDIDA INFORMATION BOOKS WITH FEW OR NO RECIPES

The Yeast Connection, William G. Crook, M.D., Professional Books, ISBN 0-933478-06-02

Candida Yeast Infection—The Silent Killer, Rupert Beebe, Healthology Association, ISBN 0-9693588-0-6

CANDIDA AND WOMEN'S HEALTH

The Yeast Connection and the Woman, William G. Crook, M.D., Professional Books, ISBN 0-933478-22-4

Take Charge of Your Body: Women's Health Advisor, Carolyn DeMarco, M.D., Well Women Press, 0-9694766-1-2 (1-800-387-4761)

ALLERGY COOKBOOKS

The All Natural Allergy Cookbook, Jeanne Marie Martin, Harbour Publishing, ISBN 1-55017-044-9

Freedom from Allergy, Ron Greenberg, M.D., and Angela Nori, Gordon Soules Book Publishers, ISBN 0-88925-905-4

The Self-Help Cookbook, Marjorie Hurt Jones, R.N., Rodale Press, ISBN 0-87857-505-7

Dr. Mandell's Allergy-Free Cookbook, Fran Gare Mandell, Simon and Schuster, ISBN 0-671-83603-X

The Allergy Cookbook: Diets Unlimited for Limited Diets, A.I.A.—Allergy Information Association Canada, ISBN 0-458-80690-0

Allergy Cooking, Marion L. Conrad, Jove Publications, ISBN 0-515-05738-X

Creative Cooking Without Wheat, Milk, and Eggs, Ruth R. Shattuck, A. S. Barnes and Co., ISBN 0-498-02047-9

The Food Intolerance Diet Book, Elizabeth Workman, Dr. Virginia Alun-Jones, and Dr. John Hunter, Martin Dunitz Ltd., ISBN 0-948269-16-2

ALLERGY INFORMATION BOOKS

Allergies—Diseases in Disguise, Dr. Carolee Bateson-Koch, Alive Books, ISBN 0-920470-42-4

The Complete Guide to Allergy and Intolerance, Dr. Jonathan Brostoff, and Linda Gamlin, Bloomsbury Publishing, ISBN 0-7475-0566-7

How to Control Your Food Allergies, Robert Forman, Ph.D., Larchmont Books, ISBN 0-915962-29-2

An Alternative Approach to Allergies, Theron G. Randolph, M.D., and Ralph W. Moss, Ph.D., Bantam Books, ISBN 0-553-20830-6

Hidden Food Allergies, Stephen Astor, M.D., Avery Publishing Group, ISBN 0-89529-369-2

Parents' Guide to Allergy in Children, Claude A. Frazier, M.D., Grosset & Dunlap, ISBN 0-448-16180-X

Tracking Down Hidden Food Allergies, William G. Crook, M.D., Professional Books, ISBN 0-933478-05-4

FOODS AND ADDITIVES

A Consumer's Dictionary of Food Additives, Ruth Winter, Crown Publishers, Inc., ISBN 0-517-531615

Empty Harvest, Bernard Jensen and Mark Anderson, Avery Publishing Group, ISBN 0-89529-416-8

Safe Food, Michael F. Jacobson, Ph.D., Lisa Y. Lefferts, and Anne Witte Garland, Living Planet Press, ISBN 1-879326-01-9

NUTRITION AND VITAMIN GUIDEBOOKS

Nutrition Almanac, Lavon J. Dunne, McGraw-Hill Publishing Co., ISBN 0-07-034912-6

Healthy Healing, Linda Rector-Page, N.D., Ph.D., Healthy Healing Publications, ISBN 0-912331-21-6

Prescriptions for Nutritional Healing, James F. Balch, M.D., and Phyllis A. Balch, C.N.C., Avery Publishing Group, ISBN 0-89529-429-X

Vitamin Bible, Earl Mindell's, Warner Books, ISBN 0-446-30626-6

Diet and Nutrition: A Holistic Approach, Rudolph Ballentine, M.D., Himalayan International Institute, ISBN 0-89389-048-0

HERB BOOKS

Back to Eden, Jethro Kloss, Back to Eden Books, ISBN 0-940676-001

The Herb Book, John Lust, Bantam Books, ISBN 0-553-23827-2

The New Age Herbalist, Richard Mabey, Collier Books, ISBN 0-02-063350-5

The Herbalist, Joseph E. Meyer, Meyer Books, 0-916638-00-6

Indian Herbalogy of North America, Alma Hutchens, Merco, 620 Wyandotte East, Windsor, Ontario, Canada

Handbook of Bach Flower Remedies, Philip M. Chancellor, C.W. Daniel Company LTD, ISBN 0-85207-002-0

Capsicum, Dr. John R. Christopher, Christopher Publications, P. O. Box 412, Springville, Utah 84663

P'au d'Arbo, Immune Power from the Rain Forest, Kenneth Jones, Healing Arts Press, ISBN 0-89281-497-7

WHOLESOME FOOD GUIDEBOOKS

The Guide to Natural and Healthy Eating, Renee Frappier, Les Editions Asclepiades Inc., ISBN 2-9801115-3-8

Shopper's Guide to Natural Foods, East West Journal Editors, Avery Publishing Group, Inc., ISBN 0-89529-233-5

The Safe Shopper's Bible, David Steinman and Samuel S. Epstein, M.D., Macmillan Publishing, ISBN 0-02-082085-2

Whole Food Facts, Evelyn Roehl, Healing Arts Press, ISBN 0-89281-231-1

The Wellness Encyclopedia of Food and Nutrition, Sheldon Margen, M.D., ISBN 0-929661-03-6

GUIDEBOOKS FOR NEW VEGETARIANS WITH RECIPES

Becoming Vegetarian, Vesanto Melina, R.D., Brenda Davis, Victoria Harrison, Macmillian Publishing, ISBN 0-7715-9045-8

The Gradual Vegetarian, Lisa Tracy, Dell Publishing, ISBN 0-440-53124-1

Vegetarian Cookbooks

For the Love of Food / The Complete Natural Foods Cookbook, Jeanne Marie Martin, Alive Books, ISBN 0-920470-70-X

Hearty Vegetarian Soups and Stews, Jeanne Marie Martin, Harbour Publishing, ISBN 1-55017-050-3

The Moosewood Cookbook, Mollie Katzen, Ten Speed Press, ISBN 0-89815-490-1

Vegetarian Times Cookbook, The Editors of Vegetarian Times, Macmillan Publishing, ISBN 0-02-010370-0

The New McDougall Cookbook, John A. McDougall and Mary McDougall, Dutton Books, ISBN 0-525-93610-6

Horn of the Moon Cookbook, Ginny Gallam, Harper Perennial, ISBN 0-06-096038-8

Cabbagetown Cafe, Julie Jordan, Crossing Press, ISBN 0-89594-192-9

The Vegetarian Feast, Martha Rose Schulman, Harper Perennial, ISBN 0-06-095001-3

Vegan Cookbooks (No Dairy, Meat, or Animal Products)

Vegan Delights, Jeanne Marie Martin, Harbour Publishing, ISBN 1-55017-079-1

Vegan Vitality, Diane Hill, Thorsons Publishing, ISBN 0-7225-1341-0

Country Kitchen Collection, Silver Hills Guest House, ISBN 0-88925-933-X

365 Plus One Vegan Recipes, Leah Leneman, Thorsons Publishing, ISBN 0-7225-1454-9

Simply Vegan, Deborah Wasserman and Reed Lazarus, Vegetarian Resource Group, ISBN 093-141-105X

Vegan Information Books

Diet for a New America, John Robbins, Stillpoint Publishing, ISBN 0-913299-54-5

Vegan Nutrition: Pure and Simple, Michael Klaper, M.D., Gentle World Inc., ISBN 0-9614248-2-6

Vegan Nutrition: A Survey Of Research, Dr. Gill Langley, The Vegan Society Ltd., ISBN 0-907337-15-5

Natural Food Cookbooks with Meat

Jeanne Marie Martin's Light Cuisine / Seafood, Poultry, and Egg Recipes for Healthy Living, Jeanne Marie Martin, Harbour Publishing, ISBN 1-55017-123-2

The New York Times New Natural Foods Cookbook, Jean Hewitt, Avon Books, ISBN 0-380-62687-X

Recipes from an Ecological Kitchen, Lorna J. Sass, William Morrow and Co., Inc., Hardcover ISBN 0-688-10051-1

Rodale's Basic Natural Foods Cookbook, Fireside Books/Simon and Schuster, ISBN 0-671-67338-6

Jane Brody's Good Food Book, Jane E. Brody, Bantam Books, ISBN 0-0553-34346-7

Books About Water

The Shocking Truth About Water, Paul C. Bragg, N.D., Ph.D., Health Science, ISBN 0-87790-000-0

The Choice Is Clear, Dr. Allen E. Banik, Acres U.S.A., ISBN 911-311-31-9

Water Can Undermine Your Health, Norman Walker, Ph.D., Norwalk Press, ISBN 0-890-19-037-2

Water: Healer or Poison?, Jan De Vries, Mainstream Publishers, ISBN 1-85158-341-6

Oxygen and Ozone

O 2 Xygen Therapies / A New Way of Approaching Disease, Ed McCabe, Energy Publications, ISBN 0-9620527-0-1

The Unmedical Miracle—Oxygen, Elizabeth Baker, Drelwood Communications, ISBN 0-937766-12-7

Sugar and Related Health Concerns (Low Blood Sugar and Candida)

Diabetes and Hypoglycemia, Michael T. Murray, N.D., Prima Publishing, ISBN 1-55958-426-2

Hypoglycemia: A Better Approach, Paavo Airola, Ph.D., Health Plus Publishers, ISBN 0-932090-01-X

Sugar Blues, William Duffy, Warner Books, ISBN 0-446-89288-2

Breaking the Vicious Cycle (Food and the Gut Reaction), Elaine Gottschall, Kirkton Press, ISBN 0-969-2768-1

FATS AND OILS

Fats That Heal, Fats That Kill, Udo Erasmus, Alive Books, ISBN 0-920470-40-8

The Facts About Fats, John Finnegan, Elysian Arts Book, ISBN 0-927425-12-2

HEALING FOODS AND RECIPES

Return to the Joy of Health, Zoltan P. Rona, M.D., and Jeanne Marie Martin, Alive Books, ISBN 0-920470-62-9

Healing Power of Foods Cookbook, Michael T. Murray, N.D., Prima Publishing, ISBN 1-55958-318-5

The Healing Cuisine / India's Art of Ayurvedic Cooking, Harish Johari, Healing Arts Press, ISBN 0-89281-382-2

Foods and Healing, Annemarie Colbin, Ballantine Books, ISBN 0-345-30385-7

Foods That Heal, Maureen Salaman, Statford Publishing, ISBN 0-913087-025

Foods That Heal, Bernard Jensen, Avery Publishing Group, ISBN 0-89529-563-3

The Healing Foods, Patricia Hausman and Judith Benn Hurley, Dell Publishing, ISBN 0-440-21440-8

Miracle Medicine Foods, Rex Adams, Parker Publishing, Inc., ISBN 0-13-585463-6

CHLOROPHYLL AND GREEN FOODS

The Healing Power of Chlorophyll from Plant Life, Bernard Jensen, Bernard Jensen Books, Route 1, Box 52, Escondido, CA 92025

Cereal Grass / What's In It for You! Edited by Ronald L. Seibold, Wilderness Community Education Foundation, ISBN 0-9628126-0-9

The Wheatgrass Book, Ann Wigmore, Avery Publishing Group, ISBN 0-89529-234-3

Green Barley Essence, Yoshihide Hagiwara, M.D., Keats Publishing, ISBN 0-87834-8-8

Chlorella, William Lee, Michael Rosenbaum, Keats Publishing, ISBN 0-87983464-1

Spirulina, Jack Joseph Challem, Keats Publishing, ISBN 0-87983-262-2

JUICING FOR HEALTH

Healing with Herbal Juices, Siegfried Gursche, Alive Books, ISBN 0-920470-34-3

Getting the Best Out of Your Juicer, William H. Lee, Ph.D., Keats Publishing, ISBN 0-87983-586-9

The Complete Raw Juice Therapy, Thorsons Editorial Board, Thorsons Publishing, ISBN 0-7225-1877-3

BOOKS ABOUT INTESTINAL PARASITES

Guess What Came to Dinner: Parasites and Your Health, Ann Louise Gittleman, Avery Publishing Group, ISBN 0-89529-570

Parasites / The Enemy Within, Hanna Kroeger, Ms.D., and Jerald Foote, Kroeger Products, 1122 Pearl St., Boulder, CO 80302

FASTING AND CLEANSING BOOKS

Detoxification, Linda Page N.D., Ph.D., Healthy Healing Publications, ISBN 1-884334-54-7

Natural Detoxification, Jacqueline Krohn, M.D., Hartley & Marks, ISBN 0-88179-127-X

7–Day Detox Miracle, Peter Bennett, N.D. and Stephen Barrie, N.D., Prima Publishing, ISBN 0-7615-1422-8

Achieve Maximum Health, Colon Flora, David Webster, Hygeia Publishing, ISBN 0-9647537-1-5

Miracle of Fasting, Paul C. Bragg, Health Science Publishers, ISBN 0-87790-002-7

How to Keep Slim, Healthy, and Young with Juice Fasting, Paavo Airola, Ph.D., Health Plus Publishers, ISBN 0-932090-02-8

Colon Health: The Key to a Vibrant Life, Norman W. Walker, Ph.D., Norwalk Press, ISBN 0-89019-069-0

Tissue Cleansing Through Bowel Management, Bernard Jensen and Sylvia Bell, Bernard Jensen Enterprises, ISBN 0-960836-07-1

Inner Cleansing, Carlson Wade, Parker Publishing Company, 0-13-465575-3

The Body Ecology Diet, Donna Gates, B.E.D. Publications, ISBN 0-9638458-8-8

How to Lower Your Fat Thermostat, Dennis Remington, M.D., Garth Fisher, Ph.D., and Edward Parent, Ph.D., Vitality House International, Inc., ISBN 0-912547-01-4

NATURAL FOOD VEGETARIAN RESTAURANT GUIDEBOOKS

Vegetarian Journal's Guide to Natural Foods Restaurants in the U.S. and Canada, Vegetarian Resource Group, Avery Publishing Group, ISBN 0-89529-571-7

The Canadian Vegetarian Dining Guide, Lynne Tomlinson, Wizard Publishing, ISBN 0-9697539-0-X

RECOMMENDED NEWSLETTERS AND WEB SITES

Dr. Zoltan Rona
1366 Yonge St., Suite 202; Toronto, Ontario; Canada M4T 3A7
toll free subscription line: 877-920-8887
Web site: www.srvitamins.com
e-mail: info@srvitamins.com

Jeanne Marie Martin, C.I.N.
P.O. Box 4391; Vancouver, British Columbia; Canada V6B 3Z8
604-878-8787
Web site: www.jeannemariemartin.com

Townsend Letter for Doctors & Patients
911 Tyler Street; Pt. Townsend, Washington 98368-6541 USA
fax: 360-385-0699
Web site: www.tldp.com
e-mail: tldp@olympus.net

Current Health News You Can Use by Dr. Joseph M. Mercola
1443 West Schaumburg; Schaumburg, Illinois 60194 USA
847-985-1777
Newsletter via e-mail: dr@mercola.com

BOOKS WRITTEN BY JEANNE MARIE MARTIN ARE AVAILABLE FROM:

The Internet at: Amazon.com

In the U.S.A. from: Nutri-Books, New Leaf Distributing Co., Bookpeople, Ingram Book Company, Partners West, and Integral Yoga Distribution

In Canada from: Health Management Books, Apple Publishing and Harbour Publishing

Bibliography

BY DR. ZOLTAN P. RONA

Ali, Majid. RDA: *Rats, Drugs, and Assumptions.* Denville, N.J.: Life Span Press, 1996, 424–62.

Baranowski, Zane. *Colloidal Silver: The Natural Antibiotic Alternative.* N.Y.: Healing Wisdom Publications, 1995.

Barnes, Broda O. *Hypothyroidism, The Unsuspected Illness.* N.Y.: Harper and Row, 1976.

Bigazzi, Pierluigi E. "Autoimmunity and Heavy Metals." *Lupus,* 1994;3:449–453.

Blaylock, Russell L., *Excitotoxins: The Taste That Kills*; Santa Fe, New Mexico Health Press, 1994.

Blumenthal, Mark. "FDA Rejects AHPA Stevia Petition." *Whole Foods,* April 1994.

Breuss, Rudolf. *Breuss Cancer Cure.* Burnaby, B.C.: Alive Books, 1995.

Calabrese, V.P. et al. "DHEA in multiple sclerosis: positive effects on the fatigue syndrome in a non-randomized study." In *The Biologic Role of DHEA* by Kalimi, M. and Regelson, W., Editors. New York: Walter De Gruyter, 1990, pp. 95–100.

Clark, Daniel G. and Wyatt, Kaye. *Colostrum, Life's First Food.* Salt Lake City:CNR Publications. 1996.

Costantini, A. V., H. Wieland, and Lars I Qvick. *Fungalbionics, The Fungal/Mycotoxin Etiology of Human Disease, Vol. 1 Atherosclerosis & Vol. II Cancer.* Freiberg, Germany: Johann Friedrich Oberlin Verlag, 1994. Available in Canada from Fungal/Mycotoxin Conference, 12 Sifton Place, Brampton, Ont. L6Y 2N8; 905-450-0445 (phone); 905-450-0559 (fax).

Crook, William G. *The Yeast Connection.* N.Y.: Random House, 1987.

———. *Detecting Your Hidden Allergies.* Jackson, Tenn.: Professional Books, 1988.

———. *Help For The Hyperactive Child.* Jackson, Tenn.: Professional Books, 1991.

———. *Chronic Fatigue Syndrome and the Yeast Connection.* Jackson, Tenn.: Professional Books, 1992.

———. *The Yeast Connection and the Woman.* Jackson, Tenn.: Professional Books, 1995.

Cruess, W.V. and Alsberg, C.L. "The bitter glucoside of the olive." *J. Amer. Chem. Soc.* 1934; 56:2115–7.

Donsbach, Kurt W. *Dr. Donsbach Tells You What You Need to Know About Candidiasis & Chronic Fatigue Syndrome.* 1993. Available by calling The Rockland Corporation at 800-421-7310.

Elliott GA et al. "Preliminary studies with calcium elenolate, an antiviral agent." *Anfimicrob. Agents Chemother.,* 1970. 173–76.

Gaby, Alan R. and Wright, Jonathan V. "Nutritional Therapy in Medical Practice. Protocols and Supporting Information." Seattle, WA, Oct. 25-28, 1996. *Wright/Gaby Seminars,* 515 W. Harrison St., Suite 200, Kent, WA 98032; 206-854-4900, ext. 166.

Gariboldi P et al, "Secoiridoids from olea europaea." *Phytochem.,* 1986, 25(4) 865–69.

Hanssen, M. *Cider Vinegar,* Northamptonshire, England: Thorsons, 1974.

Heinerman, John. *Dr. Heinerman's Encyclopedia of Anti-Aging Remedies.* Paramus:Prentice Hall, 1997; pp.85–86.

Heinze JE et al, "Specificity of the antiviral agent calcium elenolate." *Antimicrob. Agents Chemother.,* 1975: 8(4), 421–25.

Hirschman SZ, "Inactivation of DNA polymerases of Murine Leukaemia viruses by calcium elenolate." *Nature New Biology,* 1972; 238:277–79.

Jarvis, D. C. *Folk Medicine,* Greenwich, Conn: Fawcett, 1958.

Jensen, Bernard. *Colostrum: Man's First Food, The White Gold Discovery.* Escondido: Bernard Jensen, 1993.

John, Michael. "Systemic antifungals: what's new, what's tried-and-true?" *Medicine North America*, September 1995, 741–45, 791–95.

Juven B et al, "Studies on the mechanism of the antimicrobial action of oleuropein." *J. Appl. Bact.,* 1972; 35:559–67.

Kubo I et al, "A multichemical defense mechanism of bitter olive olea europaea (Oleaceae)—Is oleuropein a phytoalexin precursor?" *J. Chem. Ecol* 1985, 11(2):25163.

Lorscheider, Fritz L., M.D., et al. "The Dental Amalgam Mercury Controversy—Inorganic Mercury and the CNS; Genetic Link of Mercury and Antibiotic Resistance in Intestinal Bacteria." *Toxicology* 97 (1995): 19–22.

Lorscheider, Fritz L., et al. "Mercury Exposure From 'Silver' Tooth Fillings: Emerging Evidence Questions a Traditional Dental Paradigm." *FASEB Journal* 9 (1995): 504–08.

McCabe, Ed. *O2xygen Therapies, A New Way of Approaching Disease.* Morrisville, N.Y.: Energy Publications, 1988.

McDougall, John A. *McDougall's Medicine, A Challenging Second Opinion.* N.J.: New Century Publishers, 1985.

———. *The McDougall Report, Lifesaving Facts Your Doctor Never Told You.* Seattle: Trillium Health Products, 1992.

McDougall, John A. and Mary A. McDougall. *The McDougall Plan.* N.J.: New Century Publishers, 1983.

Moore, Neecie. *Bountiful Health, Boundless Energy, Brilliant Youth: The Facts About DHEA.* Dallas: Charis Publishing, 1994.

Murray, Michael T. *Natural Alternatives to Over-the-Counter and Prescription Drugs.* New York: William Morrow and Company, Inc., 1994.

———. *Encyclopedia of Nutritional Supplements.* Rocklin, CA: Prima Publishing, 1996.

Ornish, Dean. *Program For Reversing Heart Disease.* N.Y.: Ballantine Books, 1990.

Ornish, Dean, et al. "Can lifestyle changes reverse coronary heart disease?" *Lancet,* 21 July 1990; 336:129–33.

Panizzi L et al, "The constitution of oleuropein, a bitter glucoside of the olive with hypotensive action." *Gazz. Chim. Ital*; 1960, 90:1449–85.

Petkov V and Manolov P, "Pharmacological analysis of the iridoid oleuropein." *Drug Res.,* 1972; 22(9):1476–86.

Pitchford, Paul. *Healing with Whole Foods.* Berkeley: North Atlantic Books, 1993.

Reiter, Russel J. and Robinson, Jo. *Melatonin, Your Body's Natural Wonder Drug.* New York: Bantam Books, 1995.

Renis HE, "In vitro antiviral activity of calcium elenolate." *Antimicrob. Agents Chemother.,* 1970; 167–72.

Roberts, E. and T. J. Fauble. "Oral DHEA in multiple sclerosis: results of a phase one, open study." In *The Biologic Role of DHEA*, edited by M. Kalimi and W. Regelson. N. Y.: Walter De Gruyter, 1990, 81–93.

Rona, Zoltan, P. "Bovine colostrum emerges as immune system modulator." *American Journal of Natural Medicine*; March, 1998, pp. 19–23.

——— *Childhood Illness and The Allergy Connection.* Rocklin, California: Prima Books, 1996.

Samuelsson G, "The blood pressure lowering factor in leaves of Olea Europaea." *Farmacevtisk Revy,* 1951, 15:229–39.

Scott, C. *Cider Vinegar.* Northamptonshire, England: Athene, 1968.

Soret MG, "Antiviral activity of calcium elenolate on parainfluenza infection of hamsters." *Anfimicrob. Agenls Chemother.,* 1970: 160–66.

Spiegel, J.E., et al. "Safety and benefits of fructooligosaccharides as food ingredients." *Food Technology*, Jan. 1994; pp.85–89.

Stiles, J.C. et al. "The inhibition of Candida albicans by oregano." *J. Appl. Nutr.,* 1995;47(4):96–102.

Theiss, Barbara, and Peter Theiss. *The Family Herbal.* Rochester, Vt.: Healing Arts Press, 1989.

Thomas, Richard. *The Essiac Report.* Los Angeles: The Alternative Treatment Information Network, 1993.

Tomomatsu, Hideo. "Health effects of oligosaccharides." *Food Technology,* October 1994, 61–4.

Veer WLC et al, "A compound isolated from olea europaea." *Recueil,* 1957; 76:83940.

Werbach, Melvyn R. *Nutritional Influences on Illness.* Northamptonshire, England: Thorsons, 1989.

———. *Nutritional Influences on Illness, Second Edition.* Tarzana, Calif.: Third Line Press, 1993.

———. *Nutritional Influences on Mental Illness.* Northamptonshire, England: Thorsons, 1991.

Werbach, Melvyn R. and Michael T. Murray. *Botanical Influences on Illness.* Tarzana, Calif: Third Line Press, 1994.

Wilson, Denis E. *Wilson's Syndrome—The Miracle of Feeling Well.* Longwood, Fla: Cornerstone Publishing, 1995. Available by calling 800-621-7006.

Zand, Janet, Rachel Walton, and Bob Rountree. *Smart Medicine for a Healthier Child.* N.Y.: Avery Publishing Group, 1994.

Recipe Title Index

An alphabetical listing of every recipe by exact title

Index

Chronic vaginitis, 65–66
Cigarette smoking
    avoided for mycotoxin-
      related illnesses, 36
    cessation of, 22, 224, 487
    chronic low-grade Candida
      infection with, 68
    immune system suppressed
      by, 171, 476
    reducing cravings for, 210
Cigarettes, fungus in, 19–20
Citrus seed extracts, 85, 476
Cleaning products, 279
Cleanliness, household and per-
    sonal, 176–177, 184–185,
    287
Cleansing treatments, 3, 4,
    471–472, 479, 486–487,
    489
    foods for cleansing, 138–144
    for allergies, 480
    for bowel problems, 482
    for parasites, 77–78
    Phase II or III diet for,
      222–223, 249, 472
    regular use of, 476
Cloves, 77, 85
Coenzyme Q$_{10}$, 27, 36, 49, 51,
    64, 65, 82, 85, 105,
    109–110. *See also* Oxygen
    therapy
Colchicine, 34, 39, 42, 54, 115
Cold symptoms, 152, 156, 476
Colitis, ulcerative, 32, 39–41
Colloidal silver as natural anti-
    fungal remedy, 48, 58, 59,
    67, 86, 287
Colon cleanser, 77–78, 487
Colonic irrigation, 77, 487
Colostrum, bovine, 81, 86–93
    components of, 87–89
    dosages of, 91
    healing crises with, 91–92
    product quality of, 90–91
    uses of, 89–90
*Colostrum: Life's First Food, the
    White Gold Discovery,* 91
Condiments and special season-
    ings, 447–454
Constipation. *See* Bowel and
    Colon

Consumer Health Organization
    of Canada, 76, 147
*Consumer's Dictionary of Food
    Additives, A,* 252
Controversial foods for Can-
    dida, 132
Cookware, 278–280
Copper, 55, 60, 66
Corn and popcorn, 37, 43,
    136–137, 243, 261, 480,
    482
Cousins, Norman, 180
Cravings
    reduced by vegetarian diets,
      210
    satisfying, 300–301
    sugar, 30–31, 123, 137
    as symptom of Candida-
      related complex, 20, 21
Crying, 152
Crohn's disease, 32, 39–41
Crook, William, 38–39
Cure Is in the Cupboard, The,
    106, 107
Curcumin, 52
Cyclosporin (mycotoxin), 20

D

D-lactic acid, fungal inhibitor,
    71
Dairy products, 5, 18, 44, 58,
    425–429. *See also* Milk
    substitutes
    as allergenic, 33, 43, 79, 85,
      480, 481
    avoided in Candida diet, 71,
      483
    avoided in restaurants, 188
    enzymes needed to digest,
      134, 204
Dehumidifying home to mini-
    mize Candida growth,
    178–179
Dental fillings. *See* Mercury
    dental fillings
Department of Agriculture
    guidelines, 256
Depression, 153, 469–470
Desensitization injections, 93
Detoxification. *See* Cleansing
    treatments

DHEA (dehydroepiandros-
    terone) hormone, 43–44,
    63, 67, 103
Diabetes, 17, 73, 151
    case history of, 166
    diet for, 488
Diaper rash, 127, 142
Diarrhea, 153
Diet, antifungal
    low-carbohydrate, 50, 220
    for mercury toxicity, 74
Diet, antiparasite, 78
Diet, Candida treatment, 70–71,
    221–250
    alternative uses for,
      222–223, 478–488, 491
    for children, 198–199, 460,
      461–464
    choosing proper, 223
    consequences of cheating
      on, 471
    food combining chart for,
      211
    four-phase program for,
      222–249
    meal planning guidelines
      for, 212–213
    rotating, 33, 207, 330, 333,
      480
    tips for, 248–249
    in treatment of any fungal
      infection, 44
Diet, hypoallergenic, 41, 119,
    161, 170
Diet questions to ask your doc-
    tor (list), 249–250
Diet revision, key elements of,
    44–45
Digestion, 2, 203–209. *See also*
    Stomach acid
    Digest-Aid-Meal-In-A-Soup,
      360–361, 485
    digestive aids for, 120–127,
      155, 156, 170, 302, 332,
      339, 456, 471, 476, 481,
      485
    enjoyable foods as aiding,
      205
    indigestion problems with,
      120, 157
    of proteins, slow, 204
    rotation diet to help, 330

therapeutic, 50–51, 129–144

Foods to avoid, 45, 51, 71, 85, 251–252, 330–332, 433, 454, 484, 485, 488. *See also* Restaurant guide
    in Phase I diet, 225
    in Phase II diet, 236–238
    in Phase III diet, 240

Free radicals, 59, 74, 76

Freezing foods, 6, 258–259, 260–261, 461. *See also* Storing foods

Friendly bacteria, 16, 48, 110, 144, 171, 174

Frozen treats, 461–462

Fructo-oligosaccharides (FOS), 94, 100, 174

Fruit, 30, 34, 45, 71, 457–465, 488. *See also* Juice
    for children on Candida diet, 198–199, 460
    connection to sweets of, 16, 457
    digesting, 209–210, 225, 458–459
    fasting using, 489–490
    insomnia and raw, 164, 225
    on Phase I diet, 224–225, 458–460, 463–465, 482–483
    on Phase II diet, 229–230, 458, 460, 461
    on Phase III diet, 239–240, 458, 460–461, 463–465
    on Phase IV diet, 245–246, 458, 463–465
    subacid/tart, 144, 198, 458, 459
    sugar in, 33, 133, 457–458
    washing, 81
    yogurt combined with, 210, 212, 459–461, 465

Fungal-related complex. *See* Candida albicans

Fungus
    foods containing, 16
    localized skin infections caused by, 16
    number of species and forms of, 15

Fusarium (mycotoxin), 19–20

G

Galland, Leo, 77, 85

Garlic
    allicin as essential ingredient in, 139
    cleansing, 139
    breast milk quality improved when mother eats, 286
    buying guidelines for, 334
    eaten during meals, technique for, 139–140
    healing reactions caused by, 140
    increased in Candida diet, 71
    as insulin-lowering food, 29, 30
    as natural antifungal remedy, 36, 41, 48, 50, 58–60, 64, 67, 94, 139–140, 171, 194, 476
    raw, added to recipes, 139
    storing, 336
    to treat parasites, 77, 78, 139–140

Gas (flatulence), 273–274

Gentian formula, 94

Gentiana lutea, 52

Germanium, 51, 94, 97, 134, 483

Giardia lamblia, 77

Ginger and ginger tea, 77, 94–95, 128, 290

Ginkgo biloba extract (GBE), 26, 38, 64

Ginseng, 94, 290

Glutamic acid hydrochloride, 79, 123, 124

Glutamine, 123–134

Goiter, 72–73

Goldenseal, 58, 77, 95, 128, 290

Gottschall, Elaine (Gottschall Specific Carbohydrate Diet), 40

Gout, 24, 34–35

Grain, cereal, 19, 32, 319–320
    cooked, types of, 320–322
    tips for preparing, 320

Grain, whole
    bread made from, 454
    cereal, 319–322

cooking tips for, 270–271
    in mild cases of Candida, 243
    preparation of, 167, 207, 271–273, 483, 485
    sources for buying, 255
    storing, 6, 258

Grains avoided
    in Candida diet, 71, 454
    in MS diet, 44
    in Phase III diet, 237

Grapefruit juice effect, 293–294

Grapefruit seed extract, 50, 77

Green food supplements, 51, 95, 130–131, 481, 486
    aloe vera gel. *See* Aloe vera gel or juice
    barley green juice, 27, 76, 95, 130, 141–143
    blue green algae, 76, 82, 95, 130
    chlorella, 76, 82, 95, 130
    green drinks, 27, 76
    green kamut, 95, 130
    liquid chlorophyll, 27
    spirulina, 76, 82, 95, 130
    wheat grass juice, 27, 97, 141–143

Griseofulvin, 20, 116

Guess What Came to Dinner: Parasites and Your Health, 83

Gugulipid, 64

H

Hair loss, 72
    case history of, 165

Halitosis, 26–27, 182

Hashimoto's thyroiditis, 72

Hawthorn, 64

Headaches, 154

Healing aids, natural, 175

Healing foods for Candida, 138

Healing process
    diagnoses and treatment options overlooked in extended, 469–470
    role of immune system in, 169–186
    speeding, 175–186

Healing process (continued)
as yeast die, 2–3, 7, 138, 140, 148, 149, 301
Health hazards, 195–196
Health maintenance guidelines, 474–477
Health principles, 6–9
Healthy Healing, 207–208, 479
Heart and circulatory problems, 19, 59–65
angina and hardening of arteries, 60
foods to help reverse, 60
polycythemia, 48–49
stroke, TIA, atheroscleroses, and heart disease, 24, 32, 59–60, 93
supplemental nutrients for, 60–65
Helicobacter pylori, 15
Hemorrhoids, 35–37, 127
Herbs
for autoimmune disease, 67
for gout, 35
for hemorrhoids, 36
for immune system support, 170
increased in Candida diet, 71
for inflammatory bowel disease, 41
for parasite infestations, 77, 80
for psoriasis, 54
for rheumatoid arthritis, 55
for scalp problems, 58
for tea, 288–292. *See also* Teas
uses of fresh, 330–331
High blood pressure, case history of, 159
Holidays, tips for maintaining health during, 474–477
Home testing kits for food allergies, 119–120
Homeopathic remedies, 95, 128
Hot and cold packs, 177, 180
How to Meditate, 181
Hoxsey-like formula, 52
Hydrochloric acid. *See* Stomach acid

Hydrogen peroxide. *See* Oxygen therapy
Hyperactivity, 21, 37–39, 154
Hypoallergenic diet, 41, 119, 161, 170
Hypochlorhydria (low stomach acid), 18–19, 27, 48, 66–67, 79, 125, 133
Hypoglycemia. *See* Low blood sugar and Blood sugar
Hypothyroidism, 71–73
Hypothyroidism: The Unsuspected Illness, 72

I

Ibuprofen, 56
Idiopathic thrombocytopenic purpura (ITP), 41–42. *See also* Blood, platelets in
Immune system
attack on one's own body of, 31–32
dietary support for, 170
emotional/spiritual support for, 170
healing and, 169–186
herb and nutrient support for, 170–171
improved to minimize environment for Candida, 70, 473
process of mycotoxin attack on, 56
protection against fungal infections by, 16
relation to other systems of, 22, 169
supplements enhancing, 112, 172–175
suppressors of, 170–172
visualization/relaxation support of, 170
weakening of, 16–17
Immune system illnesses, 2, 16, 17, 31. *See also* Autoimmune diseases
Immunocal, 51
Indigestion, 154. *See also* Digestion
Infants
beverages for, 286

Candida treatments for, 127–128, 286
Inflammatory bowel disease, 39–41
Insulin, 29, 73. *See also* Diabetes
Insomnia (Sleeplessness), 156
Interferon, 95–97
boosters of, 174
Inulin, 80, 121
International Bio-Oxidative Medicine Foundation, 147
Intestinal tract. *See* Bowel and colon *and* Digestion
Iodine
hormonal imbalance and, 72
as natural antifungal remedy, 97
Iron, 39, 48
Iron deficiency, 38
Iron, stored, 61–62
Itraconazole (Sporanox), 65, 116

J

Jaffe, Russell, 37, 40
Jeanne Marie's Candida story, 9–11
Jensen, Bernard, 91–92, 136
Juice, 33, 34, 36, 60, 294–297
for asthma or eczema, 481
avoiding fruit, 71
bottled or canned, 292, 296
combinations of, 296–297
fresh, 293
high sugar content in fruit, 127
sources for buying, 255

K

Kasha, 271. *See also* Grain, whole
Kaufmann, Klaus, 44
Kelp. *See* Seaweed
Ketoconazole (Nizoral), 39, 50, 65, 116–117, 148
Key concepts in controlling Candida albicans, 4
Kidney stones, case history of, 160
Kitchen utensils, 278–279

About the Authors

Jeanne Marie Martin, C.I.N., lectures internationally on topics concerning natural foods and holistic lifestyles. She has over twenty-five years experience that has led her to write and coauthor twelve health books and cookbooks and over 300 magazine articles. Some of her titles include *For the Love of Food, All Natural Allergy Cookbook, Hearty Vegetarian Soups and Stews, Vegan Delights, Light Cuisine, Return to the Joy of Health, Eating Alive, The Power of Superfoods, Recipes for Romance,* and *Your Natural Medicine Chest.*

As a clinical nutritionist, Jeanne Marie has worked with more than thirty holistic medical doctors, naturopaths, and chiropractors whose clients have special health problems.

In addition to her nutrition consultations, Jeanne Marie teaches natural cooking and nutrition for Langara College in Vancouver, B.C., Canada, and in Washington state. She also taught for six years for Scott Community College in the U.S. Jeanne Marie lectures on nutrition for universities, schools, clinics, TV, and radio shows. For lecture information only, call 1-604-878-8787 or write to: J.M. Martin, P.O. Box 4391, Vancouver, B.C., Canada V6B 3Z8.

Jeanne Marie is also a professional floral designer, gardener, published poet, singer, arts and crafts expert, meditation teacher, and qualified yoga instructor who has trained other teachers.

Dr. Zoltan P. Rona is a graduate of McGill University Medical School (1977), and he has a Master's Degree in Biochemistry and Clinical Nutrition from the University of Bridgeport in Connecticut (1984). He is the author of three Canadian bestsellers: *The Joy of Health* (1991), *Return to the Joy of Health* (1995), and *Childhood Illness and the Allergy Connection* (1997). He is also the medical editor of the *Encyclopedia of Natural Healing* (1998), which won the Benjamin Franklin Publishing Award in 1999. Dr. Rona has had a private medical practice in Toronto for the past 23 years.

He is currently working on a series of small health books on various health topics. Already published works from this series are *Natural Alternatives to Vaccinations, Osteoarthritis,* and *Boosting Male Libido Naturally.* Titles to be published later in 2000 and 2001 include *Treating Fibromyalgia Naturally, Rheumatoid Arthritis, Bodybuilding Supplements,* and *Natural Remedies for Menopause.*